MEDICAL RADIOLOGY

Diagnostic Imaging and Radiation Oncology

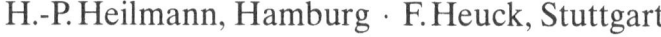

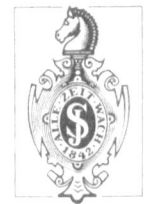

The Thymus

Diagnostic Imaging, Functions, and Pathologic Anatomy

Contributors

K.-M. Debatin · G. de Geer · W. J. Hofmann · H. F. Otto
E. Walter · W. R. Webb · H. Wiethölter · E. Willich

Edited by

E. Walter, E. Willich, and W. R. Webb

Foreword by

M. W. Donner and F. Heuck

With 127 Figures

Springer-Verlag
Berlin Heidelberg New York
London Paris Tokyo
Hong Kong Barcelona
Budapest

Professor Dr. EBERHARD WALTER
Radiologische Klinik der Universität Tübingen
Abteilung Röntgendiagnostik
Hoppe-Seyler-Straße 3
W-7400 Tübingen
FRG

Professor (em.) Dr. EBERHARD WILLICH
Klinikum der Universität Heidelberg – Kinderklinik –
Abteilung für Pädiatrische Radiologie
Im Neuenheimer Feld 153
W-6900 Heidelberg
FRG

W. RICHARD WEBB, M.D.
Department of Radiology
University of California, Medical Center
505 Parnassus Ave.
San Francisco, CA 94143
USA

MEDICAL RADIOLOGY · Diagnostic Imaging and Radiation Oncology
Continuation of
Handbuch der medizinischen Radiologie
Encyclopedia of Medical Radiology

ISBN-13: 978-3-642-84194-1   e-ISBN-13: 978-3-642-84192-7
DOI: 10.1007/978-3-642-84192-7

Library of Congress Cataloging-in-Publication Data. The Thymus : diagnostic imaging, functions, and pathologic anatomy / contributors, K. N. Debatin ... [et al.] ; edited by E. Walter, E. Willich, and W. R. Webb ; foreword by M. W. Donner and F. Heuck. p. cm. – (Medical radiology)
Includes bibliographical references and index.

1. Thymus–Imaging. 2. Thymus–Diseases–Diagnosis. 3. Thymus–Anatomy. I. Debatin, K. M. II. Walter, E., III. Willich, Eberhard. IV. Webb, W. Richard (Wayne Richard), 1945– . V. Series.
[DNLM: 1. Diagnostic Imaging. 2. Thymus Gland–anatomy & histology. 3. Thymus Gland–physiology.   WK 400 T54855] RC663.T48 1992 616.4′3–dc20 DNLM/DLC

© Springer-Verlag Berlin Heidelberg 1992
Softcover reprint of the hardcover 1st edition 1992

10/3130-5 4 3 2 1 0 – Printed on acid-free paper

List of Contributors

Priv.-Doz. Dr. K.-M. Debatin
Universitäts-Kinderklinik Heidelberg
Abteilung für Onkologie/Immunologie
Im Neuenheimer Feld 150
W-6900 Heidelberg
FRG

G. de Geer, M.D.
Department of Radiology
University Hospital of Geneva
CH-1211 Genève 4
Switzerland

Dr. W. J. Hofmann
Institut für Pathologie
der Universität Heidelberg
Im Neuenheimer Feld 220/221
W-6900 Heidelberg
FRG

Professor Dr. H. F. Otto
Institut für Pathologie
der Universität Heidelberg
Im Neuenheimer Feld 220/221
W-6900 Heidelberg
FRG

Professor Dr. E. Walter
Radiologische Klinik der Universität
Tübingen
Abteilung Röntgendiagnostik
Hoppe-Seyler-Straße 3
W-7400 Tübingen
FRG

W. R. Webb, M.D.
Professor of Radiology
University of California
Medical Center
505 Parnassus Ave.
San Francisco, CA 94143
USA

Priv.-Doz. Dr. H. Wiethölter
Neurologische Klinik der Universität
Tübingen
Abteilung Allgemeine Neurologie
Hoppe-Seyler-Straße 3
W-7400 Tübingen
FRG

Professor (em.) Dr. E. Willich
Universitäts-Kinderklinik Heidelberg
Abteilung für Pädiatrische Radiologie
Im Neuenheimer Feld 153
W-6900 Heidelberg
FRG

Foreword

Until the middle of the present century, the morphology and function of the thymus were primarily of interest to those working in the fields of pathologic anatomy, endocrinology, and pediatrics. However, during recent decades careful and refined histologic studies of the organ have expanded our knowledge. It now seems certain that the thymus plays a central role in the immune system, and some of the substances produced by this organ are considered together under the collective term of "thymic hormones".

In clinical medicine (in particular endocrinology and pediatrics, as well as surgery and radiologic oncology), the startling advances that have taken place in radiologic diagnostics with the advent of new imaging procedures such as computed tomography and magnetic resonance imaging have provided fresh impetus in the search for effective treatments for hyperplasia, tumors, and tumor-like changes of the thymus. Normal variants of the thymus, which lies concealed within the anterior superior mediastinum, have been recorded, and pathologic changes such as primary or secondary tumors can now be analyzed and correctly diagnosed.

As the editors of this series, we have succeeded in procuring as the chief authors of this volume radiologists who, in their clinical activity, have been intensively involved in the noninvasive radiologic diagnosis of the thymus and its diseases and disorders. A sound knowledge of the anatomy and pathology of the organ is both a prerequisite for and a significant supplement to diagnosis by means of modern imaging procedures. It is thus gratifying that W. J. HOFMANN and H. F. OTTO, two pathologists with proven expertise in the specific field of thymic disease, should have agreed to cover these important areas. Special mention should be made of the chapters on developmental abnormalities and tumors, which represent a successful joint approach by pathologists and radiologists. Myasthenia gravis is discussed in a separate chapter by H. WIETHÖLTER, who is an expert in this neuromuscular disorder.

The present volume is designed to contribute to a better understanding of thymic diseases and thereby to their earlier diagnosis using the new noninvasive radiologic imaging procedures. It will fill a gap in the world literature to which attention is only seldom drawn. Those working within various specialties will find the volume of value in their everyday clinical work. The excellent quality of the illustrative material is attributable to the efforts of Springer-Verlag. As editors of the *Medical Radiology* series, we hope that this volume will, like earlier volumes, be well received by our colleagues in all fields of medicine, and we would be glad to learn of any constructive criticism that might be offered.

MARTIN W. DONNER   FRIEDRICH HEUCK
Baltimore   Stuttgart

Preface

In this monograph it is the intention of the editors to review the clinical, radiologic, and pathoanatomic results of 90 years' research into the thymus. Furthermore, the individual authors discuss their own examination techniques and research findings, and also make full reference to the most recent literature. The latter feature is essential owing to the enormous progress that has taken place in respect of imaging diagnostics.

The aims of the monograph are to provide information concerning the current state of the art in thymic research, to make suggestions regarding the deployment of modern diagnostic imaging procedures, to improve the standard of thymic diagnostics, and to serve as a source of reference when special questions are being tackled. We hope that these aims have been achieved.

The idea for this book came from Prof. Dr. F. HEUCK, whom we thank.

Thanks are also due to a number of our colleagues for providing figures:
Prof. Dr. F. BALL (Frankfurt/M., FRG), Prof. Dr. G. BENZ-BOHM (Cologne, FRG), Prof. Dr. A. DÜX (Mönchengladbach, FRG), Prof. Dr. K. D. EBEL (Cologne, FRG), Prof. Dr. M. GEORGI (Mannheim, FRG), B. KIM HAN, M. D. (Cincinnati, USA), Dr. K. KLOTT and co-workers (Stuttgart-Bad Cannstatt, FRG), Prof. Dr. H. J. von LENGERKE (Münster i. W., FRG), Prof. Dr. A. OESTREICH (Cincinnati, USA), Dr. H. PETZEL (Stuttgart-Bad Cannstatt, FRG), Dr. K. RASCHKE (Cape Town, South Africa/Heidelberg, FRG), Prof. Dr. R. SCHUMACHER (Mainz, FRG), Priv. Doz. Dr. H. TSCHÄPPELER (Berne, Switzerland).

The authors also owe debt of gratitude to Dr. med. P. B. CLOSE BSc (Dinkelsbühl) and Dr. C. WÜRTENBERGER (Berlin) for their accomplishment in performing the demanding task of translation, and to the copy editor, Mr. R. MILLS, for his excellent work in applying the finishing touches.

Ms. U. N. DAVIS of Springer Verlag, Heidelberg, provided enthusiastic assistance during the passage of the manuscript from its early stages to completion. Indeed, Springer-Verlag was generous in meeting all our wishes and therefore deserve special thanks for the success of the book.

EBERHARD WALTER
EBERHARD WILLICH
W. RICHARD WEBB

Contents

1 **Introduction – Historical Background**
E. WILLICH 1

2 **Anatomy and Embryology of the Thymus**
W. J. HOFMANN and H. F. OTTO 5

2.1 Embryology 5
2.2 Normal Anatomy 5
2.3 Involution 9
References 11

3 **Immunologic Function of the Thymus**
K.-M. DEBATIN 15

3.1 Historical Overview 15
3.2 T Cell Molecules in Antigen Recognition 16
3.2.1 Accessory Molecules 17
3.3 Ontogeny of T Cells 17
3.3.1 Thymocyte Precursors 18
3.3.2 TCR Rearrangements 18
3.3.3 Maturation into Functional T Cells 18
3.3.4 Factors Governing T Cell Development Within the Thymus . . . 18
3.4 Cellular Selection in the Thymus 19
3.5 Clinical Aspects 19
3.6 Summary 20
References 20

4 **Imaging Procedures for Visualization of the Thymus**
E. WALTER, E. WILLICH, W. R. WEBB, and G. DE GEER 23

4.1 Plain Film Diagnostics
E. WALTER and E. WILLICH 23
4.1.1 Chest Radiography in Two Planes 23
4.1.2 Fluoroscopy 23
4.2 Conventional Tomography 24
4.3 Ultrasonography 24
4.4 Computed Tomography 25
4.5 Magnetic Resonance Imaging
W. R. WEBB and G. DE GEER 26
4.5.1 Principles of Magnetic Resonance Imaging 27
4.5.2 Image Production 27
4.5.3 Normal Appearances 27
4.5.4 Image Contrast and Interpretation 27
4.5.5 MRI Diagnosis of Mediastinal Masses 28
4.5.6 Image Acquisition and ECG Gating 28

4.5.7   Characterization of Mediastinal Masses   29
4.6   Nuclear Medicine
         E. WALTER and E. WILLICH   29
4.6.1   67 Gallium Citrate   29
4.6.2   75 Selenium Methionine   30
4.6.3   99m Technetium Pertechnetate   30
4.7   Esophagography   30
4.8   Angiography   30
4.8.1   Arteriography   30
4.8.2   Angiocardiography   31
4.8.3   Phlebography and Superior Venacavography   31
4.9   Obsolete Methods   32
4.9.1   Kymography   32
4.9.2   Pneumomediastinography   32
4.10   Supplementary Procedures (Mediastinography, Bronchoscopy,
         Bronchography)
         E. WILLICH   32
         References   32

5   **Diagnostic Imaging of the Normal Thymus**
         E. WILLICH, E. WALTER, W. R. WEBB, and G. DE GEER   35

5.1   Conventional Diagnostics in Children
         E. WILLICH and E. WALTER   35
5.1.1   Newborns and Infants   35
5.1.2   Preschool Age to Adolescence   40
5.1.3   Adults   40
5.2   Ultrasonography   40
5.2.1   Children   40
5.2.2   Adults   41
5.3   Computed Tomography
         E. WALTER   41
5.4   Magnetic Resonance Imaging
         W. R. WEBB and G. DE GEER   46
5.4.1   Children   46
5.4.2   Adults   48
5.5   Invasive Procedures (Pneumomediastinography, Arteriography,
         Phlebography)
         E. WALTER   50
5.6   Measurement of the Size of the Thymus
         E. WILLICH   51
5.6.1   Radiographic Method   51
5.6.2   Computed Tomography   51
5.6.3   Magnetic Resonance Imaging
         W. R. WEBB and G. DE GEER   53
         References   54

6   **Acute and Stress-Induced Involution of the Thymus**
         E. WILLICH   57

6.1   Acute Endogenous Involution of the Thymus   57
6.2   Exogenous Involution of the Thymus: the Steroid Test   57
6.3   Transplacental Influence of Steroids on the Premature Infant's Thymus .   59
         References   60

7   Developmental Abnormalities of the Thymus
       E. WILLICH, E. WALTER, H. F. OTTO, and W. J. HOFMANN 63

7.1   Aplasia, Hypoplasia, and Dysplasia
        E. WILLICH and E. WALTER 63
7.2   Dystopia 63
7.2.1   Cervical and Superior Mediastinum 65
7.2.2   Middle Mediastinum 66
7.2.3   Posterior Mediastinum 66
7.2.4   Miscellaneous 68
        References 68
7.3   Persistent Thymus
        E. WILLICH 70
7.3.1   Introduction 70
7.3.2   Pathophysiologic Causes 70
7.3.3   Clinical Features 70
7.3.4   Imaging Methods 70
7.3.5   Differential Diagnosis 70
        References 77
7.4   Hyperplasia 77
7.4.1   Introduction 77
7.4.2   Pathologic Features
        W. J. HOFMANN and H. F. OTTO 78
7.4.2.1 True Thymic Hyperplasia 78
7.4.2.2 Thymic Hyperplasia with Massive Enlargement of the Gland 78
7.4.2.3 Thymic Rebound in Childhood and Adolescence 81
7.4.2.4 True Thymic Hyperplasia in Association with Other Diseases 81
7.4.2.5 Lymphofollicular Hyperplasia of the Thymus 82
7.4.3   Clinical Features
        E. WILLICH 84
7.4.3.1 Asymptomatic Thymic Hyperplasia 84
7.4.3.2 Symptomatic Thymic Hyperplasia 84
7.4.4   Associated Diseases 89
7.4.5   Imaging Procedures and Findings 90
7.4.6   Regenerative Hyperplasia (Regrowth, Rebound Phenomenon) 92
7.4.7   Differential Diagnosis 94
7.4.8   Therapy 103
7.4.9   Follow-up 104
        References 104

8   Tumors of the Thymus
       E. WALTER, E. WILLICH, W. J. HOFMANN, H. F. OTTO, W. R. WEBB,
       and G. DE GEER 109

8.1   Introduction
        E. WALTER 109
8.2   Epithelial Tumors of the Thymus 110
8.2.1   Pathologic Features
        W. J. HOFMANN and H. F. OTTO 110
8.2.1.1 Macroscopic Appearance 110
8.2.1.2 Histologic Appearance 110
8.2.1.3 Classification 114
8.2.1.4 Immunohistology 116
8.2.1.5 Clinicopathologic Correlations 118
        References 119

8.2.2   Encapsulated and Invasive Thymomas
          E. WALTER 121
8.2.2.1   Occurrence and Clinical Symptoms 121
8.2.2.2   Association of Thymoma with Other Syndromes and Diseases 125
8.2.2.3   Diagnosis with Imaging Procedures 127
8.2.2.4   Differential Diagnosis 137
8.2.2.5   Relative Value of the Imaging Procedures 139
8.2.2.6   Therapy and Prognosis 139
          References 141
8.2.3   Carcinoma of the Thymus 145
8.2.3.1   Occurrence and Clinical Symptoms 145
8.2.3.2   Diagnosis with Imaging Procedures 146
8.2.3.3   Differential Diagnosis 147
8.2.3.4   Relative Value of the Imaging Procedures 147
8.2.3.5   Therapy and Prognosis 147
          References 147
8.3   Carcinoid Tumors of the Thymus 148
8.3.1   Pathologic Features
          W. J. HOFMANN and H. F. OTTO 148
8.3.2   Occurrence and Clinical Symptoms
          E. WALTER 149
8.3.2.1   Occurrence 149
8.3.2.2   Clinical Symptoms 151
8.3.3   Diagnosis with Imaging Procedures 152
8.3.4   Differential Diagnosis 154
8.3.5   Relative Value of the Imaging Procedures 155
8.3.6   Therapy and Prognosis 155
          References 155
8.4   Thymic Involvement in Malignant Lymphomas and Leukemia
          E. WILLICH and E. WALTER 156
8.4.1   Pathologic Features
          W. J. HOFMANN and H. F. OTTO 156
8.4.2   Hodgkin's Disease
          E. WILLICH and E. WALTER 159
8.4.2.1   Occurrence 159
8.4.2.2   Clinical Symptoms 160
8.4.2.3   Diagnosis with Imaging Procedures 160
8.4.2.4   Hodgkin's Disease of the Thymus Before and After
          Radiotherapy and Chemotherapy
          E. WALTER and E. WILLICH 164
8.4.3   Non-Hodgkin's Lymphoma 164
8.4.4   Leukemia 165
8.4.5   Non-Hodgkin's Lymphoma and Leukemia with Thymic Involvement,
          During and After Radiotherapy and Chemotherapy 170
8.4.6   Differential Diagnosis
          E. WALTER 170
8.4.7   Relative Value of the Imaging Procedures 171
          References 172
8.5   Mesenchymal Tumors (Thymolipoma)
          E. WALTER 174
8.5.1   Pathologic Features
          W. J. HOFMANN and H. F. OTTO 174
8.5.2   Occurrence and Clinical Symptoms
          E. WALTER 174

8.5.2.1 Occurrence 174
8.5.2.2 Clinical Symptoms 175
8.5.3   Diagnosis with Imaging Procedures 176
8.5.4   Differential Diagnosis 178
8.5.5   Relative Value of Imaging Procedures 178
8.5.6   Therapy and Prognosis 178
        References 179
8.6   Germ Cell Tumors and Teratomas
        E. WALTER 180
8.6.1   Pathologic Anatomy
        W. J. HOFMANN and H. F. OTTO 180
8.6.2   Seminoma
        E. WALTER 182
8.6.2.1 Occurrence and Clinical Symptoms 182
8.6.2.2 Diagnosis with Imaging Procedures 183
8.6.2.3 Differential Diagnosis and Relative Value of the Imaging Procedures . . 186
8.6.2.4 Therapy and Prognosis 186
8.6.3   Nonseminomatous, Pure or Mixed Germ Cell Tumors 186
8.6.3.1 Occurrence and Clinical Symptoms 186
8.6.3.2 Diagnosis with Imaging Procedures 187
8.6.3.3 Differential Diagnosis and Relative Value of the Imaging Procedures . . 190
8.6.3.4 Therapy and Prognosis 190
        References 191
8.7   Rare Tumors of the Thymus 192
8.7.1   Hemangioma of the Thymus 192
8.7.2   Choristoma of the Thymus 193
        References 193
8.8   Metastases to the Thymus 193
        Reference 193

9   Tumor-like (Nonneoplastic) Conditions of the Thymus
        and/or Mediastinum
        E. WALTER, E. WILLICH, W. J. HOFMANN, H. F. OTTO, W. R. WEBB,
        and G. DE GEER 195

9.1   Thymogenic Cysts 195
9.1.1   Pathologic Anatomy
        W. J. HOFMANN and H. F. OTTO 195
9.1.2   Occurrence and Clinical Symptoms
        E. WALTER and E. WILLICH 195
9.1.3   Diagnosis with Imaging Procedures 197
9.1.4   Differential Diagnosis 200
9.1.5   Relative Value of the Imaging Procedures 201
9.1.6   Therapy and Prognosis 201
9.2   Hydatidosis of the Thymus 201
9.3   Tuberculoma of the Thymus 202
9.4   Histiocytosis X of the Thymus 202
        References 202

10   Trauma and Hemorrhage of the Thymus
        E. WILLICH 205

10.1   Trauma 205
10.2   Hemorrhage 206
        References 207

11	**Thymus and Myasthenia Gravis**	
	H. WIETHÖLTER, E. WILLICH, and E. WALTER 209	
11.1	Definition of Myasthenia Gravis	
	H. WIETHÖLTER 209	
11.2	Clinical Manifestation 209	
11.2.1	Symptoms and Signs 209	
11.2.2	Classification 209	
11.2.3	Clinical Examination 209	
11.2.4	Prognosis 210	
11.3	Associated Thymic Changes 210	
11.3.1	Association of Thymic Changes with Other Diseases 211	
11.4	Pathogenesis 212	
11.5	Autoimmune Origin 212	
11.6	Diagnosis 212	
11.6.1	Radiological Diagnosis	
	E. WILLICH and E. WALTER 213	
11.7	Treatment	
	H. WIETHÖLTER 213	
	References 214	
	Subject Index 217	

1 Introduction – Historical Background

E. WILLICH

The changes that have taken place in recent decades in the interpretation of the function, pathology, and imaging of the thymus exceed those in respect of any other organ. The radical nature of these developments is witnessed even within the clinical field, where the sudden infant death syndrome used to be interpreted as "thymic death" (mors thymica: WALDBOTT 1934; FINKELSTEIN 1938; WERNE 1942; WERNE and GARROW 1947; RABSON 1949; HUSLER 1959). Furthermore, relationships were also suggested between goiter and the thymus (DUTOIT 1913) and between the goiter heart and the thymic heart (FEER 1923). "Status thymico-lymphaticus" became a routine descriptive term employed by every pediatrician [it was introduced in 1903 by HOCHSINGER and was subsequently used by PALTAUF (1919), BOYD (1927), GREENWOOD and WOODS (1927), COOPERSTOCK (1930), FINKELSTEIN (1938), and MITCHELL-NELSON (1945)] and also entered the radiologic literature (HOTZ 1928). This concept, like that of "status thymicus," introduced by ESCHERICH (1909) and PALTAUF (1919), even led to the use of radiotherapy (BIRK and SCHALL 1932). So-called stridor thymicus was also the subject of controversy for a long time (HOCHSINGER 1904; see Sect. 7.4.3.2).

Similar changes arising from misinterpretations took place within radiotherapy of the enlarged thymus between the 1920s and 1940s (KARGER 1920; MEYER 1921; SPOLVERINI 1922; FREEMAN 1923; REMER and BELDEN 1927; BIRK and SCHALL 1932).

The history of roentgenologic imaging of the thymus appears even more grotesque: In 1910 the French author SAVY was the first to describe the thymus as "superior anterior mediastinal pleuritis." This view was subsequently supported by ENGEL (1932), SCHÖNFELD (1933), SCHMID and JUNKER (1950), and KIRCHHOFF (1953), and was also later echoed by KRAUS et al. (1970) and in F. SCHMID's textbook of pediatric radiology (1973) despite the fact that autopsy findings had provided fundamental proof of the error.

In 1939 and 1941 GEFFERTH described the picture of mediastinal pleuritis as "typical and unmistakable"; however, he recognized this misdiagnosis in three cases with similar appearances, the misdiagnosis being revealed by the course of the disease and autopsy, at which a thymus was found.

For more than two decades the superior vena cava was thought to be pushed aside by the thymus and thus to border the right superior mediastinum, causing enlargement of the right-hand midshadow (BENJAMIN and GOETT 1912; GOETT 1918; ASSMANN 1934).

Upper lobe atelectasis constituted a further misdiagnosis (P. SCHMID 1956; to some extent also DIEU and MENUT 1960).

As late as 1929 CHAOUL claimed that radiologic demonstration of the thymus is not possible during infancy, with the exceptions of thymic persistence and pathologic enlargements. In 1931, however, BECKER was able to recognize the large thymic midshadow in newborns during the first few days of life by means of metal clipping of the organ in infant cadavers. He thought, however, that the thymus disappears with the development of the lung in newborns and subscribed to GOETT's theory (regarding the superior vena cava) in respect of the subsequent age periods. Not until 1948 did similar investigations by KEMP and co-workers in 44 children (twice by means of autopsy) provide proof that the thymus is the source of the wide midshadow or the paramediastinal triangular shadow in infants. This conclusion was supported by HARVEY and BROMER (1948), CAFFEY (1950), and TWINING et al. (1951), and subsequent careful investigations by DÜNNER (1954, 1956) and ESSER and HILGERT 1956) provided confirmation. It must be remembered, however, that the thymic shadow had already been positively identified by REYHER (1912, 1931), VOGT (1924), and SAUPE (1926).

The thymic tip, situated in the interlobar fissure between the right upper lobe and the middle lobe, was in the past often interpreted as "interlobar pleuritis." As early as 1933 HASLEY surmised that growth of the thymic tip into the interlobar fissure was responsible, a view shared in 1955 by GEFFERTH. Nevertheless, ENGEL and SAMSON (1933),

SCHMID (1952), and HABERMANN (1957) adhered to the diagnosis of interlobar pleuritis until ZSEBÖK proved by autopsy in 1958 that growth of the thymic tip into the interlobar fissure was indeed responsible.

References

Assmann H (1934) Die klinische Röntgendiagnostik der inneren Organe, 5th edn. FCW Vogel, Berlin, p 193 ff.

Becker J (1931) Röntgendiagnostik und Strahlentherapie in der Kinderheilkunde. J Springer, Berlin, p 103

Benjamin K, Goett T (1912) Zur Deutung des Thoraxradiogramms beim Säugling. Dtsch Arch Klin Med 107: 508

Birk W, Schall L (1932) Behandlung der Kinderkrankheiten mit Ultraviolett- und Röntgenstrahlen, 2nd edn. Urban and Schwarzenberg, Berlin

Boyd E (1927) Growth of the thymus: its relation to status lymphaticus and thymic symptoms. Am J Dis Child 33: 867

Caffey J (1950) Pediatric x-ray diagnosis, 2nd edn. Year Book Publishers, Chicago, p 322 ff.

Chaoul H (1929) Klinische Röntgendiagnostik der Erkrankungen der Brustorgane. J Springer, Berlin, p 202

Cooperstock M (1930) Present concepts of enlarged thymus and status lymphaticus: review of a decade of experience. J Michigan Med Soc 29: 21

Dieu JC, Menut G (1960) Remarques sur l'aspect radiologique du thymus du nourrisson et de l'enfant. Pédiatrie 15: 771

Dünner L (1954) Klinisch-röntgenologische Differentialdiagnostik der Lungenkrankheiten. Gustav Enke, Stuttgart

Dünner L (1956) Der paramediastinale Schatten des Thymus. ROFO 84: 18

Dutoit A (1913) Die Beziehungen des M. Basedow zur Thymushyperplasie. Dtsch Med Wochenschr 39: 272

Engel S (1932) Die Pleuritis mediastinalis superior. Z Kinderheilkd 53: 455

Engel S, Samson K (1933) Das Mediastinum. In: Engel S, Schall L (eds) Handbuch der Röntgendiagnostik und -therapie im Kindesalter. Thieme, Leipzig, p 393

Escherich T (1909) Vortr. Gesellsch. d. Ärzte 12.2. 1909. Wien Klin Wochenschr, p 7

Esser Cl, Hilgert F (1956) Zur Frage: Thymus, Atelektase oder mediastinaler Pleuraerguß? ROFO 84: 3

Feer E (1919) Lehrbuch der Kinderheilkunde, 5th edn. G. Fischer, Jena, p 185

Feer E (1923) Kropfherz und Thymusherz der Neugeborenen und Säuglinge. Monatsschr Kinderheilkd 25: 88

Finkelstein H (1938) Säuglingskrankheiten, 4th edn. Elsevier, New York, p 644

Freeman RG (1923) The symptoms and treatment of thymus hypertrophy in infancy. Arch Pédiatr 40: 665

Gefferth K (1939) Über einen Fall von beidseitiger Pleuritis mediastinalis superior anterior. Monatsschr Kinderheilkd 81: 128

Gefferth K (1941) Über Pleuritis mediastinalis anterior superior. Monatsschr Kinderheilkd 86: 264

Gefferth K (1955) Thymus? Mediastinalpleuritis? Ein Beitrag zum diagnostischen Wert der interlobären Haarlinie. ROFO 82: 462

Goett T (1918) Die Röntgenuntersuchung in der Kinderheilkunde. In: Rieder M, Rosenthal J (eds) Lehrbuch der Röntgenkunde, vol II. J. A. Barth, Leipzig, p 171

Greenwood M, Woods HM (1927) "Status thymolymphaticus" considered in the light of recent work on the thymus. J Hyg (Lond) 26: 305

Habermann P (1957) Ein Beitrag zur Differentialdiagnose Thymushyperplasie – Mediastinalpleuritis. ROFO 86: 321

Hammar JA (1930) Physiological and pathological significance of the thymico-lymphatic system. Acta Paediatr 11: 241

Harvey RM, Bromer RS (1948) Significance of triangular hilar shadows in roentgenograms of infants and children. AJR 59: 845

Hasley CK (1933) A study of the motor phenomenon of the mediastinum in infants and children. With particular reference to hyperplasia of the thymus. Radiology 21: 477

Hochsinger C (1903) Stridor thymicus infantum. Wien Med Wochenschr, pp 2106, 2162, 2214

Hochsinger C (1904) Stridor congenitus und Thymushypertrophie. Verh Dtsch Ges Kinderheilkd 20: 61

Hotz A (1928) Thymus. In: Schinz HR, Baensch W, Friedl E (eds) Lehrbuch der Röntgendiagnostik, 2nd edn. Thieme, Leipzig, p 786

Husler J (1959) In: Lust-Pfaundler-Husler: Krankheiten des Kindesalter. 21st edn. Urban and Schwarzenberg, Munich, p 107

Karger P (1920) Erfahrungen und Indikationen bei der Röntgentiefentherapie im Kindesalter. Jahrb Kinderheilkd 93: 295

Kemp FH, Morley HMC, Emrys-Roberts E (1948) A sail-like triangular projection from the mediastinum: a radiographic appearance of the thymus gland. Br J Radiol 21: 618

Kirchhoff HW (1953) Zur Differentialdiagnose der Mittelschattenveränderungen im frühen Kindesalter. ROFO 79: 557

Kraus R, Klemencic J, Keller R (1970) Erkrankungen und Tumoren des Mediastinums. In: Strnad F (ed) Röntgendiagnostik der oberen Speise- und Atemwege, der Atemorgane und des Mediastinums. Springer, Berlin Heidelberg New York (Handbuch der medizinischen Radiologie, vol IX/6, pp 268–276)

Meyer WH (1921) Roentgen therapy in intrathoracic lesions with special reference to status thymus lymphaticus. Arch Pédiatr 38: 572

Mitchell-Nelson, ed. by Nelson EW (1945) Textbook of pediatrics, 4th edn. WB Saunders, Philadelphia, p 925

Paltauf A, cited by Feer E (1919) Lehrbuch der Kinderheilkunde, 5th edn. E. Fischer, Jena, p 185

Rabson SM (1949) Sudden and unexpected natural death in infants and young children. J Pediatr 34: 166

Remer J, Belden WW (1927) Roentgen diagnosis and therapy of the thymus in children. AJR 18: 119

Reyher P (1912) Das Röntgenverfahren in der Kinderheilkunde. H. Meusser, Berlin, pp 25, 166

Reyher P (1931) Das Röntgenbild der Thymusdrüse. Ergeb Inn Med Kinderheilkd 39: 578

Saupe E (1926) Über das Thoraxröntgenbild im frühen Kindesalter. ROFO 34: 976

Savy M (1910) Les pleurésies médiastines. Progrès méd 27: 371

Schmid F (1952) Lungenhilus und Bronchialsystem. Kinderärztl Prax 20: 462

Schmid F (1973) Pädiatrische Radiologie, vol 2, Springer, Berlin Heidelberg New York, p 171 ff.

Schmid F, Junker F (1950) Die Bedeutung der Pleuritis mediastinalis im Kindesalter. Z Kinderheilkd. 67: 545

Schmid PC (1956) Thymushyperplasie oder Oberlappenatelektase? ROFO 84: 20–28

Schönfeld H (1933) Die Pleura und ihre Erkrankungen. In: Engel S, Schall L (eds) Handbuch der Röntgendiagnostik und -therapie im Kindesalter. Thieme, Leipzig, p 228 ff.

Spolverini LM (1922) Contributo al trattamento radioterapico dell'ipertrofia del timo. Riv Clin Pediatr 19: 513

Twiming EW, Shanks SC, Kerley P (1951) A textbook of x-ray diagnosis by British authors. H. K. Lewis, London

Vogt E (1924) Zur Kritik der Röntgendiagnostik des Herzens und des Thymus in der ersten Lebenszeit. ROFO 32: 75

Waldbott GL (1934) So-called "thymic death": pathologic process in 34 cases. Am J Dis Child 47: 41

Werne J (1942) Post mortem evidence of acute infection in unexpected death in infancy. Am J Pathol 18: 759

Werne J, Garrow I (1947) Sudden death of infants due to mechanical suffocation. Am J Public Health 37: 675

Zsebök Z (1958) Röntgenanatomie der Neugeborenen- und Säuglingslunge. Thieme, Stuttgart, pp 118–135

2 Anatomy and Embryology of the Thymus

W. J. Hofmann and H. F. Otto

2.1 Embryology

The thymus is an important organ of the immune system (see Chap. 3). Numerous experimental and clinicopathologic investigations have demonstrated that the immunologic function of the thymus is closely dependent on the presence of normal thymic structures.

The thymus is embryologically derived from the third and, to a lesser and inconstant degree, fourth branchial (pharyngeal) pouches during the 6th intrauterine week (Hammar 1905; Weller 1933; Norris 1938; von Gaudecker and Müller-Hermelink 1980; Ciba Foundation Symposium, No. 84, 1981; Otto 1984; von Gaudecker 1986; Suster and Rosai 1990). The thymus shares a common embryologic origin with the lower pair of parathyroid glands.

From the neck, the embryonal thymus migrates downward and medially into the anterior or anterosuperior mediastinum as epithelial tubules, plugs, or cords. The thymic epithelial cells proliferate in the mediastinum, and by the 8th (intrauterine) week, the thymus has lost its connection with the branchial clefts.

The thymus is an epithelial organ during the first 8 weeks of intrauterine life. By the end of the 2nd month, the proliferating epithelial tubules, plugs, and cords become infiltrated by lymphocytes (migrating bone marrow cells) and mesenchymal elements. The thymus grows rapidly in embryonic life, and in the neonatal period the thymus reaches its largest relative size (cf. Fig. 2.5).

Small islands of ectopic thymic tissue can be found in the neck ("cervical thymic tissue"), tympanic cavity, different areas of the mediastinum, and the lung (Rosai and Levine 1976; Otto 1984). Aberrant (ectopic) nodules of thymic tissue are found in approximately 20% of humans (Gilmour 1941). These islands of ectopic thymic tissue can be the site of origin of numerous pathologic conditions including hyperplastic lesions, cysts, tumors, and tumor-like lesions.

2.2 Normal Anatomy

The human thymus is located predominantly in the anterior (anterosuperior) mediastinum in front of the great vessels at the base of the heart and pericardium. It is a pyramid-shaped organ composed of two closely apposed lobes (Fig. 2.1). The two lobes are connected at their basis, which is situated just in front of the pericardium. The lower borders may extend down to the fourth costal cartilages; the upper borders often reach the thyroid gland or higher. Laterally the thymus may lie alongside the pleura of the lungs; mostly, however, mediastinal fat intercedes. Anteriorly it is related to the sternum, the upper four costal cartilages, and the sternohyoid and sternothyroid muscles.

Histologically, the thymus is covered by a thin fibrovascular capsule which extends into the paren-

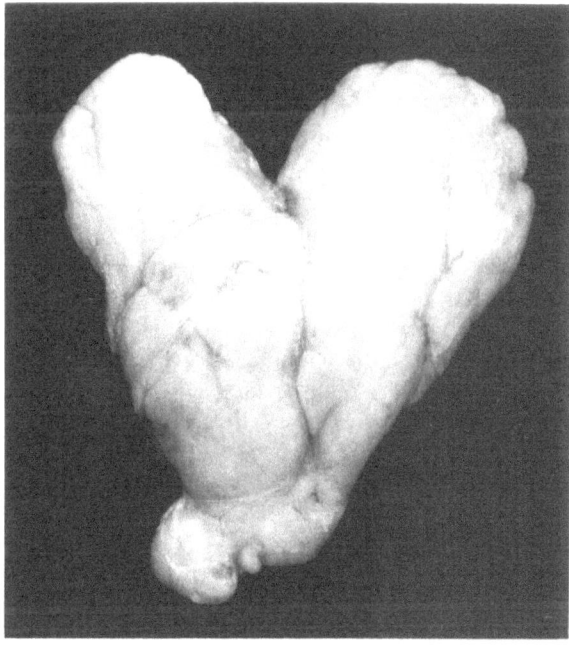

Fig. 2.1. Normal infant (10 weeks) thymus (24 g), showing its typical bilobate pyramidal shape (Otto 1984)

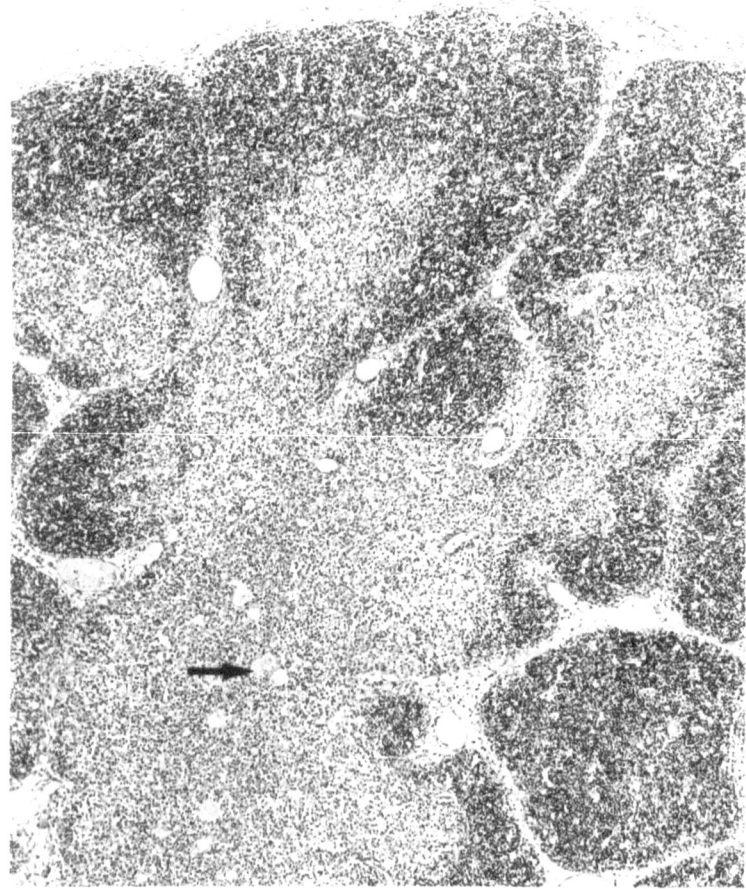

Fig. 2.2. Low power view of normal thymus showing dense cortex composed predominantly of lymphocytes (thymocytes) and less dense medulla with Hassall's corpuscles *(arrow)* and fewer lymphocytes. H & E, ×40

chyma, giving the organ its typical lobular pattern (Fig. 2.2). Within the parenchyma, two clear-cut different zones can be identified: the lymphocyte-rich and therefore darker staining cortex (Fig. 2.3) and the medulla containing Hassall's corpuscles (Fig. 2.4) and less lymphocytes than the cortex. Thus the organ can be divided into three compartments. The cortex and the medulla constitute the true thymic parenchyma (i. e., intraparenchymal zone), the third compartment, the so-called extraparenchymal zone being located within the perivascular (paraseptal) spaces of the thymus (LEVINE and ROSAI 1978; LEVINE and BEARMAN 1980; HOFMANN et al. 1984, 1988 a, b).

The thymic parenchyma is composed of three different cellular constituents:
- Epithelial cells
- Lymphocytes (thymocytes)
- Macrophages and interdigitating reticulum cells (nonepithelial nonlymphoid cells)

The epithelial cells of the thymus form a reticular network, which extends from the medulla, including Hassall's corpuscles, to the cortex. Cortical and medullary epithelial cells can be distinguished by their different cytologic appearance in light and electron microscopy (OTTO 1984; MARINO and MÜLLER-HERMELINK 1985, 1986; VON GAUDECKER 1986; SUSTER and ROSAI 1990). Cortical epithelial cells are of stellate shape and possess oval to round nuclei with prominent nucleoli. Medullary epithelial cells are more spindle shaped with oval to spindle-shaped nuclei without prominent nucleoli.

The differences in morphology are also reflected by their different antigenetic properties, which have been studied immunohistologically by many investigators using monoclonal antibodies (MCFARLAND et al. 1984; HAYNES 1984; DEMAAGD et al. 1985; VON GAUDECKER et al. 1986; GAY-BELLILE et al. 1986; TAKACS et al. 1987; NAKAHAMA et al. 1990).

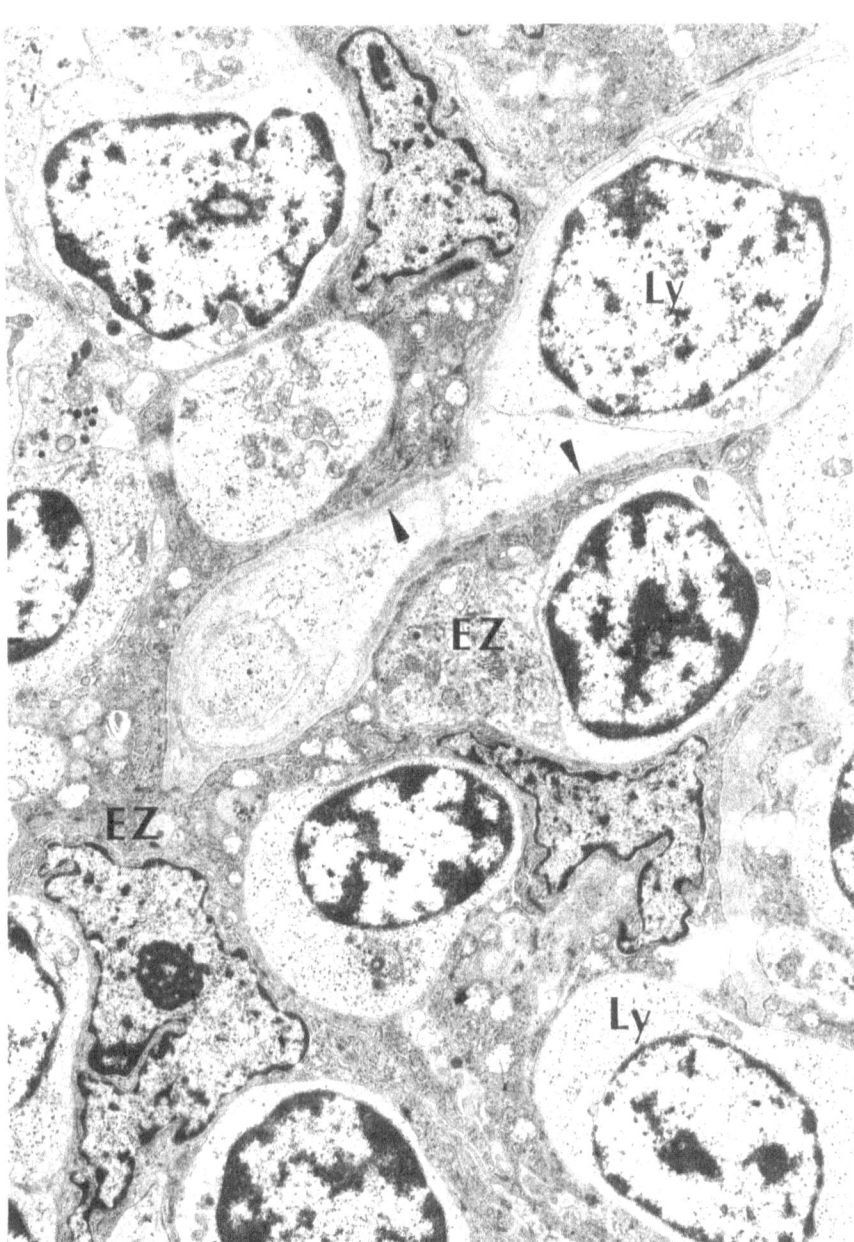

Fig. 2.3. Ultrastructure of normal thymus. Cortical epithelial cells *(EZ)*, surrounded by basal lamina *(arrowheads)*. Lymphocytes *(Ly)*. (Otto 1984) Uranyl acetate-lead citrate stain, × 7800

In our own investigation we found a complementary expression of antigens detected by the monoclonal antibodies T2/30, BG3C8, RFD-4, and L 263 and could define cortical epithelial cells as T2/30 + , BG3C8 − , RFD-4 − , L 263 − and medullary epithelial cells as BG3C8 + , RFD-4 + , L 263 + , T2/30 > + (Hofmann et al. 1989).

There are some lines of evidence that the thymic epithelial cells, besides providing the reticular framework of the organ, play an important role in maturation and differentiation of the thymocytes (see Chap. 3). Close contact exists between lymphocytes and epithelial cells which is mediated via the CD2 antigen on T lymphocytes (see below) and the LFA3 (leukocyte function molecule) expressed on the surface of epithelial cells (Singer et al. 1986). Within thymus cortex the most intimate contact is by thymic nurse cells, epithelial cells which contain numerous lymphocytes within their cytoplasm (Wekerle et al. 1980; Ritter et al. 1981).

Furthermore, the thymic epithelial cells mostly in the thymus cortex express MHC class II antigens on their surface (Rouse et al. 1982; von Gau-

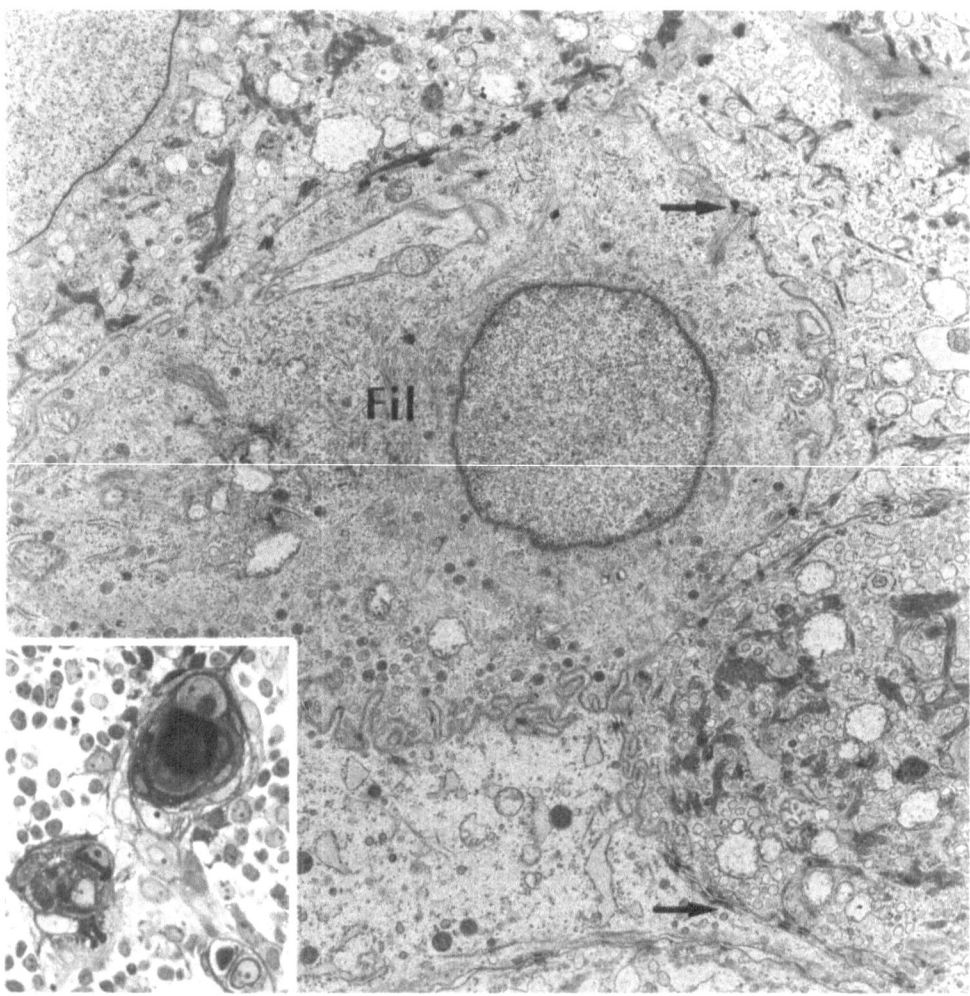

Fig. 2.4. Ultrastructure of normal thymus. Hassall's corpuscle with intertwining cell processes and desmosomes *(arrow)*. The epithelial cells contain tonofilaments *(Fil)* and membrane-coating granules. Uranyl acetate-lead citrate stain, × 11 300. *Inset:* Hassall's corpuscles. Note the concentric arrangement of the epithelial cells. Epon-embedded section stained with toluidine blue, × 720 (Otto 1984)

decker et al. 1986; Marrock et al. 1989), a fact which might be important for the acquirement of the self-MHC restrictivity of T lymphocytes which for T helper cells and class II antigens is shown to take place within the thymus (Kast et al. 1984; Kruisbeek and Longo 1985).

Lastly, thymic epithelial cells have been found to be the source of thymic hormones (Dalakas et al. 1981; Schmitt et al. 1982; Auger et al. 1987; Oates et al. 1987; Fabien et al. 1988; Fujiwara et al. 1988), which are polypeptides with immuno-

pharmacologic properties (Sztein and Goldstein 1986; Sztein et al. 1986; Serrate et al. 1987).

The above-mentioned expression of MHC class II antigens can also be found on other cells within the thymus belonging to the mononuclear phagocytosing cell system, i.e., mononuclear phagocytes (MNPs) and interdigitating dendritic cells (IDCs) (Kaiserling et al. 1974). Whereas MNPs occur both in the cortex and the medulla, IDCs are situated only in the medulla and at the corticomedullary region. In in vitro experiments those cells can be identified as dendritic cells which are able to present antigen to lymphocytes (Kyewski et al. 1986).

Thus, the thymic stromal cells, i.e., the epithelial cells, the MNPs and ICDs constitute a unique microenvironment (van Ewijk 1988; Nabarra and Papiernik 1988; Ruco et al. 1990) which is a prerequisite for the differentiation and maturation of the T lymphocytes.

Lymphocytes within the thymus mainly belong to the T cell subset although recently a small but distinct B cell population of the thymus medulla could be identified (ISAACSON et al. 1987; HOFMANN et al. 1988 a, b).

Morphology and immunophenotype of the T lymphocytes indicate cortical lymphocytes to be of an early maturation and differentiation stage and medullary lymphocytes to be mature and of the peripheral T cell type.

During ontogeny, prethymocytes from the bone marrow and liver enter the thymus, attracted by chemoattractants (CHAMPION et al. 1986; SAVAGNER et al. 1986). Within the peculiar microenvironment of the thymus cortex they start to differentiate as could be shown by rearrangement of the genes coding for the proteins of the T cell receptor (ROYER et al. 1984). This event is followed by the appearance of lymphocyte differentiation antigens on the surface of the cells, by which they can be differentiated into three maturation stages: Stage I thymocytes only express the CD2 antigen. Stage II thymocytes express CD1 antigen, which is not found on peripheral T cells, together with the CD4 and CD8 antigens. Thymocytes of stage I and II are found within the thymus cortex.

Further maturation into stage III cells results in the loss of the CD1 and either the CD4 or CD8 antigen and the expression of the CD3-Ti complex, which is the T cell antigen receptor. The stage III cells are immunocompetent and occur mostly in the medulla although a small number can also be detected within the cortex (for review see REINHERZ and SCHLOSSMAN 1980; MATHIESON and FOWLKES 1984).

Although the pathway of lymphocytes entering and leaving the thymus is not exactly known, it is believed that prethymocytes enter the cortex through the capsule and with further maturation and differentiation migrate towards the medulla, from where they leave the organ through perivascular spaces which belong to the third, extraparenchymal compartment of the organ. Different models, however, exist and have been discussed by SCOLLAY (1983).

2.3 Involution

Severe changes in thymic morphology occur during aging and this process is known as the normal age-dependent thymic involution. The first studies

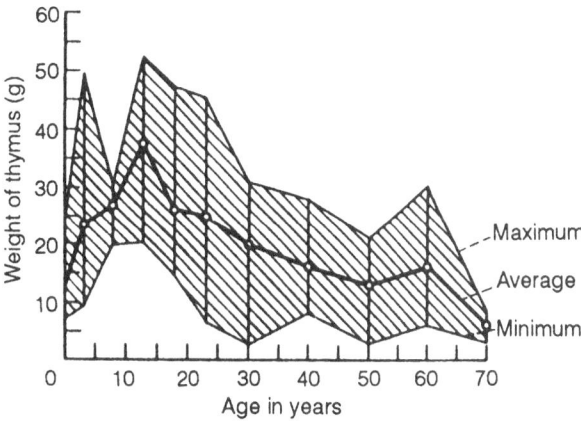

Fig. 2.5. Normal weight range of the human thymus during life, according to the findings of HAMMAR (1926). (HOFMANN et al. 1990)

about age-dependent changes stem from HAMMAR (1906, 1926), who found an increase in the weight of the organ until puberty and thereafter a continuous weight loss. The weight ranges within the different age groups, however, are very large (Fig. 2.5).

STEINMANN, however, in a more recent study, found no evidence that the thymus grows until puberty. Using the volume of the organ as the superior parameter for the size he found that the thymus grows only during the 1st year of life, at the end of which the final size of about 20 cm³ is reached. This size is kept up to 80 years of age (STEINMANN 1984, 1986).

The age-dependent weight loss is the result of changes within the organ capsule, i.e., the reduction of the lymphoid tissue and the augmentation of fat, which has a lower specific gravity than lymphatic tissue (Fig. 2.6). There is a progressive loss of lymphatic tissue of the thymus cortex and medulla whereas fat tissue within the perivascular spaces and the thymic septal spaces increases. These changes start as early as in the 1st year of life, leading to a nearly complete lipomatous atrophy of the organ in older individuals (older than 50 years). The thymus then consists predominantly of fat tissue in a fibrous capsule with only thin stripes of residual lymphatic tissue, which can be detected in vivo using computed tomography (MOORE et al. 1983). However, it is now well established that the thymus nevertheless retains the ability to serve its function in cell-mediated immunologic responses by providing new T cells even in those individuals with only remnants of lymphatic tissue (STUTMAN and GOOD 1974; VON GAUDECKER

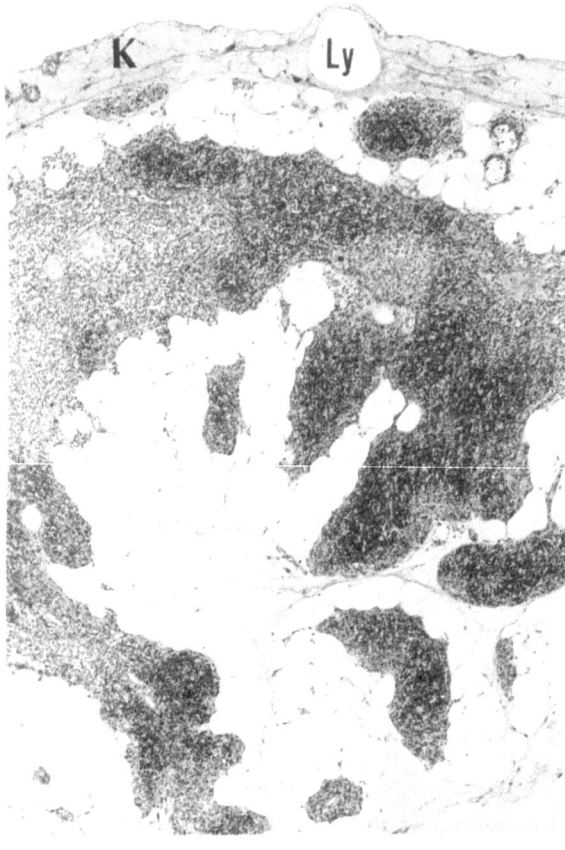

Fig. 2.6. Age involution of the thymus. Female, 27 years. This adult thymus shows involution with fat replacement. *K* capsule, *Ly* small cyst of a lymph vessel (OTTO 1984) PAS, ×50

Fig. 2.7. Accidental involution in the thymus of a 2-year-old child. There is a very marked reduction in the thymic lymphocyte population ("lymphocytic depletion"). The resultant irregular shrunken lobules are composed of spindle-shaped epithelial cells. There is loss of demarcation between cortex and medulla. Hassall's corpuscles are often cystic. (OTTO 1984) PAS, ×80
▽

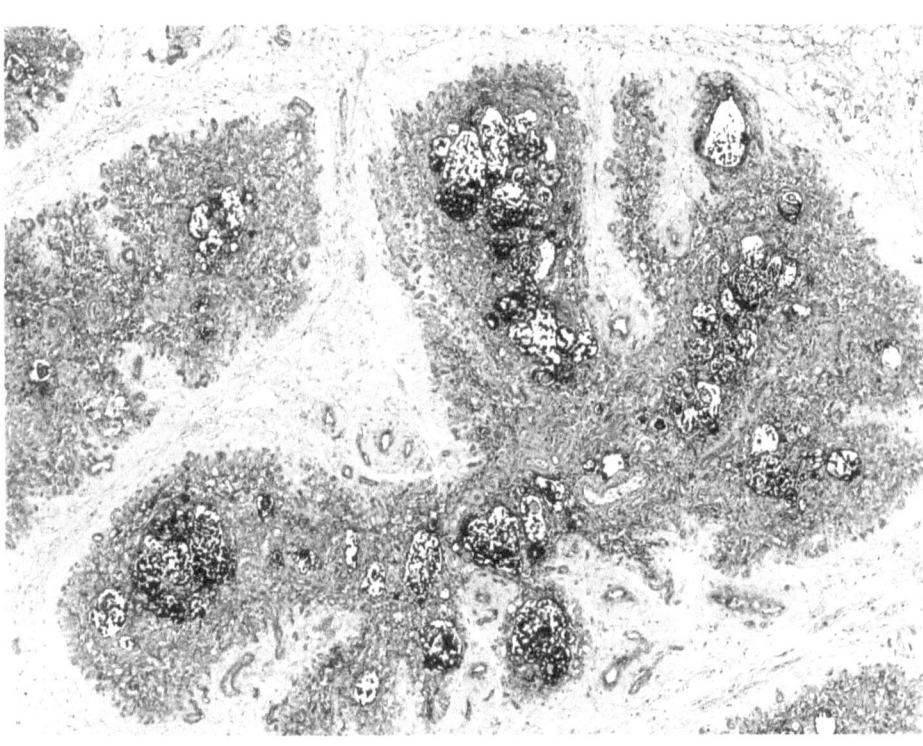

1978; KENDALL 1984; CLARKE and MacLENNAN 1986).

This normal, age-dependent thymic involution may be accelerated under certain circumstances, a fact which becomes important especially in children. This involution process is known as accidental involution or thymic atrophy and must not be confused with some aspects of thymic dysgenesis. The circumstances which may lead to such an accidental involution are any kind of stress with elevated blood levels of corticosteroid hormones, corticosteroid therapy, chemotherapy, radiotherapy of the mediastinum, and malnutrition (DOUROV 1970; VAN BAARLEN et al. 1988) (The thymus gland in seconardy immunodefiency: LINDER 1987: SCHUURMAN et al. 1989).

The histologic picture of thymic atrophy in man is similar to that described in animals after injection of glucocorticoids (DOUROV 1986). Necrosis of cortical thymocytes and their resorption by phagocytosing macrophages lead to a drastic reduction of cortical thymocytes without significant modification of the medulla. Thus, a reverse aspect of the thymus is achieved with a lymphocyte-poor cortex and a relatively dense medulla. Hassall's corpuscles generally persist and become multicystic (Fig. 2.7). The existence of Hassall's corpuscles within the atrophic thymus helps to distinguish between thymic atrophy and thymic dysgenesis, where Hassall's corpuscles are not found.

The accidental involution of the thymus to a certain degree is reversible (HENRY 1968) and may even lead to a rebound phenomenon and hyperplasia (see Sect. 7.4).

References

Auger C, Stahli C, Fabien N, Monier J-C (1987) Intracellular localization of thymosin alpha-1 by immunoelectron microscopy using a monoclonal antibody. J Histochem Cytochem 35: 181–187

Champion S, Imhof BA, Savanger P, Thiery JP (1986) The embryonic thymus produces chemotactic peptides involved in the homing of hematopoietic precursors. Cell 44: 781–790

Ciba Foundation Symposium, No. 84 (1981) Microenvironments in haemapoietic and lymphoid differentiation. Pitman, London

Clarke AG, MacLennan KA (1986) The many facets of thymic involution. Immunol Today 7: 204–205

Dalakas MC, Engel WK, McClure JE, Goldstein AJ, Asconas V (1981) Immunocytochemical characterization of thymosin alpha-1 in thymic epithelial cells of normal and myasthenia gravis patients and in thymic cultures. J Neurol Sci 50: 239–247

DeMaagd RA, Mackenzie WA, Schuurman HJ, Ritter MA, Price KM, Broekhuizen R, Kater L, (1985) The human thymic microenvironment: heterogeneity detected by monoclonal antiepithelial antibodies. Immunology 54: 745–754

Dourov N (1970) L'atrophie thymo-lymphatique chez le nourrisson après traitment prolongé à l'ACTH. Pathol Europ 5: 216–231

Dourov N (1986) Thymic atrophy and immunodeficiency in malnutrition. In: Müller-Hermelink H-K (ed) The human thymus. Histophysiology and pathology. Springer, Berlin Heidelberg New York, pp 127–150

Fabien N, Auger C, Monier J-C (1988) Immunolocalisation of thymosin alpha-1, thymopoietin and thymulin in mouse thymic epithelial cells at different ages of culture: a light and electron microscopic study. Immunology 63: 721–727

Fujiwara S, Kobayashi H, Awaya A (1988) The distribution and structure of FTS immunoreactive cells in the thymus of the mouse. Arch Histol Cytol 51: 467–472

Gay-Bellile V, Boumsell L, Caillou B, Bernard A (1986) Phenotypic characterization of the thymic microenvironment. Study of the human thymus architecture. Thymus 8: 201–223

Gilmour JR (1941) Some developmental abnormalities of the thymus and parathyroids. J Pathol Bacteriol 52: 213–218

Hammar JA (1905) Zur Histogenese und Involution der Thymusdrüse. Anat Anz 27: 23–30, 41–89

Hammar JAA (1906) Über Gewicht, Involution und Persistenz des Thymus im Postfötalleben des Menschen. Arch Anat Physiol, Anat Abt (Suppl): 91–1982

Hammar JA (1926) Der Menschenthymus in Gesundheit und Krankheit: Ergebnisse der numerischen Analyse von mehr als tausend menschlichen Thymusdrüsen. Teil 1: Das normale Organ – zugleich eine kritische Beleuchtung der Lehre des "Status thymicus". Z Mikrosk Anat Forsch 6 (Suppl): 1–570

Haynes BF (1984) The human thymic microenvironment. Adv Immunol 36: 87–142

Henry L (1968) "Accidental" involution of the human thymus. J Pathol Bact 96: 337–343

Hofmann W, Möller P, Momburg F, Moldenhauer G, Otto HF (1984) Struktur des normalen Thymus, der lymphofollikulären Thymushyperplasie und der Thymome, dargestellt mit Lectinen, S-100-Protein und Keratin-Antiseren und monoklonalen (epitheliotropen) Antikörpern. Verh Dtsch Ges Pathol 68: 504

Hofmann WJ, Möller P, Otto HF (1990) Hyperplasia. In: Givel JC (ed) Surgery of the thymus. Springer, Berlin Heidelberg New York, pp 59–70

Hofmann WJ, Momburg F, Möller P (1988a) Thymic medullary cells expressing B lymphocyte antigens. Hum Pathol 19: 1280–1287

Hofmann WJ, Momburg F, Möller P, Otto HF (1988b) Intra- and extrathymic B cells in physiological and pathological conditions. Immunohistochemical study on normal thymus and lymphofollicular hyperplasia of the thymus. Virchows Arch [A] 412: 431–442

Hofmann WJ, Pallesen G, Möller P, Kunze W-P, Kayser K, Otto HF (1989) Expression of cortical and medullary thymic epithelial antigens in thymomas. An immunohistological study of 14 cases including a characterization of the lymphocytic compartment. Histopathology 14: 447–463

Isaacson PG, Norton AJ, Addis BJ (1987) The human thymus contains a novel population of B lymphocytes. Lancet II: 1488–1490

Kaiserling E, Stein H, Müller-Hermelink HK (1974) Interdigitating reticulum cells in the human thymus. Cell Tissue Res 155: 47–55

Kast WM, deWaal LP, McLief CJM (1984) Thymus dictates major histocompatibility complex (MHC) specificity and immune response gene phenotype of class II MHC-restricted T cells but not calls I MHC-restricted T cells. J Exp Med 160: 1752–1766

Kendall MD (1984) Have we underestimated the importance of the adult human thymus? Experientia 40: 1181–1185

Kruisbeek AM, Longo DL (1985) Acquisition of MCH-restriction specificities: role of thymic stromal cells. Surv Immunol Res 4: 110–119

Kyewski BA, Fathman CG, Rouse RV (1986) Intrathymic presentation of circulating non-MHC antigens by medullary dendritic cells. J Exp Med 163: 231–246

Levine GD, Rosai J (1978) Thymic hyperplasia and neoplasia: a review of current concepts. Hum Pathol 9: 495–515

Levine GD, Bearman RM (1980) The thymus. In: Johannessen JV (ed) Electron microscopy in human medicine, vol 5. McGraw-Hill, New York, pp 214–254

Linder J (1987) The thymus gland in secondary immunodeficiency. Arch Pathol Lab Med 111: 1118–1122

Marino M, Müller-Hermelink H-K (1985) Thymoma and thymic carcinoma – relation of thymoma epithelial cells to the cortical and medullary differentiation of thymus. Virchows Arch [A] 407: 119–149

Marrock P, McCormack J, Kappler J (1989) Presentation of antigen, foreign major histocompatibility complex proteins and self by thymus cortical epithelium. Nature 338: 503–505

Mathieson BJ, Fowlkes BJ (1984) Cell surface antigen expression on thymocytes: development and phenotypic differentiation of intrathymic subsets. Immunol Rev 82: 141–173

McFarland EJ, Scearce RM, Haynes BF (1984) The human thymic microenvironment: cortical thymic epithelium is an antigenetically distinct region of the thymic microenvironment. J Immunol 133: 1241–1249

Moore AV, Korobkin M, Olanow W, Heaston DK, Ram PC, Dunnick NR, Silverman PM (1983) Age-related changes in the thymus gland. CT-pathologic correlation. AJR 141: 291

Müller-Hermelink H-K (ed) (1986) Current topics in pathology 75. The human thymus. Histophysiology and pathology. Springer, Berlin Heidelberg New York

Nabarra B, Papiernik M (1988) Phenotype of thymicstromal cells. An immunoelectron microscopic study with anti-IA, anti-MAC-1, and anti-MAC-2 antibodies. Lab Invest 58: 524–531

Nakahama M, Mohri N, Mori S, Shindo G, Yokoi Y, Machinami R (1990) Immunohistochemical and histometrical studies of the human thymus with special emphasis on age-related changes in medullary epithelial and dendritic cells. Virchows Arch B Cell Pathol 58: 245–251

Norris EH (1938) The morphogenesis and histogenesis of the thymus gland in man: in which the origin of the Hassall's corpuscles of the human thymus is discovered. Carnegie Inst Wsh Publ no 496. Contrib Embryol 27: 191–221

Oates KK, Naylor PH, Goldstein AL (1987) Localization of thymosin alpha-1 production to thymus medullary epithelial cells by use of monoclonal antibodies. Hybridoma 6: 47

Otto HF (1984) Pathologie des Thymus. In: Doerr W, Seifert G, Uehlinger E (eds) Spezielle pathologische Anatomie, vol 17. Springer, Berlin Heidelberg New York

Reinherz EL, Schlossman SF (1980) The differentiation and function of human T lymphocytes. Cell 19: 821–827

Ritter MA, Sauvage CA, Cotmore SF (1981) The human thymus microenvironment: in vivo identification of thymic nurse cells and other antigenically distinct subpopulations of epithelial cells. Immunology 44: 439–446

Rosai J, Levine GD (1976) Tumors of the thymus. In: Atlas of tumor pathology, second series, fascicle 13. Armed Forces Institute of Pathology, Washington, DC

Rouse RV, Parham P, Grumet FC, Weisman JL (1982) Expression of HLA antigens by human thymic epithelial cells. Human Immunol 5: 21–34

Royer HD, Acuto O, Fabbi M, Tizard R, Ramachandram K (1984) Genes encoding the Tib subunit of the antigen/MHC receptor undergo rearrangement during intrathymic ontogeny prior to surface T3/Ti expression. Cell 39: 261–266

Ruco LP, Pisacane A, Pomponi D, Stoppacciaro A, Pecarmona E, Rendina EA, Santoni A, Boraschi D, Tagliabue AT, Uccini S, Baroni CD (1990) Macrophages and interdigitating reticulum cells in normal human thymus and thymomas: immunoreactivity for interleukin-1 alpha, interleukin-1 beta and tumour necrosis factor alpha. Histopathology 17: 291–299

Savagner P, Imhof BA, Yamada KM, Thiery J-P (1986) Homing of hemopoietic precursor cells to the embryonic thymus: characterization of an invasive mechanism induced by chemotactic peptides. Cell Biol 103: 2715–2727

Schmitt D, Monier JC, Dardsenne M, Pleau JM, Bach JF (1982) Location of FTS (facteur thymique serique) in the thymus of normal and autoimmune mice. Thymus 4: 221–231

Schuurman H-J, Krone WJA, Broekhuizen R, van Baarlen J, van Veen P, Goldstein AL, Huber J, Goudsmit J (1989) The thymus in aquired immune deficiency syndrome. Comparison with other types of immunodeficiency diseases, and presence of components of humanimmunodeficiency virus type 1. Am J Pathol 134: 1329–1338

Scollay R (1983) Intrathymic events in the differentiation of T lymphocytes: a continuing enigma. Immunol Today 4: 282–286

Serrate SA, Schulof RS, Leonaridis L, Goldstein AL, Sztein MB (1987) Modulation of natural killer cell cytotoxic activity, lymphokine production, and interleukin 2 receptor expression by thymic hormones. J Immunol 139: 2338

Singer KH, Wolf LS, Lobach DF, Denning SM, Tuck DT, Robertson AL, Haynes BF (1986) Human thymocytes bind to autologous and allogeneic thymic epithelial cells in vitro. Proc Natl Acad Sci USA 83: 6588–6592

Steinmann GG (1984) Altersveränderungen des menschlichen Thymus. Habilitationsschrift, Faculty of Medicine, University of Kiel

Steinmann GG (1986) Changes in the human thymus during aging. In: Müller-Hermelink H-K (ed) The human thymus. Histophysiology and pathology. Springer, Berlin Heidelberg New York, pp 43–88

Stutman O, Good RA (1974) Duration of thymic function. Semin Hematol 7: 504–523

Suster S, Rosai J (1990) Histology of the normal thymus. Am J Surg Pathol 14: 284–303

Sztein MB, Goldstein AL (1986) Thymic hormones – a clinical update. Springer Semin Immunopathol 9: 1–18

Sztein MB, Serrate SA, Goldstein AL (1986) Modulation of interleukin 2 receptor expression on normal human lymphocytes by thymic hormones. Proc Natl Acad Sci USA 83: 6107–6111

Takacs L, Savino W, Monostori E, Ando I, Bach J-F, Dardenne M (1987) Cortical thymocyte differentiation in thymomas: an immunohistologic analysis of the pathologic microenvironment. J Immunol 138: 687–698

van Baarlen J, Schuurman H-J, Huber J (1988) Acute thymus involution in infancy and childhood: A reliable marker for duration of acute illness. Hum Pathol 19: 1155–1160

van Ewijk W (1988) Cell surface topography of thymic microenvironments. Lab Invest 59: 579–590

von Gaudecker B (1978) Ultrastructure of the age-involuted adult human thymus. Cell Tissue Res 186: 507–525

von Gaudecker B (1986) The development of the human thymus microenvironment. In: Müller-Hermelink HK (ed) The human thymus. Histophysiology and pathology. Springer, Berlin Heidelberg New York, pp 1–41

von Gaudecker B, Müller-Hermelink HK (1980) Ontogeny and organization of the stationary non-lymphoid cells in the human thymus. Cell Tissue Res 207: 287–306

von Gaudecker B, Steinmann GG, Hansmann M-L, Harpprecht J, Milicevic NM, Müller-Hermelink H-K (1986) Immunohistochemical characterization of the thymic microenvironment. A light-microscopic and ultrastructural immunocytochemical study. Cell Tissue Res 244: 403–412

Wekerle H, Ketelson VP, Ernst M (1980) Thymic muscle cells. Lymphoepithelial complexes in neuronic thymuses: morphological and serological characterization. J Exp Med 151: 925–944

Weller GL (1933) Development of the thyroid, parathyroid, and thymus glands in man. Carnegie Inst Wsh Publ no 443. Contrib Embryol 24: 93–143

3 Immunologic Function of the Thymus

M. DEBATIN

3.1 Historical Overview

"No structure of the body is less understood, nor, with few exceptions, has had more functions attributed to it, than the thymus gland" (NELSON 1950). This statement in the 5th edition of the *Textbook of Pediatrics* by W. E. NELSON summarizes the state of the art in thymus research as it was until 30 years ago. Prior to 1960 clinical discussions especially among pediatricians were mainly preoccupied with a condition, so-called status thymolymphaticus, in which an acutely enlarged thymus was found in children with sudden and unexpected death (FINKELSTEIN 1938; VON PFAUNDLER 1949; WALDBOTT 1934). It was argued that the large thymus caused a critical obstruction of the respiratory tract. There were, however, no substantial data to confirm a significant causative role of the thymus (RABSON 1949). The term "status thymolymphaticus" and its implication as a cause of thymic death certainly inhibited an adequate search for the real cause of death in many cases. Despite the controversy regarding thymic enlargement as a cause of airway obstruction, roentgen treatment of an enlarged thymus was widely used, entailing the long-term risk of development of thyroid carcinomas (McCONAHEY and HAYLER 1976). Another clinical condition in which a causative role of the thymus was postulated was myasthenia gravis. It had been suggested that myasthenia gravis was an autoimmune disease on the basis of experimentally induced thymic lesions in animals (EATON and GLAGETT 1955). The improvement in some instances following thymectomy supported this view.

A remarkable clinical observation related to the size of the thymus was the extraordinary flexibility of the organ during life and under several conditions. It had been recognized that the size of the thymus, in relationship to body weight, was largest in childhood and that the thymus undergoes progressive involution in adults (BOYD 1927). In addition the wider use of x-ray diagnostics revealed that temporary changes in the size of the thymus occur in a variety of conditions. For example, nutritional status as well as severely debilitating diseases influence the thymic size, reducing the weight of the thymus within a few days. Pharmacologic influences such as steroid treatment were found to cause a dramatic temporary involution of the thymus. In addition fluctuation of the size of the thymus in relationship to adrenal function was observed. The most important interrelationship was the inverse relation between the size of the thymus and adrenocortical activity in fetal, newborn, and adult animals. Therefore it was suggested that the thymus may have an endocrine function. However, an endocrinologic clinical syndrome has not been observed after human thymectomy and extirpation experiments in animals done at that time did not provide conclusive proof of endocrine function.

The lack of knowledge about the true function of the thymus was perpetuated by the preoccupation of immunologists over the decades with the most easily accessible molecules explaining immunologic reactivity and specificity, namely the immunoglobulins. The wide application of serologic methods and the restriction of more cellular approaches to classic histologic methods obscured rather than revealed the function of the thymus and the function of lymphocytes as the primary immunologically relevant cells. However, the search for immunocompetent cells in the 1950s and especially carefully performed studies in experimental animals in the 1960s led to dramatic progress in our understanding of the immune system in general, and more recently of the molecules and genes involved in the development of the immune system. This research has caused the thymus to be attributed a central role within the whole immune system.

In the 1960s it was shown by various groups (MILLER 1961; GOOD et al. 1962; SZENBERG and WARNER 1962; COOPER et al. 1965) that the thymus is the central breeding organ for a particular subsets of lymphocytes, the so-called T lymphocytes. On the other hand B lymphocytes, which are the antibody-producing cells, are derived from a different breeding organ, the bursa of Fabricius in birds or fetal liver and bone marrow in mammals. The identification of T lymphocytes and B lymphocytes as the cellular components of the immune system was followed by the identification of different T cell subpopulations, T helper cells and T suppressor/killer cells, which are involved in different regulatory networks in the immune system (REINHERZ et al. 1979; REINHERZ and SCHLOSSMANN 1980). From these studies it has also become clear that T cells are also involved in antibody formation by providing necessary helper factors for B cells. The last 10 years have brought even more major breakthroughs in respect of principal questions posed by immunologists as well as molecular biology in general. Thus the recognition structures by which T cells interact with antigen have been identified (MEUER et al. 1983; ACUTO and REINHERZ 1985), and more recently molecular techniques have yielded new experimental evidence about the cellular selection in the thymus and the ways by which the immune system distinguishes between "self" and "nonself" (for review see VON BOEHMER 1988).

In summary, the last 30 years have shown that the thymus plays a central role in the development of the immune system because it is the only organ which generates T lymphocytes. The most important function of T cells, namely the discrimination between "self" and "nonself," ist acquired during their maturation in the thymus. Therefore the size of the thymus is largest at a time when the immune system has its strongest developmental forces, i.e., in early childhood. From this point of view the term "status thymolymphaticus" more closely reflects the normal thymic size and the small sizes which have been considered to be representative of normal glands are in actuality those of glands reduced in size by inanition and disease.

The following sections provide a brief summary of our present knowledge on T cell molecules involved in antigen recognition, on the ontogeny of T cells and the T cell development within the thymus, and on the mechanisms by which cellular selection in the thymus occurs (for a review of the literature see VON BOEHMER 1988; FOWLKES and PARDOLL 1989; HAYNES et al. 1989). In addition a few clinical aspects related to the physiology of the thymus will be discussed.

3.2 T Cell Molecules in Antigen Recognition

To exert their particular function, lymphocytes have to be able to recognize antigen specifically. This is achieved by clonally distributed antigen recognition molecules. B lymphocytes recognize soluble antigens and they use immunoglobulin molecules as antigen recognition structures. T cells recognize antigen in the context of HLA-encoded surface structures on other cells. For this purpose they are equipped with two different sets of recognition structures: the antigen receptor structure (antigen receptor CD3 complex) and recognition molecules (CD4, CD8) for HLA molecules on antigen-presenting cells.

The antigen receptor complex of T cells consists of clonally distributed highly polymorphic disulfide-linked heterodimers which are noncovalently associated on the cell surface with five invariant chains (CD3 complex). In the vast majority of mature T cells, the T cell antigen receptor complex (TCR) has α/β heterodimers. A minority (less than 5%) of mature T cells express γ/δ heterodimers.

Like antibody molecules in B lymphocytes, the TCR molecules in T cells are encoded by gene segments which undergo extensive somatic recombinations (WALDMANN 1987). Each chain of the TCR complex is encoded by a set of gene segments. For example, for the β-chain the segments are called V (variability), D (diversity), J (joining), and C for the constant part of the chain. During T cell development in each T cell one of the various V segments is combined with a particular D and J segment. Thus the enormous variability of antigen recognition molecules is not encoded as a universe of receptor structures within the germline but instead is created by recombination of a limited number of genes during somatic development of T cells. The discovery that the antigen receptors on immune cells are created by multiple recombinations of gene clusters during somatic development of the precursor cells has been one of the major breakthroughs in immunology and molecular biology during the last 15 years.

The TCR heterodimer is associated with an invariant membrane complex termed CD3. Because CD3 cross-linking can mimic antigenic stimulation of T cells and because all of the CD3 proteins have large intracytoplasmatic portions, the CD3 complex is considered to be involved in signal transduction that is initiated when the TCR complex is stimulated by antigen.

3.2.1 Accessory Molecules

T cells do not respond to soluble antigen but instead recognize antigen in the context of structures encoded by the major histocompatibility complex (MHC, the HLA system in man) on the surface of antigen-presenting or antigen-bearing cells.

The HLA system is a highly polymorphic system of membrane proteins which differ between individuals. The MHC complex has two different sets of elements: class I molecules (A, B, C) and class II molecules (D, DR, DP, DQ). Class I molecules are widely distributed on nearly all cells of the body, whereas class II molecules have a restricted pattern of expression on certain cells involved in immune responses (B cells, cells of hemopoietic lineage, activated T cells).

Several years ago it was recognized that the T cell system has two different types of cells: T helper cells, which regulate T or B cell responses mainly by the production of regulatory factors (lymphokines), and T suppressor- or T killer cells, which downregulate immune responses or function as cytotoxic T cells for, for example, virally infected cells. The responses of T helper cells have been shown to be restricted to T cells which recognize antigen in the context of HLA class II molecules; T killer cell responses require the presence of HLA class I molecules on the surface of the antigen-presenting cell.

The CD4 molecule, which is the characteristic hallmark of the T helper cells, is the recognition molecule for class II antigens. The CD8 molecule, which is characteristic for T cells of the killer type, is the recognition structure for class I molecules on the surface of the target cells.

In addition to the recognition molecules a number of functionally important or lineage-specific T cell molecules have been identified by monoclonal antibodies. These molecules are either constitutively (CD1, CD2, CD5, CD7) or temporarily (CD25) expressed on mature T cells. During development in the thymus these surface structures are sequentially acquired. The CD2 molecule, for a long time known as the receptor for sheep red blood cells on T lymphocytes, is the receptor for subsets (LFA-3) of molecules involved in lymphocyte interactions. The CD25 molecule is a part of the interleukin-2 receptor complex, which is expressed on mature T cells after activation. Inter-

leukin-2 is the essential growth factor in the proliferative responses of mature T cells. Interleukin-2 and the expression of the interleukin-2 receptor may also play a role in the development of thymocytes (see below).

3.3 Ontogeny of T Cells

The vast majority of T cells found in the periphery originate in the thymus, where T lymphocytes are formed from hemopoietic precursor cells which enter the thymus throughout life. The thymus continuously releases T cells with mature phenotypes which are fully equipped to function in antigen recognition. No further maturation occurs in the periphery; therefore all maturation events in the development of T cells must occur pre- or intrathymically. However, small numbers of T lymphocytes may differentiate ectopically and account for the few T cells found in athymic mice. T cell maturation in the thymus starts early in gestation (around 10 weeks), has its highest intensity during childhood, and declines during further life. This dynamic of T cell development as part of the age-dependent dynamic of the lymphoid system in general is reflected by the size of the thymus in different phases.

After colonization of the thymic rudiment during fetal and embryonic life, three steps of T cell development can be distinguished:

1. Immigration of precursor cells into the thymus
2. Acquisition of T lineage specific surface molecules with rearrangement and expression of TCR
3. Maturation and diversification into CD4$^+$ or CD8$^+$ subsets with the acquisition of effector functions

The different steps of maturation can be described by the sequence in which the arrangement of TCR genes and expression of recognition structures occur. Therefore thymocytes are grouped into categories of cells with respect to expression of the recognition structures, i.e., expression of TCR α/β or TCR γ/δ, the CD3 complex, and the CD4- and CD8 molecules, beginning with the most immature phenotypes. Within the thymus the different groups of thymocytes show a different distribution: the more immature cells are localized in the thymic cortex whereas the more mature cells are localized within the thymic medulla, from which they appear to leave the thymus as functional peripheral T cells.

3.3.1 Thymocyte Precursors

The thymic precursor cells originate in the pluripotent stem cell of the hemolymphopoietic lineage localized in the bone marrow. In man at around the 10th week of gestation the thymic rudiment becomes colonized by the first immature T cell precursors. These cells are characterized by the expression of a hemopoietic stem cell marker (CD34) and CD7, the first surface structure to be expressed on T cells. This cell population migrates from bone marrow to the thymus. The early immigrants lack all recognition structures (TCR, CD3, CD4, CD8) and are therefore called "triple-negative" cells (CD3$^-$, CD4$^-$, CD8$^-$). These cells represent a very minor subset in the adult thymus. The following steps of development involve the sequential expression of the recognition structures, namely the TCR complex, the CD3 complex, and the CD4- and CD8 molecules.

3.3.2 TCR Rearrangements

Approximately 100% of thymocytes from the earliest days of fetal ontogeny are triple-negative, whereas less than 50% of adult thymocytes possess this phenotype. Further developmental steps of T lymphopoiesis start from this population. The vast majority of thymocytes in the adult thymus are so-called double-positive thymocytes because they express both CD4 and CD8 molecules. It is this population in which the strongest proliferation within the thymus takes place. The acquisition of the coexpression of CD4 and CD8 recognition structures is paralleled by the arrangements of the T cell receptor complex and the CD3 complex. About half of the double-positive (CD4$^+$, CD8$^+$) thymocytes express the CD3 complex and TCR α/β chains. In mouse and man there is an ordered sequence in which the rearrangements occur in the different gene clusters. The triple-negative thymocytes which have entered the thymus do not have any rearrangements of the T cell receptor genes. The first loci to undergo rearrangement are β, γ, and probably δ. Productive γ and δ rearrangements result in a CD3-associated γ/δ heterodimer and these cells are the first functional cells to be formed in the thymus.

If β rearrangement is successful before γ rearrangement this signals a cell to start the rearrangement of the α gene segments. Thus, depending on which loci productive rearrangements occur first, the cell will end as an α/β or γ/δ expressing cell. T cells which express a γ/δ receptor structure do not express CD4 or CD8 molecules but apparently may leave the thymus as mature T cells. However, they represent less than 1% of thymocytes and also less than 1% of peripheral T cells in adult life. The function of these cells is presently not entirely understood; they may represent an unique T cell subpopulation. Nearly all T cell receptor expressing T cells within the thymus express an $\alpha\beta$ recognition structure. This is also found on nearly all T cells in the periphery. Cells which start to rearrange the α gene segment apparently become double-positive during this developmental step. Whenever the rearrangements of the T cell receptor genes are successful, the CD3 complex which is associated with the T cell receptor complex will be expressed. Within the double-positive TCR α/β positive and CD3 positive population the selection processes take place (see below).

3.3.3 Maturation into Functional T Cells

The next population to appear in T cell development after the double-positive cells are CD4$^+$8$^-$ followed by the CD4$^-$8$^+$ thymocytes (single-positive cells). Single-positive thymocytes are similar to peripheral CD4$^+$ and CD8$^+$ cells in both phenotype and function. However, evidence is mounting that these populations may be more heterogeneous than previously believed. Within the thymus these cells are located in the medulla. A number of functional differences, such as requirements for activation and differences in mitogen stimulation and lymphokine responsiveness, have been described between single-positive thymocytes and mature peripheral T cells.

3.3.4 Factors Governing T Cell Development Within the Thymus

The above-mentioned developmental steps are controlled by interactions of thymocytes with the elements of the thymus stroma. The stroma is a heterogeneous population of epithelial cells and cells derived from the hemopoietic lineage such as macrophages and dendritic cells. The interaction with these cells appears to be very important for the selection processes within the thymus (see below). In addition to cellular interactions, thymocytes respond to a variety of mainly T cell derived lymphokines (interleukin-1, interleukin-2, interleukin-3, interleukin-4, interleukin-6, and interleukin-7). Although some of these factors also act on mature T cells, the responsiveness of thymocytes is somewhat different. It is believed that these cytokines are crucially involved especially in the abundant proliferation which occurs within the thymus. Also certain steps of developmental maturation may be induced or maintained by these factors.

In addition to T cell derived cytokines, several peptides called thymic hormones have been isolated from thymic extracts. These factors may induce phenotypic or functional changes in thymic or post-thymic cells. Four peptide hormones have been characterized and chemically synthesized: thymulin, thymosin α-1, thymosin β-4, and thymopoietin. Many other materials isolated from thymus extracts have been studied in vitro and in vivo. The uncertain role of these hormones has been widely discussed.

A remarkable finding in the ontogeny of T lymphocytes and T lymphocyte precursors is the enormous proliferation which apparently is necessary to generate mature T cells. In the mouse it has been calculated that the daily production rate for the cortical double-positive thymocytes is 5×10^7 cells, which is approximately 5% of the total T cell compartment in the mouse. On the other hand only 2×10^6 medullary single-positive cells are generated. These 2×10^6 cells represent the mature thymic emigrants leaving the young adult thymus every day. Therefore most cortical cells do not become medullary cells and since they are not leaving the thymus they must die intrathymically. Indeed, the thymus is considered one of the organs in the body in which the most extensive cell death occurs (MCPHEE et al. 1979). The dying cells most probably represent cells which have not passed the filters during the selection processes (see below).

3.4 Cellular Selection in the Thymus

T cells acquire intrathymically their antigen receptors as well as their potential to become effector cells after antigenic stimulation. Since T cells recognize antigen in the context of self-MHC struc-

tures, it follows that the thymus must be the main organ where developing T cells adjust to "self" antigens and learn "self-nonself" discrimination. During development in the thymus, T cells with a strong antiself reactivity may arise, and those self-reactive T cells have to be eliminated before they leave the thymus as mature effector cells. This deletion of antiself-specific T cells has long been a central question in T cell research. Although the selection mechanisms are still not entirely clear, the current interpretation, which is supported by experimental data, is that selection processes involve three different mechanisms. First T cells which are not able to productively rearrange their T cell receptor genes die within the thymus. Thus all CD3$^-$, CD4$^+$, CD8$^+$ cells die intrathymically. In addition most of the CD3$^+$, CD4$^+$, CD8$^+$ T cells also die. This is due to additional active selection processes. T cells which have productively rearranged their T cell receptor genes and have become CD3$^+$ cells are rescued from cell death provided their α/β receptors bind to MHC antigens on epithelial cells. Depending on whether their α/β receptors bind to class I or class II MHC antigens, the expression of either CD4 or CD8 is suppressed. These positively selected cells are then screened by hemopoietic cells and those expressing sufficiently high affinity for self-antigens are clonally eliminated. All these selection processes appear to occur in the double-positive (CD4$^+$, CD8$^+$) population.

In summary, a developing T cell that expresses a T cell receptor on its surface is able to pass through the selection stage. Thymocytes must pass through two selection filters based on the T cell receptor they express. Positive selection favors the development of thymocytes expressing T cell receptors that preferentially recognize foreign antigens in association with self-MHC molecules. Negative selection eliminates thymocytes that express self-reactive T cell receptors and that could therefore cause autoimmunity.

3.5 Clinical Aspects

As mentioned earlier, during the last 20 years the role of the thymus as the central organ for T lymphopoiesis has been established. Based on these developments in basic research there are only a few situations left which are clinically important: lack or deficiency of thymic functions and enlargement of the thymus above the normal size.

From the preceding sections it is evident that any disturbance of the thymic function eventually leads to severe disturbances of the T cell arm of the immune system, thereby causing immunodeficiency. Thus the absence of a thymus is characteristic for immunodeficiency diseases grouped as severe combined immunodeficiency, in which low numbers of mature lymphocytes are found. These immunodeficiency diseases may affect T and B cells similarly. A pure thymic defect is found in DiGeorge syndrome, where B cells are formed in normal numbers but the number of T cells is dramatically reduced due to the absence of a thymic organ. This condition in its extreme form reflects what is found in athymic nude mice or what can be experimentally produced by neonatal thymectomy in mice. There has also been much speculation regarding deficient thymic function in cases of T cell immunodeficiency where T cells are produced in normal numbers but do not function properly. To date there has been no definite identification of such a functional defect within the thymus. However, several thymic peptides have been used clinically for the treatment of putative or definitely diagnosed T cell immunodeficiencies.

The other extreme of thymic pathology is the enlargement of the thymus above the size which is normally found at a given age. As stated earlier, the size of the thymus is subject to extensive variation both during life and between different individuals. The normal thymus, which is largest in early childhood, is rarely the cause of any pathologic situation, including airway obstruction.

Whenever considerable enlargement of the thymus, also called thymic mass, is found on an x-ray an underlying malignant condition has to be ruled out. Beside the rare thymomas, malignant neoplasms of the immune system itself are a major cause of thymic enlargement (HENZE et al. 1981; POPLACK 1989). In childhood by far the most important condition is the involvement of the thymus in acute lymphoblastic leukemias or high-grade malignant non-Hodgkin's lymphomas. The T cell subtypes of these diseases usually have an enlarged thymus which can cause severe problems, including airway obstruction. In these cases, the thymus can also be considered as the primary organ in which the tumor or the leukemia arose since the phenotypes which are found in acute T cell leukemias or non-Hodgkin's lymphomas T cell type usually represent differentiation stages of T cell precursors usually found in the thymus. Thus one may speculate that the malignant cells represent precursors which have escaped the normal control

mechanism for the different steps of T lymphocyte development within the thymus. Otherwise the thymus is rarely an organ for metastasizing tumors. On the other hand germ cell tumors, for example, may mimic a thymic mass in the anterior mediastinum. Another pathologic condition involving the thymus or deficient thymus function is myasthenia gravis, which is discussed in Chap. II.

3.6 Summary

Research over the last 20 years has made dramatic progress in elucidating the normal function of the thymus and the possible relationships to abnormal clinical conditions. The thymus has been established as the central organ for T lymphocyte development. The molecular mechanisms underlying T cell differentiation have been elucidated during recent years, and one of the most important questions in cellular immunology, namely how the thymus selects T cells, has been clarified.

References

Acuto O, Reinherz EL (1985) The human T-cell receptor. Structure and function. N Engl J Med 312: 1100–1111

Boyd E (1927) Growth of the thymus. Its relation to status thymolymphaticus and thymic symptoms. Am J Dis Child 33: 867–879

Cooper MD, Peterson RDA, Good RA (1965) Delineation of the thymic and bursal lymphoid systems in the chicken. Nature 205: 143–146

Eaton LM, Glagett OT (1955) Symposium on myasthenia gravis: present status of the thymectomy in the treatment of myasthenia gravis. Ann J Med 19: 703

Editorial (1983) Which thymic hormone? Lancet I: 1309–1311

Finkelstein H (1938) Erkrankungen des Thymus und Status thymolymphaticus. In: Finkelstein H (ed) Säuglingskrankheiten, 4th edn. Elsevier, New York, pp 644–654

Fowlkes BJ, Pardoll DM (1989) Molecular and cellular events of T cell development. Adv Immunol 44: 207–264

Good RA, Dalmasso AP, Martinez C, Arber OK, Pierce JC, Papermaster BW (1962) The role of the thymus in development of immunological capacity in rabbits and mice. J Exp Med 116: 773–796

Haynes BF, Denning SM, Singer KH, Kurtzberg J (1989) Ontogeny of T cell precursors: a model for the initial stages of human T cell development. Immunol Today 10: 87–91

Henze G, Langermann HJ, Kaufmann U, Ludwig R, Schellong G, Stollmann B, Riehm H (1981) Thymic involvement and initial white blood count in childhood acute lymphoblastic leukemia. Am J Pediatr Hematol Oncol 3: 369–376

Lawton AR, Cooper MD (1989) Ontogeny of immunity. In: Stiehm ER (ed) Immunological disorders in infants and children. Saunders, Philadelphia, pp 1–14

McConahey WM, Hayler MB (1976) Radiation to the head, neck and upper thorax of the young and thyroid neoplasia. J Clin Endocrinol 42: 1182

McPhee D, Pye J, Shortmann K (1979) The differentiation of thymocytes. V. Evidence for intrathymic death of most thymocytes. Thymus 1: 151

Meuer SC, Fitzgerald DA, Hussey RT, Hodgdan JC, Schlossmann SF, Reinherz EL (1983) Clonotypic structures involved in antigen specific human T cell function: relationship to the T3 molecular complex. J Exp Med 157: 705–719

Miller JFAP (1961) Immunological function of the thymus. Lancet II: 748–749

Nelson WE (1950) The thymus gland. In: Nelson WE (ed) Textbook of pediatrics, 5th edn. Saunders, Philadelphia, pp 1164–1166

Owen JJT, Raff MC (1970) Studies on the differentiation of thymus derived lymphocytes. J Exp Med 132: 1216–1232

Poplack DG (1989) Acute lymphoblastic leukemia. In: Pizzo PA, Poplack DG (eds) Principles and practice of pediatric oncology. Lippincott, Philadelphia, pp 323–366

Rabson SM (1949) Sudden and unexpected natural death in infants and young children. J Pediatr 34: 166–173

Reinherz EL, Schlossmann SF (1980) The differentiation and function of human T lymphocytes. Cell 19: 821–827

Reinherz EL, Kung PC, Goldstein G, Schlossmann SF (1979) Separation of functional subsets of human T cells by a monoclonal antibody. Proc Natl Acad Sci USA 76: 4061–4065

Szenberg A, Warner NL (1962) Immunological function of the thymus and bursa of Fabricius. Dissociation of immunological responsiveness in fowls with hormonally arrested development of lymphoid tissues. Nature 194: 146–148

von Boehmer H (1988) The developmental biology of T-lymphocytes. Ann Rev Immunol 6: 309–326

von Pfaundler M (1949) Status thymicus. In: Lust F, von Pfaundler M (eds) Krankheiten des Kindesalters 3rd edn, Urban und Schwarzenberg, Berlin; p 101

Waldbott GJ (1934) So-called "thymic death." Am J Dis Child 47: 41–60

Waldmann TA (1987) The arrangement of immunoglobulin and T cell receptor genes in human lymphoproliferative disorders. Adv Immunol 40: 247–322

4 Imaging Procedures for Visualization of the Thymus

E. Walter, E. Willich, W. R. Webb, and G. de Geer

4.1 Plain Film Diagnostics

E. Walter and E. Willich

4.1.1 Chest Radiography in Two Planes

Chest radiography in the sagittal and lateral planes remains the essential diagnostic method in respect of the thymus despite all the modern imaging methods now available.

In *infants and young children* up to the 2nd year of age, the examination is usually performed in a plastic casing (a so-called Babix casing), since the restlessness of such children makes it impossible to obtain radiographs that are precise and amenable to interpretation. Unlike in adults, radiography is performed usually with about 50–60 kV of tube voltage; in older children the kV level is raised because of the increased height.

In the anteroposterior projection which is usually employed in infants and young children (but seldom after the 3rd year of age), the thymus appears on the radiograph as a paramediastinal shadow. Although the thymus does not attain its greatest volume until puberty, it no longer overlaps the mediastinal border from the 2nd–3rd year onward (Oliva 1973; Parker et al. 1985). In order to evaluate the thymus a radiograph in the lateral projection then becomes necessary; this also holds true for infants when the anteroposterior projection yields unclear findings.

Chest radiography in adults is mainly performed in two planes with hard rays (> 100 kV). This technique is also sometimes indicated in children to examine tracheal obstruction or an ectopic thymus (Bar-Ziv 1984). In adolescents and adults the thymus is normally not visible on the posteroanterior chest radiograph because of the involution of the organ. Therefore the posteroanterior radiograph reveals pathologic processes only from a certain size upward; such visualization occurs if the contour of the mediastinum is changed. Therefore the lateral view is often indispensable, being of prime and often decisive diagnostic importance.

The thymus lays retrosternally on the heart and can fill the entire anterior mediastinum in infants. The shadow density in the so-called thymus space can reach or exceed that of the heart shadow. In children the lower margin of the thymus sometimes can be well distinguished as the horizontal border. The lateral radiograph is also of significance in differentiating heart and thymus, given that a large thymus can resemble cardiomegaly and, vice versa, an enlarged heart can be masked by a large thymus.

The lateral chest radiograph is of greater diagnostic value than the posteroanterior radiograph in adults too. For example, in the experience of Dewes et al. (1986) 7.7% of thymomas are visible only in the lateral view, being covered by the mediastinal shadow on the posteroanterior projection because of their small size. Left and right anterior oblique views also have a particular importance (Ellis et al. 1988).

4.1.2 Fluoroscopy

If there are vague findings in the anterior superior mediastinum that remain unclear on the lateral view, fluoroscopy can be helpful. In spot films in the first and second oblique projections, the thymus is seen in its typical form and position. During expiration or, better, in a crying child, thymic enlargement is seen on fluoroscopy, whereas during inspiration a diminution in its size is observed. In cases of stridor the constancy of tracheal obstruction can be viewed on inspiration and expiration spot films. Respiratory-induced tracheal collapse may be detected in the presence of harmless congenital stridor.

4.2 Conventional Tomography

Conventional tomography in the anteroposterior
or lateral projection has been employed in the past
as a supplement to chest radiograph in two planes.
Its utility in respect of orthotopically located thymogenic masses has, however, proved disappointing: it is capable of showing the configuration of
the tumor margin against the lungs, but not of deli-
neating space-occupying lesions against the mediastinal structures. The differences in absorption
between the various anatomic structures in the mediastinum are too small to appear on conventional
tomograms (in contrast to computed tomograms)
as recognizably different gray values. Consequently conventional tomography cannot yield any decisive information over and above that provided by
chest radiography in two planes (KEESEY et al.
1980; DEWES et al. 1986; WALTER 1988). Only LIVE-
SAY et al. (1979) believe that a thymoma can be
better recognized on a lateral tomogram than on
chest radiographs in two planes. On the other
hand, calcifications (found in 20%–30% of cases
of thymoma) or bones and teeth (as found with teratomas) are supposed to be more easily distinguishable on conventional tomograms than on
plain radiographs.

Compression or displacement of the trachea by
thymogenic masses is better demonstrated than on
chest radiographs, and this is especially true in respect of the cervically situated thymus and thymomas in the middle or posterior mediastinum. This
finding can, however, also be visualized by computed tomography, which is particularly well
suited for diagnosis of space-occupying lesions in
the mediastinum and the neck.

The additional diagnostic/differential diagnostic
information supplied by conventional tomography
in comparison with the other radiodiagnostic techniques is thus negligible. Computed tomography
shows all the findings recognizable on conventional tomography at least as well, and in some
cases better, while simultaneously providing further information. Consequently conventional tomography is no longer necessary nowadays.

4.3 Ultrasonography

Ultrasonography plays a valuable role in thymic
diagnosis in *young children,* since the lack of ossification of the sternum and costal cartilage can be

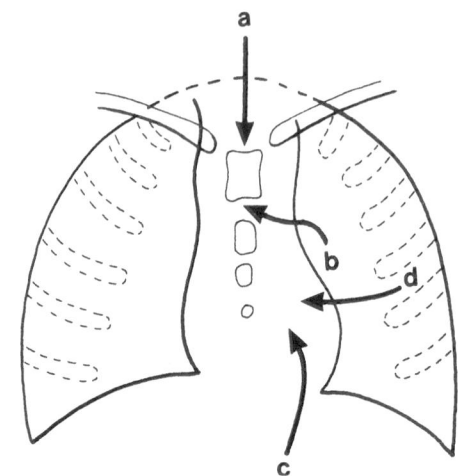

Fig. 4.1. Ultrasonographic scanning techniques in infants
and small children. *a,* suprasternal;   *b,* transosseous,
through the nonossified sternum; *c,* transcardiac or subxiphoid;   *d,* intercostal or parasternal.   *a, c* = usual approach; *b, d* = additional approaches. (HALLER et al. 1980;
CLAUS and COPPENS 1984)

used as an ultrasound window for suprasternal, left
or right parasternal access. Caudally, subxiphoid
or transcardiac access can be used for vertical
transducer management. For the horizontal scan,
transsternal and intercostal access is especially
helpful in newborns and infants, because the thymus can be imaged completely in this way
(Figs. 4.1, 4.2).

The possibility of ultrasonographic access to the
thymus decreases with age because of age-related
proportional displacements of mediastinal organs
and thymic diminution on the one hand and increasing calcification of bony structures on the
other.

Normally, 5- or 7.5-MHz transducers are used
(CLAUS and COPPENS 1984; KIM HAN et al. 1989;
LEMAITRE et al. 1987; VON LENGERKE and SCHMIDT
1988).

Ultrasonography is not usually used as a primary
diagnostic procedure; rather it is employed when
chest radiography reveals unclear appearances,
e.g., when there is a hyperplastic, dystopic, cervicomediastinal thymus or for the differential diagnosis of tumors and clarification of their structure –
especially the case of thymic cysts (GOSKE RUDICK
and WOOD 1980), thymolipomas (because of their
good echogenicity), and other solid masses such as
teratomas and malignant lymphomas (MILLER
1985).

Ultrasonography of the thymic surroundings in
adults can be performed using jugular access.
Transducers with frequencies of 3.5, 5, and

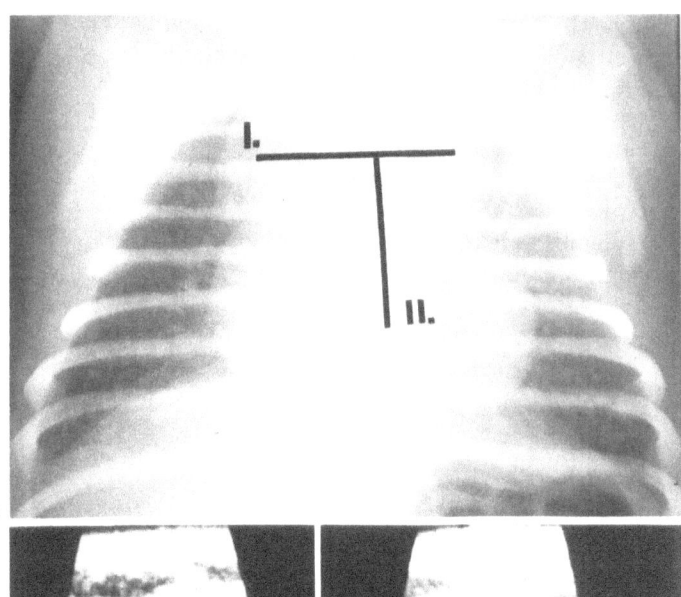

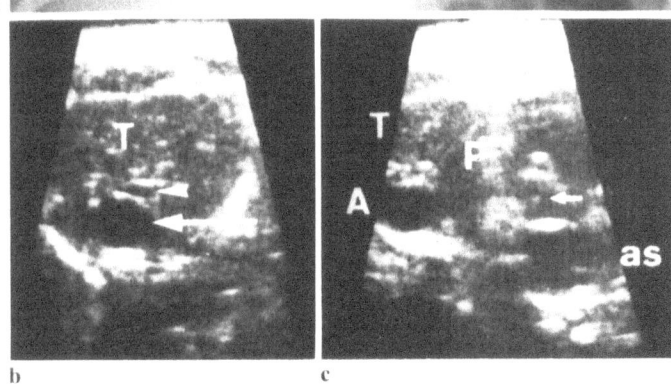

Fig. 4.2 a–c. Ultrasonography of the thymus of a 6-day-old newborn. **a** Plain anteroposterior chest radiograph with directions of scans. **b** Horizontal ultrasonography. *T*, thymus; *arrowhead*, brachiocephalic vein; *arrow*, brachiocephalic trunk. **c** Left paramedian scan (longitudinal). *T*, thymus, retrosternal; *arrow*, aortic valve; *P*, pulmonary artery; *A*, aorta; *as*, left atrium. (Courtesy of Prof. Dr. R. Schumacher, Mainz, FRG)

7.5 MHz and a short focus are used. Transverse scans with a vertically applied transducer (near 0°) and angles of inclination of 30° and 45° in relation to the longitudical axis of the body makes possible the imaging of vessels of the anterior superior mediastinum (subclavian vein, inferior thyroid vein, brachiocephalic vessels, aortic arch, jugular veins, carotid arteries), the trachea, the thymus, and the thyroid gland (Helzel 1985).

In general, however, the diagnostic value of ultrasonography is limited and positive definition of a pathologic process, e.g., in leukemia or non-Hodgkin's lymphoma with thymic infiltration, or of another tumor is not always possible (Haller et al. 1980).

4.4 Computed Tomography

The introduction of computed tomography (CT) considerably improved the differential diagnosis of space-occupying lesions in the anterior mediastinum, including those of the thymus.

Usually the CT examination is performed with a slice thickness of 8 mm and an interslice interval of 8–10 mm, although a smaller slice thickness and smaller interslice interval can be appropriate given the often relatively small size of the organs. Such reductions in the settings, however, reduce the image quality unless the signal to noise ratio is improved by increasing the mAs; this has the disadvantage of increasing the radiation dose to the patient.

Because of their restlessness, children below the age of 4 years require sedation and immobilization (Siegel et al. 1982; Salonen et al. 1984; Abel 1985). For this reason plain radiography and ultrasonography take priority in this age group, and particularly during the 1st year of life.

The advantage of CT over the conventional procedures derives from its higher resolution of anatomic structures with differing absorption properties and from the axial plane images:

1. The axial projection of the thorax, and thereby of the mediastinum, permits the anatomic region, including the thymus, to be visualized without overlapping.

2. The higher density resolution of the individual anatomic structures with the help of the window technique allows the differentiation of fat, parenchymatous organs, calcification, fluid, etc.; as a result the mediastinal structures can be easily distinguished and at the same time characteristic tissue structures within space-occupying lesions can be recognized. This is primarily of benefit with regard to differential diagnosis.

3. After administration of contrast medium, vessels and pathologic vascular processes are particularly well visualized. Dynamic CT enables conclusions to be drawn regarding the vascularity of a tumor. Depending on age, 30–50 ml of a water-soluble contrast medium (iodine content generally 300 mg/ml) is administered as a bolus via a cubital vein.

By virtue of its above-mentioned advantages, CT for the first time permits the age-dependent structural changes in the thymus to be observed in adults in a noninvasive manner.

Invasive thymomas can be distinguished from noninvasive forms, which aids operative planning and facilitates preoperative prognostic statements. Despite these and other diagnostic improvements, however, CT has not solved all differential diagnostic problems. Thus even on CT scans thymomas, solitary lymphomas, and carcinoid tumors can resemble one another, rendering differential diagnosis difficult or even impossible (see relevant sections for more details). In such cases CT nevertheless does allow guided fine needle biopsy of mediastinal and also hilar and pulmonary lesions; the technique has been described by BETTENDORF and BAUER (1981), vanSONNENBERG et al. (1983), and others. Since the position of the needle tip can be exactly determined with CT, this method is superior to fine needle biopsy guidance by fluoroscopy.

The younger the child, the narrower are the *indications for CT*. Therapeutic consequences should be taken into consideration. Indications include the following:

- Mediastinal enlargement on radiographs without clear indications as to diagnosis
- Suspicion of tumors in the mediastinum or clearly visible masses
- Differentiation between thymic hyperplasia or persistent thymus and a tumor
- Normal mediastinum on radiography, but with underlying disease such as leukemia, malignant lymphoma, or myasthenia gravis that points to the possibility of thymic involvement

- Pleural effusion with suspicion of mediastinal involvement
- "Clarification" of the extension of radiographically diagnosed mediastinal tumors in the presence of known malignant underlying disease (non-Hodgkin's lymphoma, Hodgkin's lymphoma, thymoma) and/or a pathologic x-ray finding in respect of the lungs
- Identification of a density in the middle or posterior mediastinum as being of a dystopic or accessory nature
- Detection of thymic cysts, hemorrhages, and trauma
- Follow-up after conservative, operative, or radiation treatment

At a beam voltage of 125 kV the radiation dose with modern CT apparatus is ca. 6.8 mGy/100 mAs (corresponding to 0.68 rad/100 mAs). With standard examination parameters (125 kV, 230 mAs) the resulting dose to the skin is 15.6 mGy (1.56 rad). This is within the range of conventional tomography, but well below that of angiocardiography and higher than that of plain chest radiography in two planes (SIEGEL et al. 1982).

A further advantage of CT lies in the dose distribution. Use of the collimated fan beam allows the radiation dose to be reduced drastically in the immediate vicinity of the plane of section, so that chest examinations by CT deliver a far lower radiation dose to the gonads than does conventional tomography.

Today the aforementioned advantages of CT mean that it ranks second among diagnostic procedures in adults, behind plain radiography; in children, however, ultrasonography ranks above CT. In the entire age range from late infancy to adulthood, a large number of investigative methods have been rendered superfluous by CT; examples are esophagography, conventional tomography, tracheobronchography, angiocardiography, and pneumomediastinography.

4.5 Magnetic Resonance Imaging

W. R. WEBB and G. DE GEER

In order to understand the magnetic resonance imaging (MRI) appearances of the normal and abnormal thymus, it is necessary to have some basic understanding of the phenomenon of MRI, and how an MR image is produced.

4.5.1 Principles of Magnetic Resonance Imaging

Magnetic sesonance imaging takes advantage of physical properties of matter radically different from those which result in radiographic contrast, and therefore has the potential to provide unique diagnostic information. Any atomic nucleus having an odd number of nucleons (protons and neutrons) will act as though it is a weak magnet and will tend to align itself with a strong magnetic field. If the nucleus is then perturbed by a specific radiofrequency signal, which alters its relationship to the external magnetic field, the nucleus will generate a radio signal having the same frequency as the signal that perturbed it. This generated signal is the basis of MRI.

Many nuclei can be used for MRI. These include hydrogen, phosphorus 31, sodium 23, and carbon 13. Of these, hydrogen is most commonly used because of its abundance in tissue and high sensitivity to the MR phenomenon.

4.5.2 Image Production

An MR image is constructed of individual pixels, each of which reflects the strength (intensity) of the MR radiofrequency signal generated from a small volume of the sample. The MR intensity of each pixel is governed by several factors, primarily hydrogen density, two magnetic relaxation times called T1 and T2, and motion, if any, of hydrogen protons in the volume being imaged.

The effect of hydrogen density is easy to understand. The greater the hydrogen density, the more hydrogen nuclei will be available to produce an MR signal, and the more intense the MR signal will be. Tissues such as cortical bone and air-filled lung, which contain very little hydrogen, will generate little or no MR signal.

A detailed explanation of T1 and T2 would exceed the bounds of this book. Stated simply, these two parameters quantify alterations in MR signal strength which occur as a result of interactions between the nuclei being studied and their surrounding physical and chemical environment. These factors influence the rate at which nuclei align themselves with the external magnetic field following perturbation (T1) and the rate at which the radiofrequency signal emitted by the nuclei decreases or decays following radiofrequency stimulation (T2).

The last factor influencing MR intensity is gross motion of the hydrogen protons during the imaging sequence. In thoracic imaging, this generally reflects blood flow or cardiac pulsation.

4.5.3 Normal Appearances

In general, fat is very intense on MR images and appears white, while air in lung, rapidly flowing blood, and bone appear black. Muscle, thymus, and soft tissue masses appear as varying shades of gray, depending on the image sequence used. However, the contrast between different soft tissues can be changed depending on the imaging sequence used. This is discussed in detail below.

4.5.4 Image Contrast and Interpretation

Generally speaking T1 and T2 are more important than hydrogen density in determining MR intensity. Although the hydrogen density of most soft tissues varies over a range of only 20%, the T1 and T2 values can vary by over 1000%. However, different imaging techniques, such as the spin-echo technique, can change the degree to which T1 and T2 values affect the image. Spin-echo techniques are both T1 and T2 sensitive.

4.5.4.1 The Spin-Echo Technique

With spin-echo imaging, the operator can alter the degree to which T1 and T2 affect the image produced by changing two determinants of image acquisition called the repetition time (TR) and echo time (TE) GAMSU and SOSTMAN 1989; GEFTER 1988; WEBB et al. 1984a; WEBB 1989).

The TE value is measured in milliseconds (often ranging between 20 and 80 ms) and affects the image intensity relative to T2. As stated above, T2 is a measurement of the rate at which the MR radiofrequency signal decreases from its maximum; TE is the time after maximum at which the MR signal strength is measured. Thus, with a long TE (80 ms), the signal from tissue having a short T2 value decays significantly, while the signal from a tissue with a long T2 value decays to a lesser degree and is therefore stronger. Because of this, images produced with a long TE tend to discriminate tissues having different T2 values, and such images can be said to be *T2 weighted*. On the other hand, when a short TE value (20 ms) is used, the signal from tissues with a short T2 has less time to decay, and thus is more nearly the same as that produced by tissues having a longer T2. Such images are therefore relatively T2 independent and contain much less contrast on the basis of T2. With the technique we use, images with both short and long TE values are obtained at each level scanned, and by comparing the intensities of a given area on the two images, information about T2 can be inferred or measured.

The TR affects the importance of T1 in the image. T1 is a measurement of the rate at which nuclei align themselves with the external magnetic field following perturbation, and TR is the time between perturbations. With clinical imaging, the TR value is usually determined by the length of the cardiac cycle, because these images are ECG gated. If a short TR (0.5 s or gated to every heart beat) is used, tissues having a long T1 do not have sufficient time to align themselves to the external magnetic field before being perturbed again, and their signal decreases in strength relative to that of tissues having a short T1. Thus, images performed with a short TR are said to be *T1 weighted,* and enhance image contrast relative to T1. On images performed with a long TR (2 s or gated to every other heart beat), T1 effects are lessened and tissues with both short and long T1 values can be similar in intensity. Thus, images with a long TR are said to be T1 independent. By comparing images having short and long TR values, T1 can be measured or its value can be inferred. This will be discussed in greater detail when we discuss the MR diagnosis of mediastinal masses.

4.5.5 MRI Diagnosis of Mediastinal Masses

In general, the relationship between a mediastinal mass and adjacent vessels, and vascular compression or obstruction, is better demonstrated using MRI than it is with contrast-enhanced CT. This is largely a result of the excellent mass/vessel contrast. Because blood within mediastinal vessels is flowing rapidly, it results in little or no significant signal on MR images – the so-called *flow-void effect.*

The differentiation of tumor from normal mediastinal fat can usually be accomplished by taking advantage of their differences in T1 (WEBB et al. 1984a). Although the T2 values of tumors and mediastinal fat tend to overlap, their T1 values are usually quite different, with fat having a much shorter T1. Thus, if we first examine the image of a patient with a mediastinal mass obtained using a long TR (an image with little T1 contrast), both

tumor and mediastinal fat will produce an intense signal and can be difficult or impossible to distinguish. However, on an image obtained with a short TR, fat remains intense because of its short T1, but tumor, having a longer T1 value, decreases in relative intensity.

Although the large majority of mediastinal masses differ significantly in intensity from mediastinal fat on T1-weighted images, as described above, this is not always the case. Some tumors will appear quite similar to fat in intensity, being recognizable only because of alterations in mediastinal contours or displacement of vascular structures.

The diagnosis of a mediastinal mass depends not only on the contrast between mass and fat, which is excellent on MRI, but also on spatial resolution. In general, the spatial resolution of MRI is less than that of CT, and small structures or the edges of large mediastinal masses are often less well defined on MR images.

4.5.6 Image Acquisition and ECG Gating

In general, when scanning the chest using MRI, transaxial imaging is performed using two different spin-echo sequences (GAMSU and SOSTMAN 1989; GEFTER 1988; WEBB et al. 1984a; WEBB 1989); when thymic pathology is suspected, this same protocol is also used. First, a multislice, ECG-gated, single-echo (20–30 ms), T1-weighted sequence is always obtained. The T1-weighted images are most helpful in diagnosing mediastinal masses and in defining vascular anatomy in relation to a mass. This sequence is usually followed by a T2-weighted sequence gated to every other heart beat, with two echoes (20–30 ms and 60–80 ms). The T2-weighted images are helpful in showing fluid collections and distinguishing tumor from fibrous tissue or chest wall musculature. Gating images to the ECG greatly improves spatial resolution and, in most patients, gated images have replaced ungated images with a short TR value (TR 0.5 s) in our institution. Depending on the site and nature of the suspected abnormality, an additional ECG-gated series in the sagittal or coronal plane will often be obtained.

4.5.6.1 Sagittal and Coronal Imaging

An advantage of MRI relative to CT is that it allows direct imaging in the sagittal or coronal plane (BATRA et al. 1988; O'DONOVAN et al. 1984;

WEBB et al. 1985; WEBB 1984 b). In our experience, sagittal or coronal MRI can provide information not available on transaxial CT or MR images in some patients who have a mediastinal mass. The benefits of sagittal or coronal MRI are several. First, structures oriented longitudinally in the sagittal or coronal planes can be imaged along their axes. Such structures include the trachea, superior vena cava, and aorta. Secondly, imaging in a second plane reduces the chance of misinterpretation of findings as a result of volume averaging. This is particularly important in areas of the chest where a correct (or confident) interpretation requires the resolution of the edges of structures which lie in or near the transaxial plane. The thymus is best seen and resolved from adjacent vasculature in the transaxial and sagittal planes. The coronal plane is only occasionally of value in diagnosis.

4.5.7 Characterization of Mediastinal Masses

In most patients with benign mediastinal lesions, values of T1 and T2 do not appear to differ significantly from those of patients with malignant tumors (GAMSU et al. 1984). However, fluid-filled or necrotic masses can be detected on the basis of long T1 and T2 values (GAMSU and SOSTMAN 1989; GEFTER 1988, WEBB et al. 1984a; WEBB 1989). In patients with fluid-containing lesions, scans performed with long TR and TE values (a T2-weighted image) result in a significant increase in signal from the fluid components of the mass and can demonstrate inhomogeneity invisible with short TR and TE values. In some patients, cystic or fluid-filled masses can be diagnosed on MRI when they cannot on CT.

4.6 Nuclear Medicine

E. WALTER and E. WILLICH

Three isotopes are available for nuclear medical examinations of the thymus and thymic tumors:

4.6.1 67 Gallium Citrate

67 Gallium citrate has particularly been used by SWICK et al. (1976), MIN et al. (1978), POLANSKY et al. (1979), and DONAHUE et al. (1981). DONAHUE et al. (1981) found that 67 gallium citrate was stored in normal thymus in 15% of children younger than 5 years and 11% of children older than 5 years, while HIBI et al. (1987) gave figures of 61% for children less than 2 years old and 15% for children more than 2 years old – in other words, storage decreases with age.

Uptake of the nuclide has been described in benign thymomas (PATEL et al. 1978) but also in malignant forms. In children with benign, i.e., noninvasive thymomas, storage of the nuclide in the anterior mediastinum is observed in 80% of cases (MILLER 1985); TEATES et al. (1978) found a true-positive 67 gallium citrate scintiscan in 82% of cases of thymoma.

Bone metastases of malignant thymomas can be demonstrated with both 67 gallium citrate and technetium phosphate (CANCROFT et al. 1978). Uptake of the isotope in the thymus has also been reported in reactive hyperplasia (YULISH and OWENS 1980; DONAHUE et al. 1981).

Differentiation between hyperplasia, thymoma, and Hodgkin's disease in the thymus is not possible scintigraphically. Since gallium 67 is also stored in thymic cysts (JENSEN et al. 1980), differential diagnosis between thymoma and cysts or thymoma with cystic degeneration is also impossible. KAPLAN et al. (1988) nevertheless regard the use of gallium 67 as suitable for detection of residual or metastatic thymic tissue in patients with malignant thymoma.

Increased uptake of 67 gallium citrate by the normal thymus is also to be reckoned with in diseases not primarily located in the thymus. Thus JOHNSON et al. (1978) observed uptake of activity in the thymus of a 4-year-old boy during pneumonia; 21 months after the illness this uptake was no longer demonstrable. HANDMAKER and O'MARA (1977) observed uptake during the course of meningitis, as did HIBI et al. (1987) in children with Hodgkin's disease (uptake occurred in 39% of cases), Wilms' tumor, teratoma, neuroblastoma, and other space-occupying lesions.

Last but not least, it should be pointed out that this radiopharmaceutical can also be stored in other pathologic processes. This holds true for malignant tumors such as bronchial carcinoma, malignant lymphoma, carcinoma of the breast, carcinoma of the paranasal sinuses, esophageal carcinoma, stomach cancer, and hepatoma (HIGASI and NAKAYAMA 1972; O'MARA and MATIN 1977), but also for benign diseases such as histiocytosis X, abscesses, pulmonary tuberculosis, pneumonia, and sarcoidosis (LAVENDER et al. 1971; HIGASI and

NAKAYAMA 1972; HOPKINS and MENDE 1975; HOF-
FER 1980; HIBI et al. 1987) and for cerebral infarction (ZEIDLER 1978).

67 Gallium citrate thus displays no specificity,
being stored in normal thymus as well as in inflammatory tissue and thymogenic and nonthymogenic
tumors (DAY and GEDGAUDAS 1984). Therefore
gallium uptake in the thymus does not automat-
ically justify the assumption that a mediastinal thymoma is present; rather the findings must be interpreted in conjunction with clinical and radiologic
data (JOHNSON et al. 1978).

4.6.2 75 Selenium Methionine

Selenium methionine is preferentially incorpo-
rated, via protein synthesis, in tissue with increased
metabolism; radioactive selenium is thereby con-
centrated in metabolically active lesions. As a consequence this isotope is also stored in the thymus:
this is true in respect of thymic hyperplasia (DJAJA
and BUMBIC 1965; TESTA and ANGELINI 1979) but
also for thymoma (COWAN et al. 1971; HARE and
ANDREWS 1970; MIN et al. 1978; TESTA and ANGELI-
NI 1979). However, findings are not always regular
and unequivocal. For example, TESTA and ANGELI-
NI (1979) found than in patients with myasthenia
gravis, only five of six with thymomas (83%) and
8 of 12 with hyperplasia (67%) showed tracer uptake in the thymus. MIN et al. (1978), also, report
on a thymoma that did not store 75 selenium methionine. It is noteworthy in this context that the latter authors additionally cited a case of malignant
thymoma in which the gallium scintiscan failed to
reveal isotope uptake even though 75 selenium
methionine was taken up by the tumor.

Since selenium methionine is stored, via protein
synthesis, in tissues with increased protein metabolism, uptake is also observed in numerous other tumors such as bronchogenic, thyroid, and parathyroid carcinomas, and malignant lymphoma of the
mediastinum (DAY and GEDGAUDAS 1984). Thus,
like 67 gallium citrate, 75 selenium methionine is
nonspecific: a positive scintiscan is not pathognomonic for a thymoma. On the other hand, this isotope occasionally identifies a thymoma in a patient
with myasthenia gravis that has not been revealed
by noninvasive methods, i.e., tracer uptake in the
thymus in such patients points to the presence of a
thymoma.

4.6.3 99m Technetium Pertechnetate

With this isotope it is possible to diagnose ectopic
gastric mucous membrane in mediastinally situated gastric duplicatures (gastro- and enterogenic
cysts). Since these are predominantly located in
the posterior mediastinum, differential diagnosis
includes the possibility of dystopic thymic tissue.
LEONHARD (1982) reported on storage of ^{99m}Tc-
gluceptate in the thymus, but the organ was not
examined histologically.

In summary, the use of 67 gallium citrate and
75 selenium methionine does not yield uniform results. As regards the demonstration of thymomas,
both false-positive and false-negative results have
been reported.

4.7 Esophagography

Visualization of the esophagus with barium sulfate
or a water-soluble contrast medium can be diagnostically important for two reasons: First, especially when the thymus occupies an ectopic position in the region of the neck or posterior
mediastinum, esophagography serves to distinguish between compression-related dysphagia or
dysphagia occurring in connection with infiltration
of the esophagus by an invasive thymoma. Second,
the topographic relations of the mass to the esophagus can be assessed on the basis of the esophageal displacement.

4.8 Angiography

4.8.1 Arteriography

During the 1960s and 1970s, the arteriographic
demonstration of pathologic processes in the anterior mediastinum achieved a certain importance
(CASTELLANOS et al. 1971; BOIJSEN and REUTER
1966; DÜX 1977), but since the introduction of CT
it has to a large extent lost its significance. Arteriography was ranked above phlebography in diagnostic importance.

Arterial supply to the thymus has been described in detail by DI MARINO et al. (1987). The
thymus is usually supplied by the left and right internal thoracic arteries or their branches (e.g., the
pericardial arteries). Additionally, the organ can

be supplied by branches of the superior and inferior thyroid arteries. Posterior thymic arteries derive from the brachiocephalic trunk or the arch of the aorta, but this form of supply is witnessed in only 8% of patients (DI MARINO et al. 1987). Normally a dense arterial network is seen in the thymus, the caliber of the vessels not exceeding 1 mm (DI MARINO et al. 1987).

Selective arteriography is usually performed by means of a catheter inserted into the femoral artery utilizing the Seldinger technique; however, an approach via the axillary artery has also been employed (BOIJSEN and REUTER 1966; GÖTHLIN et al. 1977).

Typically, 10 ml contrast medium suffices for *selective visualization of the internal thoracic artery*. If selective catheterization of the internal thoracic artery is unsuccessful, 20 ml contrast medium injected close to the orifice of the internal thoracic artery is necessary for visualization (BOIJSEN and REUTER 1966). A differential diagnostic classification of space-occupying lesions in the anterior mediastinum was undertaken on the basis of vascularization, displacement of vessels, luminal narrowing, arteriovenous shunts, and accumulation of contrast medium in the lesion. Thus thymic cysts display stretched, smooth vessels without central neovascularization, whereas thymomas have been described as variably well or poorly vascularized. As regards the arterial vessels themselves, displacement, arteriovenous shunts, and stenoses can be recognized; contrast accumulation in the tumor is evident. According to DÜX (1977) differential diagnosis is possible between benign and malignant lesions.

4.8.2 Angiocardiography

In the past angiocardiography was employed when an alteration in the cardiac silhouette, causing suspicion of cardiac pathology, was caused by a large thymus in childhood or a thymic mass in adulthood. It was generally employed in isolated cases only, but CASTELLANOS et al. (1971) used it on a larger scale and reported successful differentiation between thymic hyperplasia, pericardial tumors, and cardiomegaly. In one case reported by KOOK SANG OH (1971) a 15-year-old girl underwent thoracotomy and was found to have a normal thymus, despite the fact that angiocardiography had been performed. ZANCA et al. (1965) excluded a cardiac abnormality by this method, and were able to identify a thymic cyst.

Today, if the need arises, angiocardiography is still employed for differential diagnosis against primary vascular processes; aneurysmal dilatations can, however, also be diagnosed by dynamic CT.

4.8.3 Phlebography and Superior Venacavography

Phlebography was introduced into thymic diagnosis by KREEL in 1967. While KREEL selected the left median basilic vein as the point of access, YUNE nad KLATTE (1970) used the transfemoral approach. Using a specially curved catheter, they catheterized the 2–3 cm long main thymic vein of Keynes, which arises from the union of the lateral veins of the left and right thymic lobes. Its orifice lies 1–2 cm proximal to the junction of the superior vena cava and the left brachiocephalic vein, and it has a caliber of ca. 3 mm (DI MARINO et al. 1987).

The described venous drainage is, however, present in only 25% of patients. According to the detailed anatomic investigations of DI MARINO et al. (1987), extensive variation in the venous drainage is to be expected, which considerably complicates venography. Thus venous drainage of the thymus may occur into the inferior thyroid vein (41.6%), the middle thyroid vein (20%), the internal thoracic vein (16.6%), the right jugular vein (6.6%), and the region of confluence between the jugular veins and the subclavian vein (2.3%).

The normal thymus has a homogeneous network of numerous small veins (DI MARINO et al. 1987). Conclusions as to the presence of pathologic processes are drawn on the basis of vascular density, displacement, and irregularities. Thus vascular occlusions, stenoses, and corkscrew-like appearances are typical of carcinoma (YUNE and KLATTE 1970). Since the introduction of modern imaging procedures, phlebography of the thymus has completely lost its former significance. Only superior vena cavography has retained its importance: When there is a clinical picture of a blockage of the superior vena cava it serves to distinguish between tumor-related vascular narrowing and thrombosis of the superior vena cava, which is especially often observed when there is infiltration by a malignant tumor or subtotal compression.

In children the value of superior vena cavography was seen as consisting in the determination of tumor extension and the evaluation of tumor-related vascular compression and displacement, thus facilitating the choice of operative procedure

(OTTO et al. 1972; OPPERMANN and BRANDEIS 1975; OPPERMANN et al. 1977; OPPERMANN and WILLICH 1978).

4.9 Obsolete Methods

4.9.1 Kymography

Kymography (area kymography or electrokymography) was formerly used for the differential diagnosis of solid masses in the mediastinum, including the thymus. The aim of kymography was the differentiation between conducted pulsation, as found in the case of masses unrelated to vessels, and normal vessel pulsation, which provides evidence of vascular processes (GREMMEL and VIETEN 1961). Kymography was also used in conjunction with pneumomediastinography.

4.9.2 Pneumomediastinography

Before the introduction of CT, pneumomediastinography was used in the differentiation of masses in the mediastinum. This examination was performed in large series of patients in the 1950s and 1960s (LISSNER 1959; POHLENZ 1968; FISHER and CREMIN 1975; KABELKA et al. 1977; SONE et al. 1980), based on the original investigations by CONDORELLI et al. (1935). The technique was described in detail by HAUGER (1975).

According to IRVINE and SUMERLING (1965) a thymus measuring more than 6 cm² is pathologically enlarged. Bulging of the surface of the thymus is highly suspicious for thymomas and other masses. Differential diagnosis between cystic and solid tumors was usually not possible by means of pneumomediastinography. If changes on the organ surface could not be demonstrated, no diagnosis could be made. If distinction from the neighbouring organs was not possible, an infiltrative growth and therefore inoperability had to be assumed.

Complications were in general seldom. POHLENZ (1968) described only one severe complication in 120 examinations. HAUGER (1975) found anginal symptoms and emphysema only once in 75 patients.

Pneumomediastinography was especially used in children of all age groups for differential diagnosis between persistent thymus and tumor (HARRIS et al. 1980; SONE et al. 1980; DOBREV 1967; FISHER and CREMIN 1975). A congenital cardiac

murmur can be excluded in children presenting with a prominent pulmonary segment on chest radiography, and a persistent thymic lobe could be diagnosed by this method (POHLENZ et al. 1966; POHLENZ 1968; LISSNER 1963).

This method was further used when there were special problems pertaining to operative indications in small infants with thymic hyperplasia (TISCHER 1967; DOBREV 1967). This special indication was also present in seven of eight infants with stridor, especially in connection with accessory thymic lobes (KABELKA et al. 1977).

As an accompanying finding a thymus tip lifted by trauma or inflammation could sometimes be found in pneumomediastinum.

4.10 Supplementary Procedures (Mediastinography, Bronchoscopy, Bronchography)

E. WILLICH

Bronchography (TISCHER 1967; THAL 1972) and bronchoscopy (THAL 1972) have been recommended as further techniques for thymic diagnosis. Today their use is considered only exceptionally, when there is suspicion of an infiltrative mediastinal malignoma or possibly a thymoma causing invasion of the tracheobronchial system (SPAHR and FRABLE 1981; ASAMURA et al. 1988).

Mediastinoscopy, which frequently causes complications and occasionally even death when employed in children with malignant systemic diseases (OPPERMANN et al. 1977), actually displays some advantages in the diagnosis of thymogenic disorders: it does not involve x-rays, and it permits the possibility of exploratory excision with simultaneous resection of an enlarged thymus as well as the combination of diagnosis with subsequent pneumomediastinography.

References

Abel M (1985) Prämedikation und Risiken bei der Computertomographie im Neugeborenen- und Säuglingsalter. Radiologe 25: 599
Asamura H, Morinaga S, Shimosato Y, Ono R, Naruke T (1988) Thymoma displaying endobronchial polypoid growth. Chest 94: 647
Bar-Ziv J, Barki Y, Itzchak Y, Mares AJ (1984) Posterior mediastinal accessory thymus. Pediatr Radiol 14: 165
Batra P, Brown K, Steckel RJ, Collins JD, Ovenfors CO, Aberle D (1988) MR imaging of the thorax: a comparison

of axial, coronal, and sagittal imaging planes. J Comput Assist Tomogr 12: 75

Bettendorf U, Bauer K-H (1981) Thymomdiagnostik unter besonderer Berücksichtigung der computertomographisch gesteuerten perthorakalen Biopsie. Dtsch Med Wochenschr 106: 84

Boijsen E, Reuter SR (1966) Subclavian and internal mammary angiography in the evaluation of anterior mediastinal masses. AJR 98: 447

Cancroft ET, Montorfano D, Goldfarb CR (1978) Metastases to bone from malignant thymoma detected by technetium phosphate and gallium-67 scintigraphy. Clin Nucl Med 3: 312

Castellanos A, Pereiras R, Garcia O (1971) Angiocardiography in huge hypertrophy of the thymus. AJR 112: 40

Claus D, Coppens JP (1984) Sonography of mediastinal masses in infants and children. Ann Radiol 27: 150

Condorelli L, Francaviglia A, Catalano A, Capua O, Caputi G (1935) Il pneumomediastino anteriore diagnostico. Radiol Fisica Med II: 163

Cowan RJ, Maynard CD, Witcofski RL, Janeway R, Toole JF (1971) Selenmethionine Se 75 thymus scans in myasthenia gravis. JAMA 215: 978

Day DL, Gedgaudas E (1984) The thymus. Radiol Clin North Am 22: 519

Dewes W, Schrappe-Bächer M, Focke-Wenzel EK, Schmitz-Dräger H-G (1986) Zur Röntgendiagnostik invasiver Thymome. ROFO 144: 388

Di Marino V, Argeme M, Brunet C, Coppens R, Bonnoit J (1987) Macroscopic study of the adult thymus. Surg Radiol Anat 9: 51

Djaja M, Bumbic S (1965) Tumoroid hyperplasia of the thymus in a seven-year-old child. Srp Arh Celok Lek 93: 647

Dobrev P (1967) Die Bedeutung der Pneumomediastinographie in der Diagnostik von Thymuserkrankungen im Kindesalter. Z Tuberk Erkr Thoraxorg 126: 291

Donahue DM, Leonard JC, Basmadjian GP et al. (1981) Thymic gallium-67 localization in pediatric patients on chemotherapy: concise communication. J Nucl Med 22: 1043

Düx A (1977) Differentialdiagnose pathologischer Mediastinalprozesse. In: Teschendorf W, Anacker H, Thurn P (eds) Röntgenologische Differentialdiagnostik, vol I,2, 5th edn. Thieme, Stuttgart

Ellis K, Austin JHM, Jaretzki III A (1988) Radiologic detection of thymoma in patients with myasthenia gravis. AJR 151: 873

Fisher RM, Cremin BJ (1975) The extent of the inferior border of the thymus: a report of two cases in infants. Br J Radiol 48: 814

Gamsu G, Sostman D (1989) Magnetic resonance imaging of the thorax. Am Rev Respir Dis 139: 254

Gamsu G, Stark DD, Webb WR et al. (1984) Magnetic resonance imaging of benign mediastinal masses. Radiology 151: 709

Gefter W (1988) Chest applications of magnetic resonance imaging: an update. Radiol Clin North Am 26: 573

Goske Rudick M, Wood BP (1980) The use of ultrasound in the diagnosis of a large thymic cyst. Pediatr Radiol 10: 113

Göthlin J, Jonsson K, Lunderquist A, Rausing A, Alburquerque LM (1977) The angiographic appearance of thymic tumors. Radiology 124: 47

Gremmel H, Vieten H (1961) A propos de l'étude clinique et radiologique de tumeurs du thymus. Ann Radiol 4: 669

Haller JO, Schneider M, Kassner EG, Friedman AP, Waldroup LD (1980) Sonographic evaluation of the chest in infants and children. AJR 134: 1019

Handmaker H, O'Mara RE (1977) Gallium imaging in pediatrics. J Nucl Med 18: 1057

Hare WSC, Andrews JT (1970) The occult thymoma: radiological and radioisotopic aids to diagnosis. Aust Ann Med 1: 30

Harris VJ, Ramilo J, White H (1980) The thymic mass as a mediastinal dilemma. Clin Radiol 31: 263

Hauger W (1975) Zur Wertigkeit des Pneumomediastinum bei der Diagnostik von Tumoren im vorderen Mediastinum. ROFO 122: 423

Helzel M (1985) Sonographische Topographie des oberen vorderen Mediastinums. Ultraschall Med 6: 101

Hibi S, Todo S, Imashuku S (1987) Thymic localization of gallium-67 in pediatric patients with lymphoid and nonlymphoid tumors. J Nucl Med 28: 293

Higasi T, Nakayama Y (1972) Clinical evaluation of 67 gallium-citrate scanning. J Nucl Med 13: 196

Hoffer P (1980) Gallium and infection. J Nucl Med 21: 484

Hopkins GB, Mende CW (1975) Gallium 67 for the diagnosis and localization of subphrenic abscesses. West J Med 122: 281

Irvine WJ, Sumerling MD (1965) Radiological assessment of the thymus in thyroid and other diseases. Lancet I: 996

Jensen SR, Rao BR, Winebright JW, O'Reilly R (1980) Gallium-67 uptake in a benign thymic cyst. Clin Nucl Med 5: 67

Johnson PM, Berdon WE, Baker DH, Fawwaz RA (1978) Thymic uptake of gallium-67 citrate in a healthy 4 year old boy. Pediatr Radiol 7: 243

Kabelka M, Sintáková B, Zítková M (1977) Dysontogenetic accessory lobe of the thymus. A new clinical entity? Z Kinderchir 20: 116

Kaplan IL, Swayne LC, Widmann WD, Wolff M (1988) CT demonstration of "ectopic" thymoma. J Comput Assist Tomogr 12: 1037

Keesey J, Bein M, Mink J et al. (1980) Detection of thymoma in myasthenia gravis. Neurology 30: 233

Kim Han B, Babcock DS, Oestreich AE (1989) Normal thymus in infancy: sonographic characteristics. Radiology 170: 471

Kook Sang Oh, Weber AL, Borden S (1971) Normal mediastinal mass in late childhood. Radiology 101: 625

Kreel L (1967) Selective thymic venography. New method for visualization of the thymus. Br Med J 1: 406

Lavender JP, Lowe J, Barker JR et al. (1971) Gallium 67 citrate scanning in neoplastic and inflammatory lesions. Br J Radiol 44: 361

Lemaitre L, Marconi V, Avni F, Remy J (1987) The sonographic evaluation of normal thymus in infants and children. Eur J Radiol 7: 130

Leonhard JC (1982) Thymic localization of Tc-99m gluceptate. Clin Nuc Med 7: 577

Lissner J (1959) Der Wert des Pneumomediastinums bei der Differentialdiagnose mediastinaler Erkrankungen. ROFO 91: 445

Lissner J (1963) Die röntgenologische Diagnostik der Thymustumoren. Radiologe 3: 31

Livesay JJ, Mink JH, Fee HJ, Bein ME, Sample WF, Mulder DG (1979) The use of computed tomography to evaluate suspected mediastinal tumors. Ann Thorac Surg 27: 305

Miller JH (ed) (1985) Imaging in pediatric oncology. Williams and Wilkins, Baltimore, p 152

Min K-W, Waddell CC, Pircher FJ, Granville GE, Gyorkey F (1978) Selective uptake of 75-Se-Selenmethionine by thymoma with pure red cell aplasia. Cancer 41: 1323

O'Donovan PB, Ross JS, Sivak ED et al. (1984) Magnetic resonance imaging of the thorax: the advantages of coronal and sagittal planes. AJR 143: 1183

Oliva L (1973) Erkrankungen des Mediastinums. In: Schinz HR, Baensch WE, Frommhold W, Glauner R, Uehlinger E, Wellauer J (eds) Lehrbuch der Röntgendiagnostik, vol IV, 2, 6th edn. Pleura, Mediastinum und Lunge. Thieme, Stuttgart

O'Mara RE, Matin P (1977) Tumor and inflammatory lesion localization. In: Matin B (ed) Handbook of clinical nuclear medicine. Medical Examination Publishing, New York, p 283

Oppermann HC, Brandeis WE (1975) Konnatales Thymom. Z Kinderchir 16: 366

Oppermann HC, Willich E (1978) Zur Röntgendiagnostik und Differentialdiagnose der Mediastinaltumoren im Kindesalter. Radiologe 18: 218

Oppermann HC, Ulmer HE, Vogt-Moykopf J (1977) Thymom: seltene Ursachen einer akuten respiratorischen Insuffizienz im Kindesalter. Z Kinderchir 21: 178

Otto R, Flückiger A, Candardjis G (1972) Indikationen zur Darstellung der oberen Hohlvene und ihrer Hauptäste. ROFO 117: 514

Parker LA, Gaisie G, Scatliff JH (1985) Computerized tomography and ultrasonographic findings in massive thymic hyperplasia. Clin Pediatr 24: 90

Patel D, Mitnick J, Braunstein P, Genieser NB (1978) 67 Gallium scan in thymoma. Clin Nucl Med 3: 339

Pohlenz O (1968) Röntgenologische Thymusdiagnostik. Med Klin 63: 1255

Pohlenz O, Feindt HP, Hauch HJ, Nitschke M (1966) Zur Differentialdiagnose des prominenten Pulmonalisbogens mit Hilfe des Pneumomediastinum. ROFO 104: 486

Polansky SM, Barwick KW, Ravin CE (1979) Primary mediastinal seminoma. AJR 132: 17

Salonen OL, Kivisaari ML, Somer JK (1984) Computed tomography of the thymus of children under 10 years. Pediatr Radiol 14: 373

Siegel MJ, Sagel SS, Reed K (1982) The value of computed tomography in the diagnosis and management of pediatric mediastinal abnormalities. Radiology 142: 149

Sone S, Higashihara T, Morimoto S et al. (1980) Normal anatomy of thymus and anterior mediastinum by pneumomediastinography. AJR 134: 81

Spahr J, Frable WJ (1981) Pulmonary cytopathology of an invasive thymoma. Acta Cytol 25: 163

Swick HM, Preston DF, McQuillen MP (1976) Gallium scans in myasthenia gravis. Ann NY Acad Sci 274: 536

Teates CD, Bray S, Williamson BRJ (1978) Tumor detection with 67 gallium citrate: a literature survey (1970–1978). Clin Nucl Med 3: 456

Testa GF, Angelini C (1979) Assessment of the value of thymic scan in myasthenia gravis. J Neurol 220: 21

Thal W (1972) Kinderbronchologie. Barth, Leipzig, p 187

Tischer W (1967) Diagnostische und therapeutische Möglichkeiten bei Thymushyperplasie im Säuglingsalter. Kinderarztl Prax 35: 333

VanSonnenberg E, Lin AS, Deutsch AL, Mattrey RF (1983) Percutaneous biopsy of difficult mediastinal, hilar and pulmonary lesions by computed tomographic guidance and a modified coaxial technique. Radiology 148: 300

von Lengerke H-J, Schmidt H (1988) Mediastinalsonographie im Kindesalter. Ergebnisse bei 310 Untersuchungen. Radiologe 28: 460

Walter E (1988) Erkrankungen und Tumoren des Thymus im Erwachsenenalter. In: Diethelm L, Heuck F, Olsson O, Strnad F, Vieten H, Zuppinger A (eds) Röntgendiagnostik der oberen Speise- und Atemwege, der Atemorgane und des Mediastinums. Springer, Berlin Heidelberg New York (Handbuch der medizinischen Radiologie, vol IX, part 5c, p 391)

Webb WR (1989) The role of magnetic resonance imaging in the assessment of patients with lung cancer: a comparison with computed tomography. J Thorac Imag 4: 65

Webb WR, Gamsu G, Stark DD et al. (1984a) Evaluation of magnetic resonance sequences in imaging mediastinal tumors. AJR 143: 723

Webb WR, Jensen BG, Gamsu G et al. (1984b) Coronal magnetic resonance imaging of the chest: normal and abnormal. Radiology 153: 729

Webb WR, Jensen BG, Gamsu G, Sollitto R, Moore EH (1985) Sagittal MR imaging of the chest: normal and abnormal. J Comput Assist Tomogr 9: 471

Yulish BS, Owens RP (1980) Thymic enlargement in a child during therapy for primary hypothyroidism. AJR 135: 157

Yune HY, Klatte EC (1970) Thymic venography. Radiology 96: 521

Zanca P, Chuang TH, DeAvila R, Galindo DL (1965) True congenital mediastinal thymic cyst. Pediatrics 36: 615

Zeidler U (1978) Hirnszintigraphie. In: Diethelm L, Heuck F, Olsson O, Strnad F, Vieten H, Zuppinger A (eds) Nuclearmedizin. Springer, Berlin Heidelberg New York, Handbuch der medizinischen Radiologie, vol XV, part 2, p 1 ff

5 Diagnostic Imaging of the Normal Thymus

E. WILLICH, E. WALTER, W. R. WEBB, and G. DE GEER

5.1 Conventional Diagnostics in Children

E. WILLICH and E. WALTER

5.1.1 Newborns and Infants

The thymus is by far the most frequent cause of an enlarged mediastinal shadow in newborns and infants. It varies enormously in size and shape (Fig. 5.1) and in general is well differentiated on chest radiographs up to the 2nd year of age or beyond.

In newborns the thymus, in conjunction with the relatively large cardiac shadow, occasionally gives rise to a shadow that occupies the entire hemithorax and totally obscures the cardiac silhouette (so-called cardiomegaly type; "giant thymus"; Fig. 5.2a). This phenomenon is indicative of an uncomplicated perinatal period. In contrast a small thymic shadow, or its total absence, indicates pre-, peri-, or postnatal stress situations, e.g., respiratory distress syndrome, and is very seldom caused by thymic aplasia (Fig. 6.1).

In a series of 1020 unselected *newborns,* TAUSEND and STERN (1965) did not detect any enlargement of the mediastinal shadow due to thymic tissue in ca. 50%. Prominence of the right thymic lobe was present in 25%; the left lobe was thus affected in 8%, and bilateral prominence was described in 17%. Control radiographs performed in individual cases after 2–4 weeks revealed both enlargements and reductions in the thymic shadow.

In *infants* the thymus is usually easily visible. The following radiodiagnostic criteria should be considered and facilitate recognition of the thymus:

1. Position. The thymus is usually located in the upper half of the anterior mediastinum, though it sometimes extends to the lower half. Very seldom the thymus or an accessory thymic lobe is present in the middle or posterior mediastinum (see Sect. 7.2).

2. Side. The thymic shadow is more often located on the right side (44%) than on the left (6%). A thymic outline exists on both sides in 50% of in-

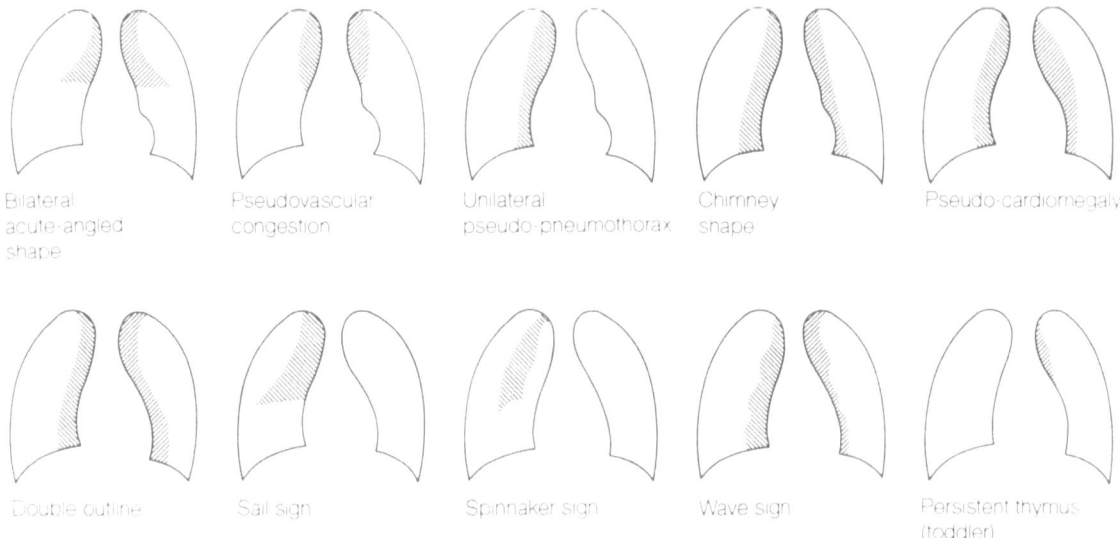

Fig. 5.1. Thymic shapes

Bilateral acute-angled shape

Pseudovascular congestion

Unilateral pseudo-pneumothorax

Chimney shape

Pseudo-cardiomegaly

Double outline

Sail sign

Spinnaker sign

Wave sign

Persistent thymus (toddler)

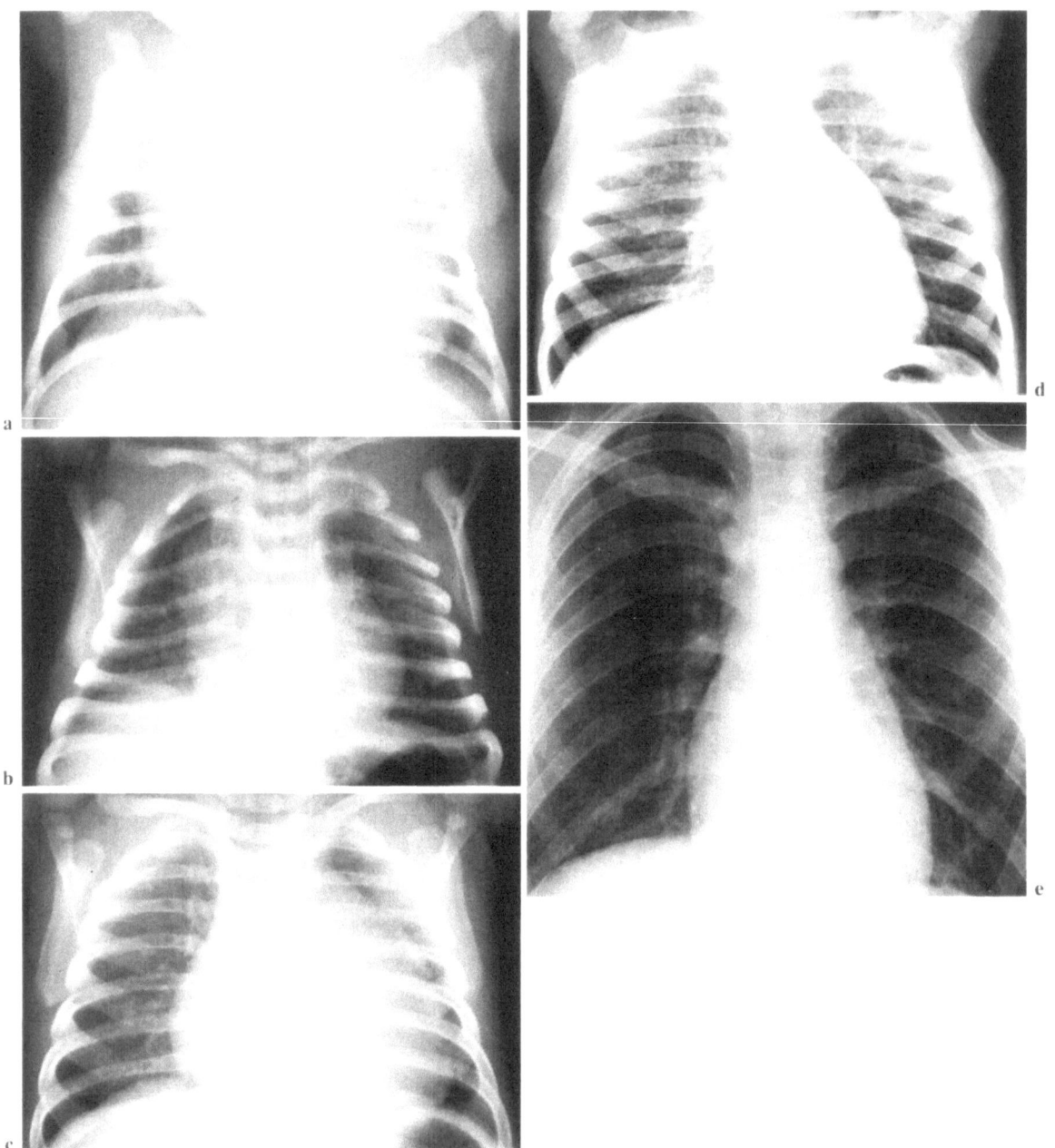

Fig. 5.2 a–e. Thymic hyperplasia: follow-up series in a male from birth until 12 years of age. **a** First day of life. The thymus occupies the whole left hemithorax and more than half of the right hemithorax. **b** 9 days old: After steroid administration, there is distinct diminution in the size of the thymus, which overlaps the mediastinum and the heart on both sides. **c** 3 months old: Recurrent enlargement of the thymus, especially on the left (rebound phenomenon). **d** At the age of 2 years the persistent thymus simulates a prominent pulmonary segment and sinking apex of the heart. **e** 12 years old: The thymus causes an "effaced heart waist"

fants (data from selected patients with a visible thymus: SCHNELL 1975) (Fig. 5.3).

3. Outline. The outline is sharp and ranges from laterally convex, concave, or straight to slightly undulating and sometimes even wavy.

The *sail sign,* a triangular shadow of the thymic tissue (KEMP 1950), is found in 3%–15% of all cases (OTLANI 1958; TAUSEND and STERN 1965). It originates from the superior mediastinum, is more often seen on the right side than on the left or bilaterally, and is usually acute angled (Fig. 5.4).

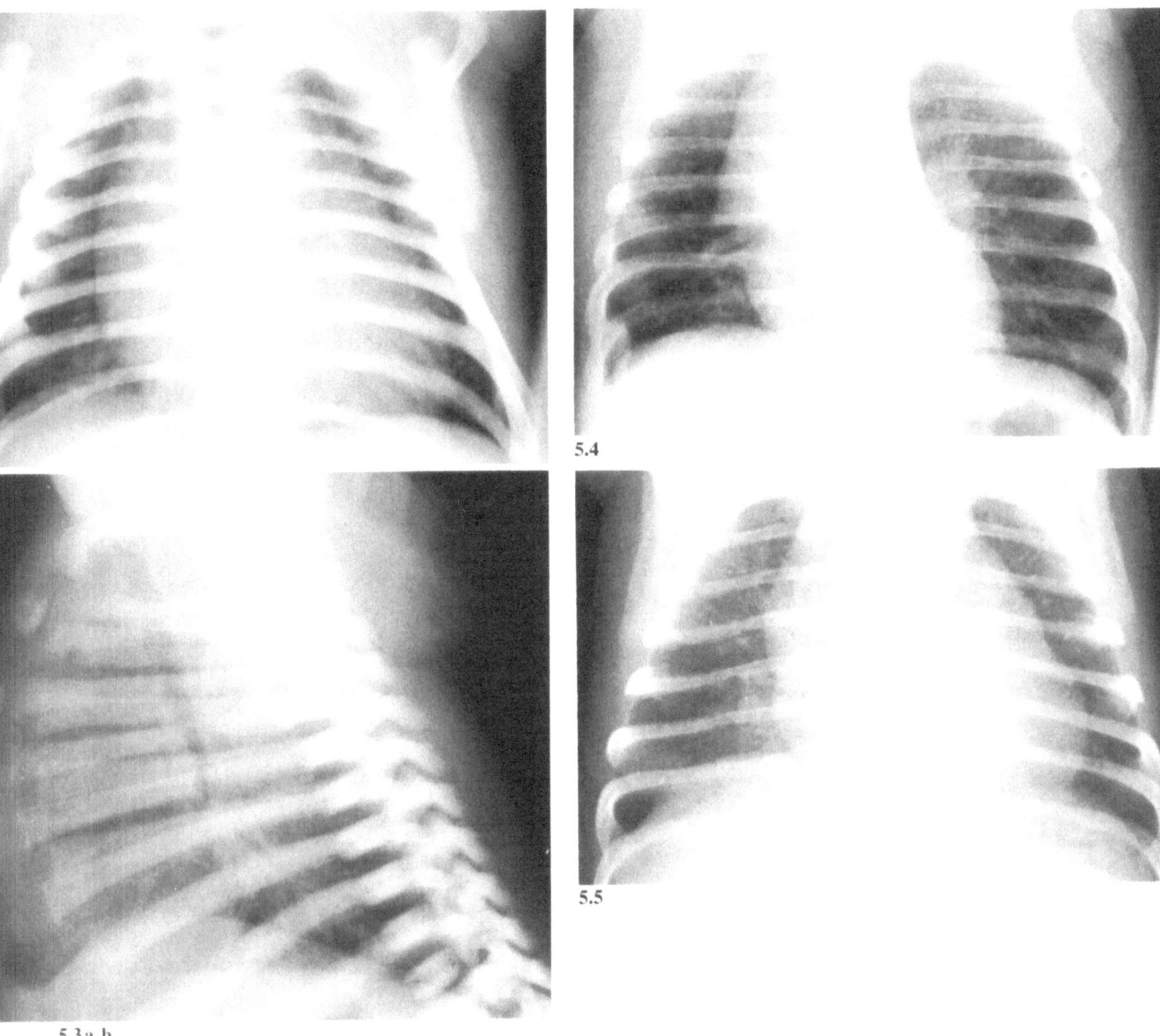

5.4

5.5

5.3 a, b

The *wave sign* (MULVEY 1963) is thought to be pathognomonic. It represents the wavy lateral thymic border brought about by compression of the soft thymic tissue by anterior ribs. It is most often found on the left side (Fig. 5.5). The frequency ranges from 5% to 8% (MULVEY 1963; SCHNELL 1975).

The *notch sign* represents an interruption of the cardiac silhouette. It may be present unilaterally or bilaterally, but is more frequently left-sided. It discloses the lower border of the thymus by way of a "step" in the shadow (Fig. 5.6). Often this step ap-

Fig. 5.3 a, b. Normal thymus of a 10-day-old infant. **a** Frontal chest radiograph. **b** Lateral view: homogeneous shadowing of the anterior mediastinum in the upper part by the thymus, and in the lower part by the heart

Fig. 5.4. Sail sign of the thymus (4-month-old infant)

Fig. 5.5. Wave sign of the thymus (1-month-old infant; Fig. 10.1 pertains to the same child)

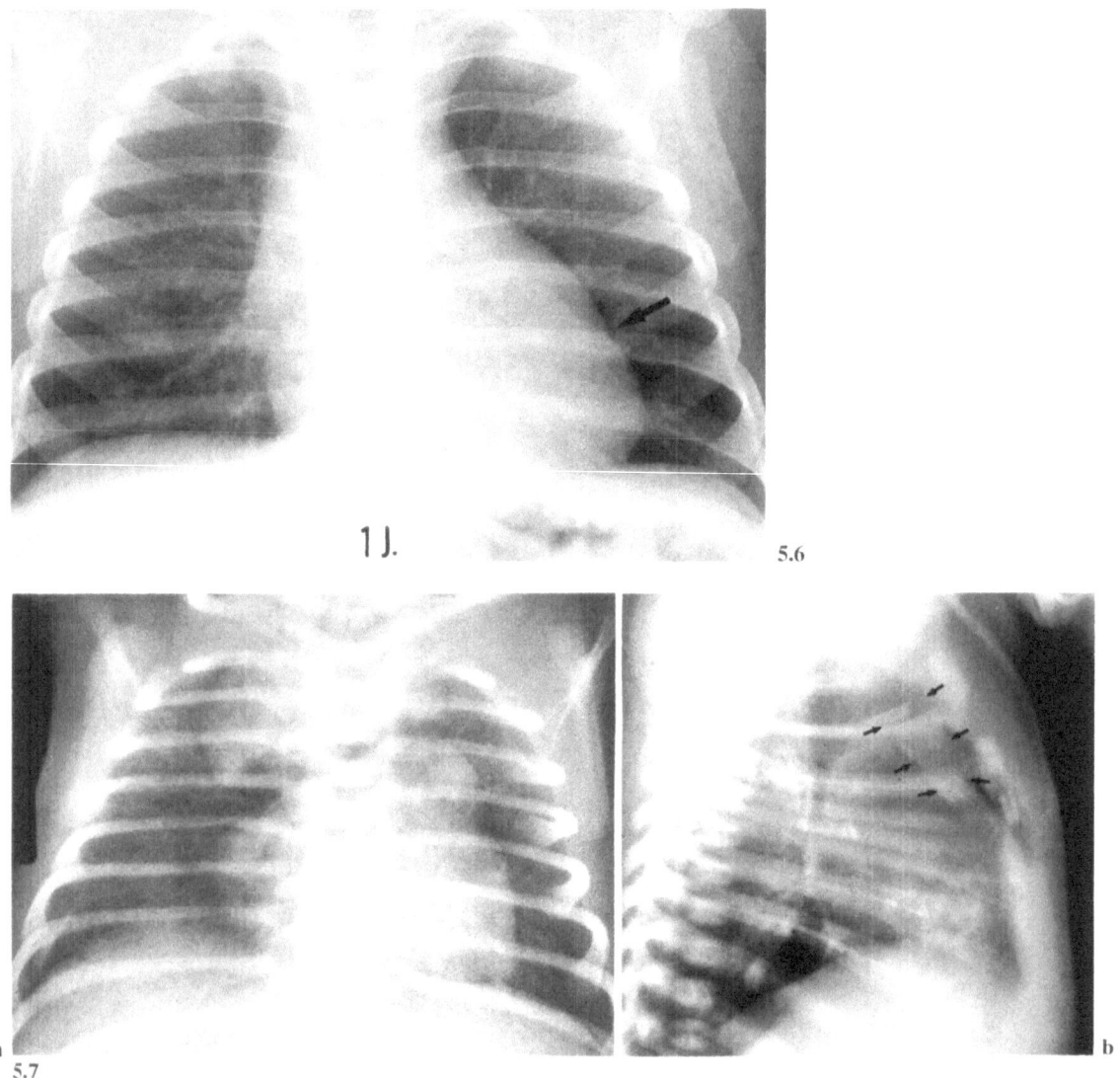

pears like a triangular figure ("paramediastinal triangular shadow," AMANN 1962).

The *spinnaker sign* (MOSELEY 1960) represents a thymus lifted from the midshadow as a result of a pneumomediastinum; the appearance is that of a sail raised from a mast (Fig. 5.7). The sign appears only on the right side of the thoracic cavity (except in the case of dextrocardia, when it appears on the left). The invariably convex outline melts into the cardiac silhouette without any disruption (see also Chap. 10).

4. Density. The thymus shows a low density because of the thin tissue layers. The underlying lung vessels are consequently visible through the semi-transparent organ. Because of the overlapping cardiac silhouette, the density decreases laterally.

Fig. 5.6. Notch sign of the thymus. The notch is situated on the left heart edge *(arrow)* in a 1-year-old girl with trilogy of Fallot. There is only a little thymic expansion on both sides. Hilar vessels cover the subhilar step on the right side. Paravertebrally on the right, the descending aorta causes a straight shadwo (condensation). See also the radiographic findings in the same child at 3 years of age: Fig. 7.11. (Courtesy of Prof. Dr. F. Ball, Department of Pediatric Radiology, University of Frankfurt/Main, FRG)

Fig. 5.7 a, b. Spinnaker sign of the thymus in a 1-day-old newborn. **a** Chest radiograph: the thymus is lifted mediastinally by insufflated air (pneumomediastinum) and therefore limited caudally. **b** The lateral view shows the tongue-shaped and raised thymus surrounded by air *(arrows)*

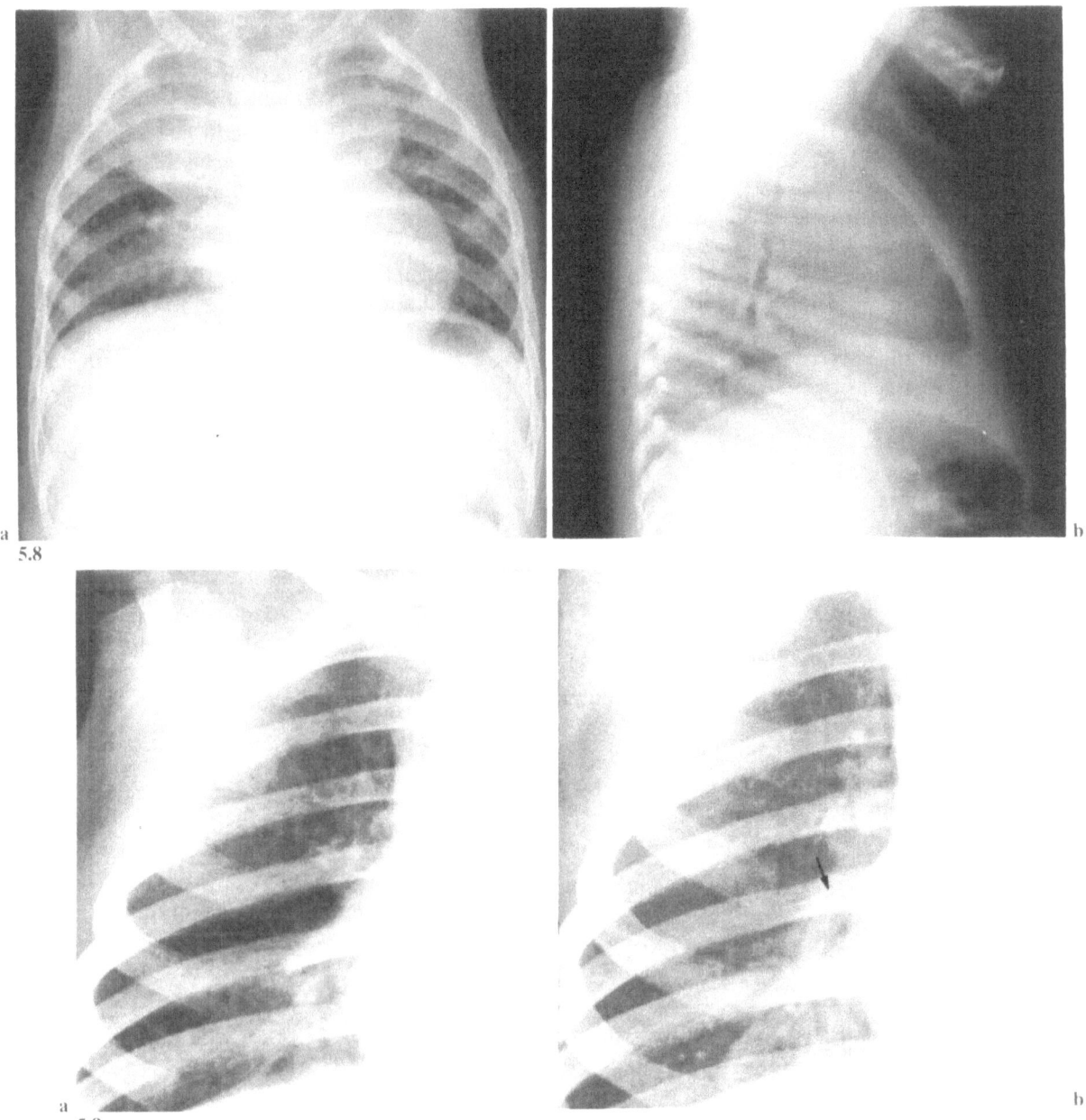

Fig. 5.8 a, b. Unusual thymus in a 4-month-old male infant. **a** Anteroposterior chest radiograph: Approximately symmetric "pseudotumor" (rounded masses) situated paramediastinally in the upper fields of the thorax. Pneumonic infiltrations are present in the right lower lobe. **b** The frontal view shows the substernal mass and the lower margin of the thymus. (Courtesy of Dr. K. Raschke, Cape Town, South Africa/Heidelberg, FRG)

Fig. 5.9 a, b. Growth of the thymic tip into the small interlobar fissure. **a** Radiographic finding at the age of 2 years and 8 months: The tip continues to grow into the condensed lobe fissure. **b** 5 years of age: The thymic tip has disappeared; the interlobar fissure only resembles a pencil scratch in the medial part *(arrow)*

The absence of an air bronchogram can serve as a differential diagnostic sign against pneumonic infiltration. Computed tomography, unlike conventional roentgenography, permits exact attenuation measurements (see Sect. 5.6).

5. Shape. The possible thymic shapes are illustrated in Fig. 5.1. There are pronounced variations in shape; the shape also alters with changes in posture and during the respiratory phase owing to the very soft and elastic nature of the thymic tissue. Sometimes the thymus appears as a circular shadow or resembles a pigeon's egg, being laterally convex (Fig. 5.8).

The lateral view usually clarifies the anatomic situation if (a) the "tumor" is situated in the anterior mediastinum, (b) the child is below 2 years of age, (c) the substrate does not show any growth potential, and (d) displacement or compression of neighboring structures is not visible. The inverted triangular-shaped thymus can simulate upper lobe pneumonia or atelectasis (LANNING and HEIKKINEN 1980; HOEFFEL et al. 1984). Translucency on the lateral margin in conjunction with pronounced irregularity in shape is caused by fat storage in the thymus. As regards the shapes seen on CT scans, see Fig. 5.12.

6. Size. Sometimes, for example in newborns, the thymus may totally shadow a hemithorax (or even the entire thoracic cavity) and overlap the cardiac silhouette in such a manner that differentiation of the organs becomes impossible. With respect to measurement of the size of the thymus, see Sect. 5.6.

7. Interlobar Involvement. If the lower thymic tip grows into the small interlobar fissure, the radiologic appearance will simulate interlobular pleurisy or mediastinal pleurisy with interlobar involvement (SWISCHUK 1980) (Fig. 5.9).

As long ago as 1955 GEFFERTH illustrated the possibility of confusion by reference to two cases. That the thymus is indeed capable of forcing apart the lobes of the lung was proved by ZSEBÖK (1958) radiologically and also on the basis of autopsy findings.

8. Biologic Behavior. The thymus is visible on radiographs during the 1st year of life but it decreases in size continuously thereafter. Under conditions of stress, e.g., during infections involving fever, during pneumonia, following surgery, and during administration of adrenal hormone substitutes (ACTH, cortisone) or cytostatics, the thymus can disappear within a few days (Figs. 5.2b, 7.4c). During reconvalescence (Fig. 7.17) or after discontinuation of steroid or cytostatic therapy, the thymus may reappear and sometimes even exceeds its original size (see Sect. 7.4.6).

According to SCHNELL (1975) 45% of 100 examined radiographs did not show any of the abovementioned radiologic signs. STERN and POPOW (1977) verified the cited radiologic signs in 70 cadavers of children up to 15 years of age by pathoanatomic means.

5.1.2 Preschool Age to Adolescence

Although, as already pointed out, the thymus usually disappears totally on chest radiographs after the initial years of life, it may persist in children older than 2 years and can then lead to diagnostic difficulties, which sometimes call for thoracotomy to exclude a tumor (Fig. 7.5; see Sect. 7.3).

From the 2nd to 3rd year of life onward, the thymus normally no longer overlaps the lateral mediastinal border (OLIVA 1973; PARKER et al. 1985). However, a small thymic tip can persist, which causes an "effaced heart waist" or a prominent pulmonary segment on chest radiographs (see Sect. 7.3.5). The persistence of a normal or an enlarged thymus may lead to incidental detection in late infancy or at school age (given that clinical symptoms are lacking). Differentiation of a persistent thymus from hyperplasia or thymomas is almost impossible (LACK 1981: two patients, 11 and 14 years old; Figs. 7.7, 7.12), often leading to surgical extirpation; alternatively there is sometimes a striking resemblance to disease of the lymphatic system.

5.1.3 Adults

In adults the thymus is no longer visible on radiographs in two planes; this can be explained by the increasing atrophy of the thymic tissue, which is replaced by fat cells (fatty infiltration of the thymus).

Even conventional tomography fails to reveal the thymus in adults, as it is hidden behind the mediastinal shadow.

5.2 Ultrasonography

5.2.1 Children

Ultrasonography is a suitable procedure for thymic diagnosis in young children, since the lack of ossification of the sternum and costal cartilage means that suprasternal access and left and right parasternal access, as well as subxiphoid or transcardiac access from caudally, can be employed for longitudinal scans. For transverse scans, transosseous access through the sternum and the intercostal spaces is suitable. In this way the thymus can be completely visualized in young children.

With increasing age during childhood, however, the possibility of ultrasonographic visualization declines owing to age-related changes in the

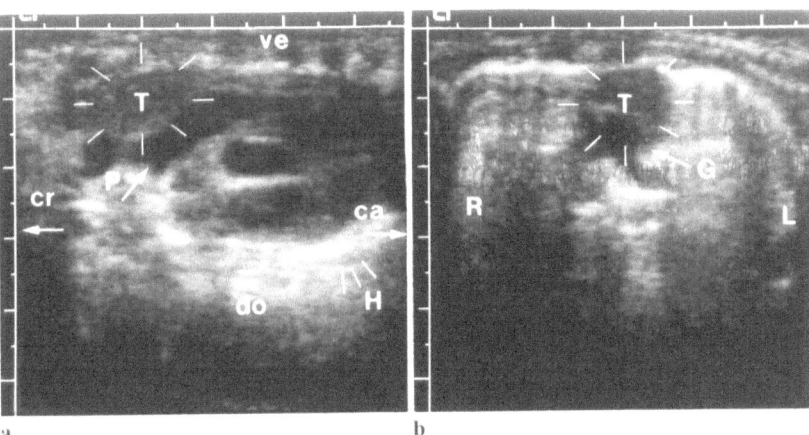

Fig. 5.10 a, b. Ultrasonography of the mediastinum in a 9-day-old infant. **a** Transverse scan. **b** Longitudinal scan. *T*, Thymus; *G*, great vessels; *H*, heart; *P*, pulmonary artery; *Cr*, cranial; *ca*, caudally; *ve*, ventrally; *do*, dorsally. (Courtesy of B. KIM HAN, M. D., and Prof. A. E. OESTREICH, M. D., Children's Hospital, Cincinnati, USA)

relative size of the mediastinal organs and atrophy of the thymus on the one hand, and to increasing calcification of the osseous structures on the other.

On longitudinal scans the normal thymus appears triangular or drop-shaped, while on transverse scans it is usually trapezoid or bilobate. The position of the thymus in front of the great vessels, caudally on to the heart and sometimes even to the diaphragm, can be clearly determined. The thymus can clasp itself around the great vessels and the heart without deforming or impressing them. The extension cervically must be determined in order to recognize accessory ectopic thymus glands or a totally cervical organ. During severe screaming by infants and young children or expiration, "cervical herniation" sometimes takes place (LEMAITRE et al. 1987).

In infancy the smooth contours of the thymus adapt to the neighboring organs. The deformation of the organ during vasomotion and during the respiratory-dependent shift towards the heart and vessel configurations is easily visible. The echo texture of the thymus resembles that of the spleen or liver in being homogeneous and coarsely reticular, while its echogenicity is slightly lower than that of the thyroid gland (REITHER 1984; WEITZEL et al. 1984; KIM HAN et al. 1989). Therefore the main criteria of recognition consist in the plasticity of the thymus and in its structural homogeneity (VON LENGERKE and SCHMIDT 1988) (Figs. 5.10, 5.11).

5.2.2 Adults

In adults ultrasonography of the thymus is of less importance, especially in the case of the normal organ. Ultrasonography is sometimes performed in cases of suspected tumor, usually employing suprasternal access (HELTZEL 1985; WERNECKE et al. 1986); however, the diagnostic value of computed tomography is superior.

5.3 Computed Tomography

E. WALTER

With computed tomography (CT) we now have at our disposal a radiologic technique that permits visualization, on plain films, of the normal thymus in all its age-dependent variations (i.e., it can also be depicted in adults).

The thymus is typically seen as a mass of homogeneous density in the anterior superior mediastinum, located between the root of the aorta, the brachiocephalic vein, the sternum, the ascending thoracic aorta, and the right and left pulmonary lobes (HEIBERG et al. 1982; SALONEN et al. 1984; WALTER 1988).

In early childhood the typically well-defined border of the thymus is normally biconvex (Fig. 5.13 a), but in older children it tends to be straight or even biconcave. In young children the thymus displays a round or quadrilateral configuration whereas at school age and especially after puberty it shows an arrowhead-like configuration (Fig. 5.12). The heart and great vessels fashion the normal borders of the thymus and only in individual cases has displacement of the aorta to the rear been reported (SALONEN et al. 1984).

During childhood the normal thymus is bilobate caudally; occasionally two totally separated lobes or only one lobe can be seen (Fig. 5.12). Apart from the normally smooth configuration there may also be an acute-angled outline at the lateral mar-

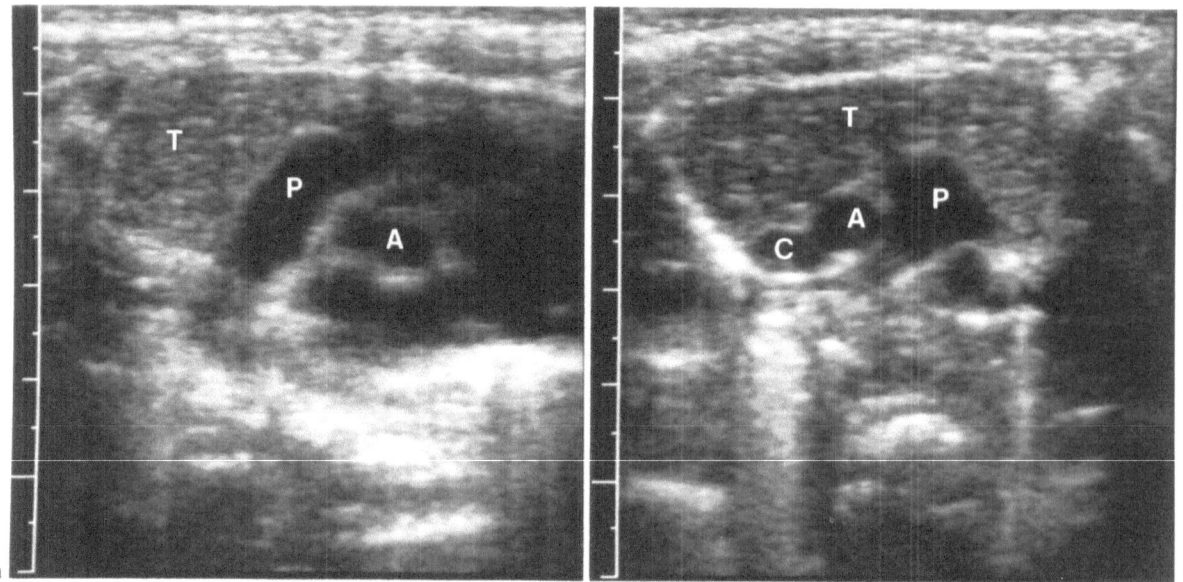

Fig. 5.11 a, b. Ultrasonography of the thymus in an 11-month-old infant. **a** Longitudinal scan. **b** Transverse scan. *T*, thymus; *P*, pulmonary artery; *A*, aorta; *C*, vena cava. (Courtesy of Prof. Dr. R. Schumacher, Dept. of Pediatric Radiology, University Children's Hospital, Mainz, FRG)

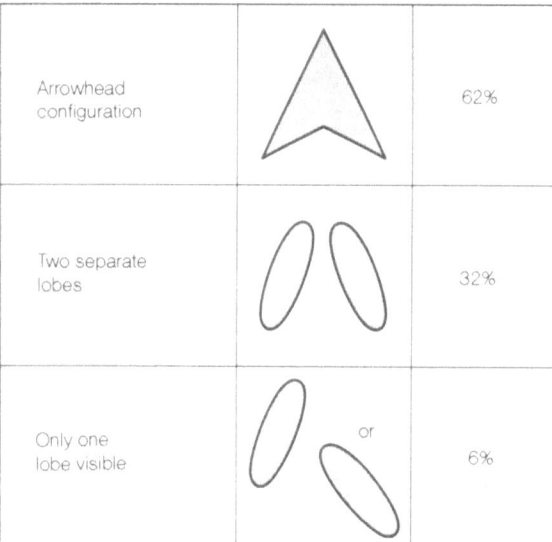

Fig. 5.12. Shapes of the thymus on CT scans (BARON et al. 1982)

gin of the thymus or a localized protuberance in the left lobe that is reminiscent of the roentgenologic sail sign (Fig. 5.13 e) although patients with this CT finding do not display the sail sign on radiographs (HEIBERG et al. 1982). Nevertheless, this CT sign represents a helpful indication that a normal thymus is present. The anterior edge extends towards the chest wall (Fig. 5.13 a, b). Differentiation into cortex and medulla is not possible on the basis of CT. Until puberty the structure is homogeneous; thereafter it is inhomogeneous, especially as a consequence of age-dependent increases in fatty infiltration.

With advancing age the morphology of the thymus changes. By the age of 16 years the spherical organ becomes a flame- or arrow-shaped, or possibly concave, homogeneous, solid mass in the anterior mediastinum (HEIBERG et al. 1982; AMOUR et al. 1987); in the process the thymus follows the contours of the mediastinal structures (as in early childhood) without impressing or displacing them (Fig. 5.13 c–e).

In adults the increasing involution of the thymus, combined with the fatty degeneration of the individual lobes, usually permits differentiation of the thymus in the anterior mediastinum from the great vessels and the sternum (Figs. 5.14, 5.15). According to the observations of BARON et al. (1982) and 54 healthy subjects, three morphologic manifestations of the thymus are thereby possible. Most frequently (in 62%) these authors observed an arrow-shaped organ (cf. also FRANCIS et al. 1985; WALTER 1988), a dorsal indentation situated in the

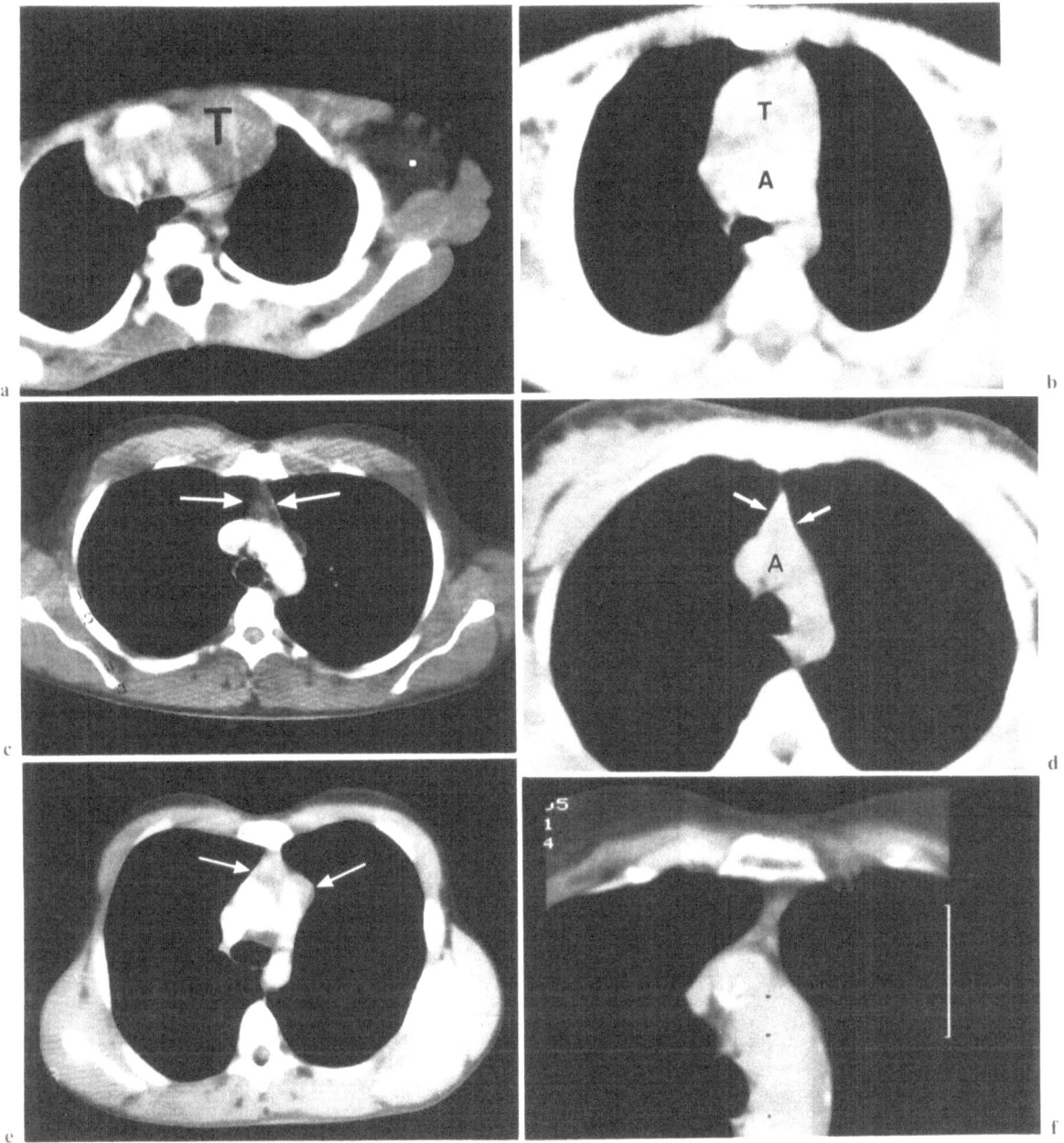

Fig. 5.13 a–f. Development of the thymus from infancy to adolescence as seen on CT. **a** $2^1/_2$-month-old infant. Large oval thymus (*T*), broadly resting on the sternum. (Indication for this investigation: lymphangioma of the left armpit; see *white point*). **b** 3-month-old infant with normal thymus (*T*). *A*, ascending aorta thoracica. **c** 10-year-old boy. The thymus becomes smaller ventrally. Its shape is triangular *(arrows)*. Scan after injection of contrast medium. **d** 15-year-old girl. Triangular thymus *(arrows)*. The left and right lobes cannot be differentiated. **e** 16-year-old with myasthenia gravis. Investigation for tumor. Bulging of the left thymic contour is present. The contrast medium is inhomogeneously taken up by the thymus. Only a narrow connection exists between the thymus and the retrosternal wall. Normal finding. – Thoracotomy: histologically normal thymic parenchyma. **f** 19-year-old with a persistent thymus. The right and left thymic lobes can be differentiated. Dorsal notching is evident

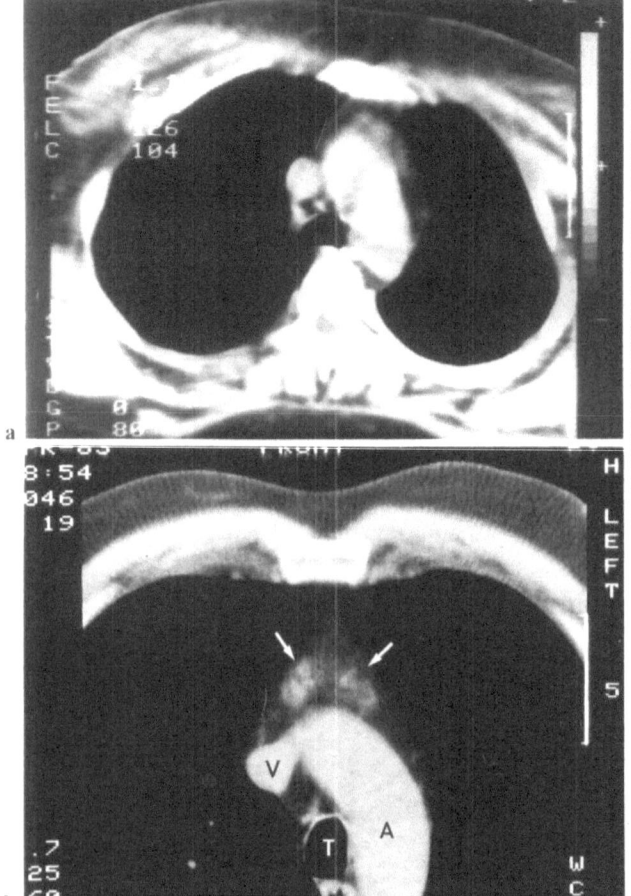

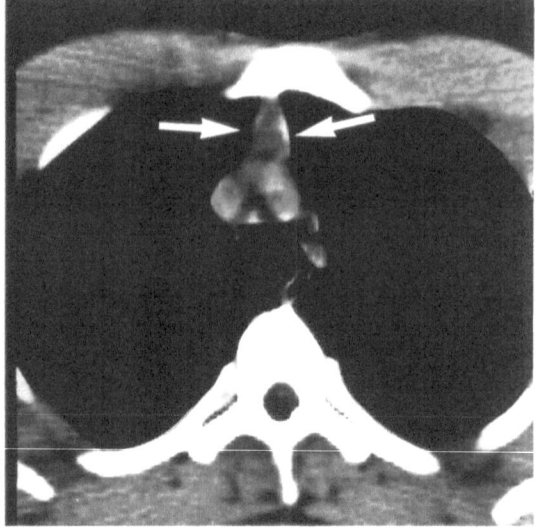

Fig. 5.14a–c. Development of the thymus during early adulthood. **a** 28-year-old female. The thymus is visible as a small, lipomatous, fat-infiltrated organ; the right and left thymic lobes are separated and homogenously dense. **b** 36-year-old patient. Involution of the thymus, typical at this age. Both thymic lobes are well visible within the fat of the anterior mediastinum. They are infiltrated by fat *(arrows)*. *V*, superior vena cava; *A*, aortic arch; *T*, trachea. **c** 32-year-old patient. Narrowing and reduction of density of the thymus are present; there is only a narrow connection to the retrosternal chest wall

middle indicating the division between the right and left lobes of the thymus. In 32% of cases, BARON et al. (1982) found two isolated thymic lobes which in each instance were oval or crescent shaped. In 6% of cases only a right or a left lobe could be demonstrated (Fig. 5.12). As already mentioned, with advancing age the thymic remnants are increasingly infiltrated by fat (Fig. 5.14), whereby large solid areas can also be found up until the 40th year of life.

Such thymic remnants in the anterior superior mediastinum subsequently decrease in frequency. Thus BARON et al. (1982) were able the recognize the thymus on CT scans in 100% of patients below 30 years old, in 73% of those aged 30–49 years, and in only 17% of those aged above 49 years.

In contrast to BARON et al. (1982), MOORE et al. (1983), and FRANCIS et al. (1985), WALTER (1988) reported three different findings in the anterior superior mediastinum which should be classified as normal and which, in correspondence with the lipomatous atrophy of the thymus described by

STEINMANN (1986), were to be observed with varying frequency depending on age. The three findings in question were (Fig. 5.16):

1. Solid tissue structures, as described by BARON et al. (1982) and FRANCIS et al. (1985), among others. Such structures can be clearly identified as thymic tissue on CT scans.
2. Fine reticular structures that no longer display a configuration reminiscent of thymic lobes. Such structures may represent residual thymic tissue (Fig. 5.15 a).
3. An anterior superior mediastinum displaying complete fatty infiltration on CT scans, without any recognizable solid residual structures (Fig. 5.15 b).

Owing to the increasing fatty infiltration and involution of the thymus, thymic attenuation values can in general be measured with precision only during childhood. During infancy, when the thymus is of homogeneous density and without fatty infiltration, values of ca. 50–60 HU are recorded,

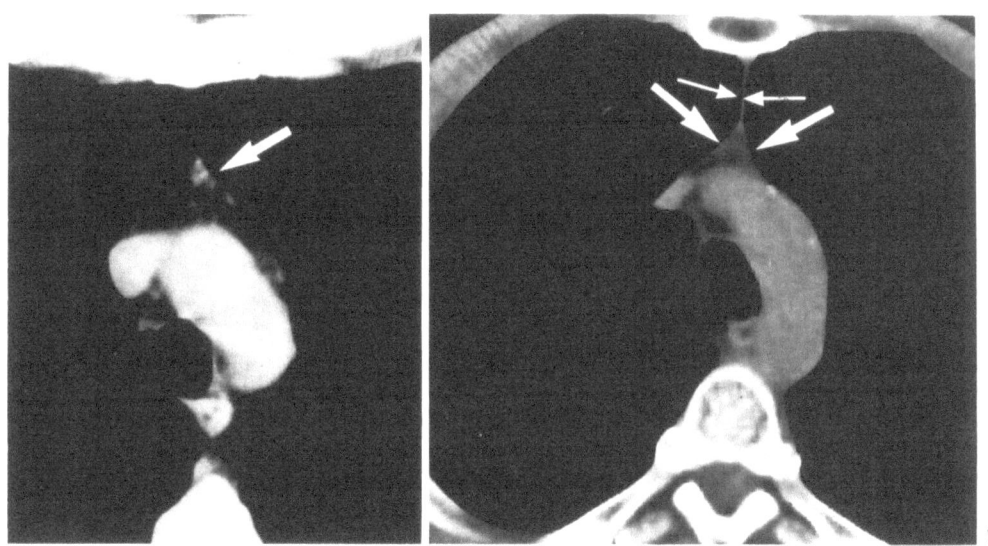

as compared with ca. 35 HU in children of school age (SALONEN et al. 1984). HEIBERG et al. (1982) reported very heterogeneous values ranging from 20 to 119 HU. WALTER (1988) agreed with SALONEN et al. (1984) that the attenuation values lie within a narrower range, namely between 35 and 50 HU with a standard deviation of ± 10 HU.

HEIBERG et al. (1982) reported that after administration of water-soluble contrast medium the attenuation values increased to 28–185 HU, while SALONEN et al. (1984) cite an increase to ca. 70 ± 7.3 HU.

In adults, also, the attenuation values of thymus not infiltrated by fat exceed 30 HU, thus corresponding to the values of the chest wall musculature (BARON et al. 1982; MOORE et al. 1983). Nor do these values change with advancing age (BARON et al. 1982). Nevertheless, in most instances the determination of attenuation values proves difficult in adults due to the fatty infiltration. In patients older than 40 years, 40% fatty degeneration is to be expected, while in patients older than 50 years the figure exceeds 50% (FRANCIS et al. 1985). Correspondingly, the correlation between attenuation values of the thymus (in EMI units) and the percentage of residual thymic tissue described by DIXON et al. (1981) displays a typical curve: with the percentage increase in fatty tissue there is a decline in CT attenuation values; when there is less than 30% residual thymic tissue the latter are in the negative range.

Figure 5.16 shows the age-dependent frequency of the typical CT findings in respect of the thymus.

As regards determination of the size of the thymus, see Sect. 5.6.

Fig. 5.15 a, b. Development of the thymus in humans older than 40 years. **a** 63-year-old man with uncharacteristic densities in the anterior mediastinum *(arrow)*. Residual parenchyma of the thymic islet. **b** 64-year-old patient. Completed thymic involution. A small triangular shadow *(thick arrows)* is seen. There is a narrow membranous connection to the retrosternal space *(thin arrows)*

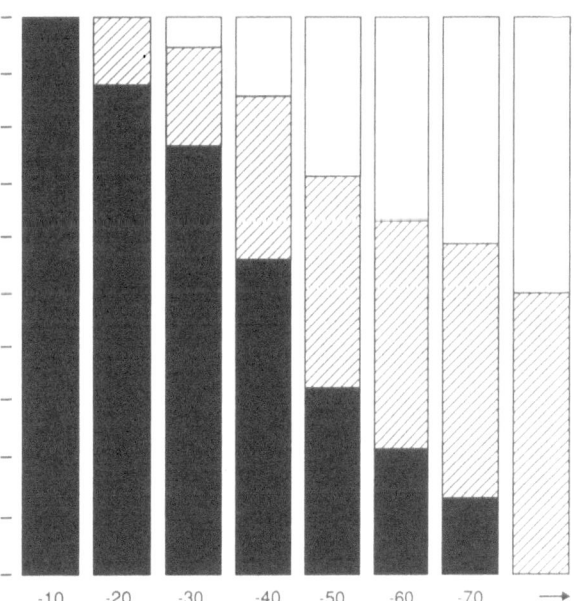

Fig. 5.16. Age-dependent frequency of the typical findings in respect of the thymus. No solid structures in the anterior mediastinum except fat tissue. Non characteristic densities in the anterior mediastinum. For thymus typical solid or lipomatous structures. ■ typical thymic structures, ▨ reticular structures, which may represent thymic remnants, □ complete fatty anterior mediastinum without any thymic remnants

5.4 Magnetic Resonance Imaging

W. R. WEBB and G. DE GEER

5.4.1 Children

The thymus is visible on magnetic resonance (MR) images in all young patients, occupying nearly all of the prevascular or anterior mediastinum (Fig. 5.17). It appears homogeneous on MR images, and there is no distinction between cortex and medulla. The thymus is proportionately largest in children less than 5 years of age. In young children, the lateral margins of the thymus, and therefore the anterior mediastinum, are characteristically convex when viewed in the transaxial plane (Fig. 5.18); in patients less than 5 years old, the thymus appears quadrilateral in shape.

In older children, the thymus is appears smaller and is more typically triangular (SIEGEL et al. 1989). The right lobe is usually smallest and is sometimes difficult to see (DE GEER et al. 1986). Often, the thymus appears to be a different shape on MRI than on CT. On MRI, the edges of the thymus appear more convex and it appears proportionately larger. This probably reflects the lower lung volumes at which MR images are obtained. CT is performed at full inspiration, while MRI is done during quiet breathing.

The thymus, as seen on MRI, generally extends from just below the left brachiocephalic vein, inferiorly to the point at which the superior vena cava enters the right atrium (Fig. 5.18) (DE GEER et al. 1986; SIEGEL et al. 1989). This anatomy is very well shown on sagittal images (Fig. 5.19). Inferiorly the thymus is closely applied to the pericardium, which can be clearly seen on MRI as a very low intensity band, because of its fluid contents and because of cardiac pulsations transmitted to the fluid (DE GEER et al. 1986). In an occasional patient, the thymus can be seen above the brachiocephalic vein, and in this location it can sometimes mimic a mediastinal mass or enlarged lymph node (SIEGEL et al. 1989).

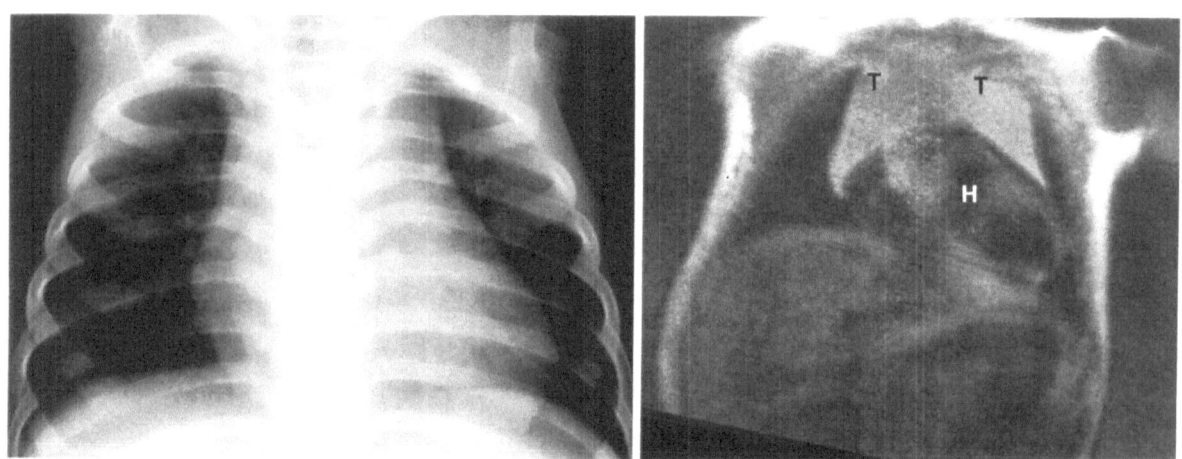

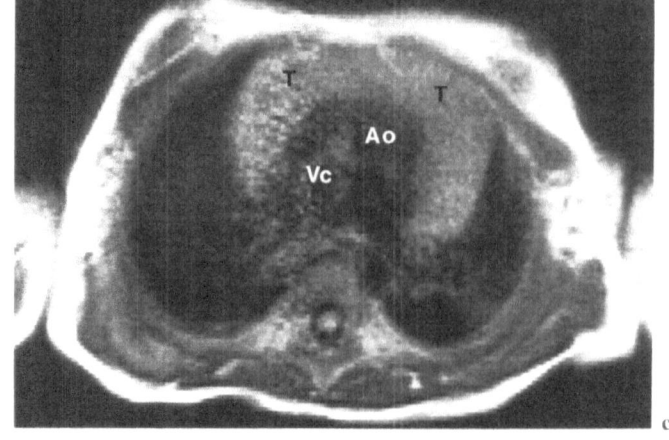

Fig. 5.17a–c. MRI of the mediastinum in a 5-month-old infant with a suspected cardiac tumor. a Chest radiograph: the upper borders of the mediastinum are formed by the thymus. b Coronal and c transverse MRI scans (TE 50 ms, TR 500 ms). The heart (*H*) and the great vessels (*Vc*, vena cava; *Ao*, aorta) are surrounded by the thymus (*T*) in both planes in a horseshoe-like fashion. The thymus can be distinguished from the great vessels by virtue of its high signal. (Courtesy of Prof. Dr. G. BENZ-BOHM, Dept. of Pediatric Radiology, University Institute of Radiology, Cologne, FRG)

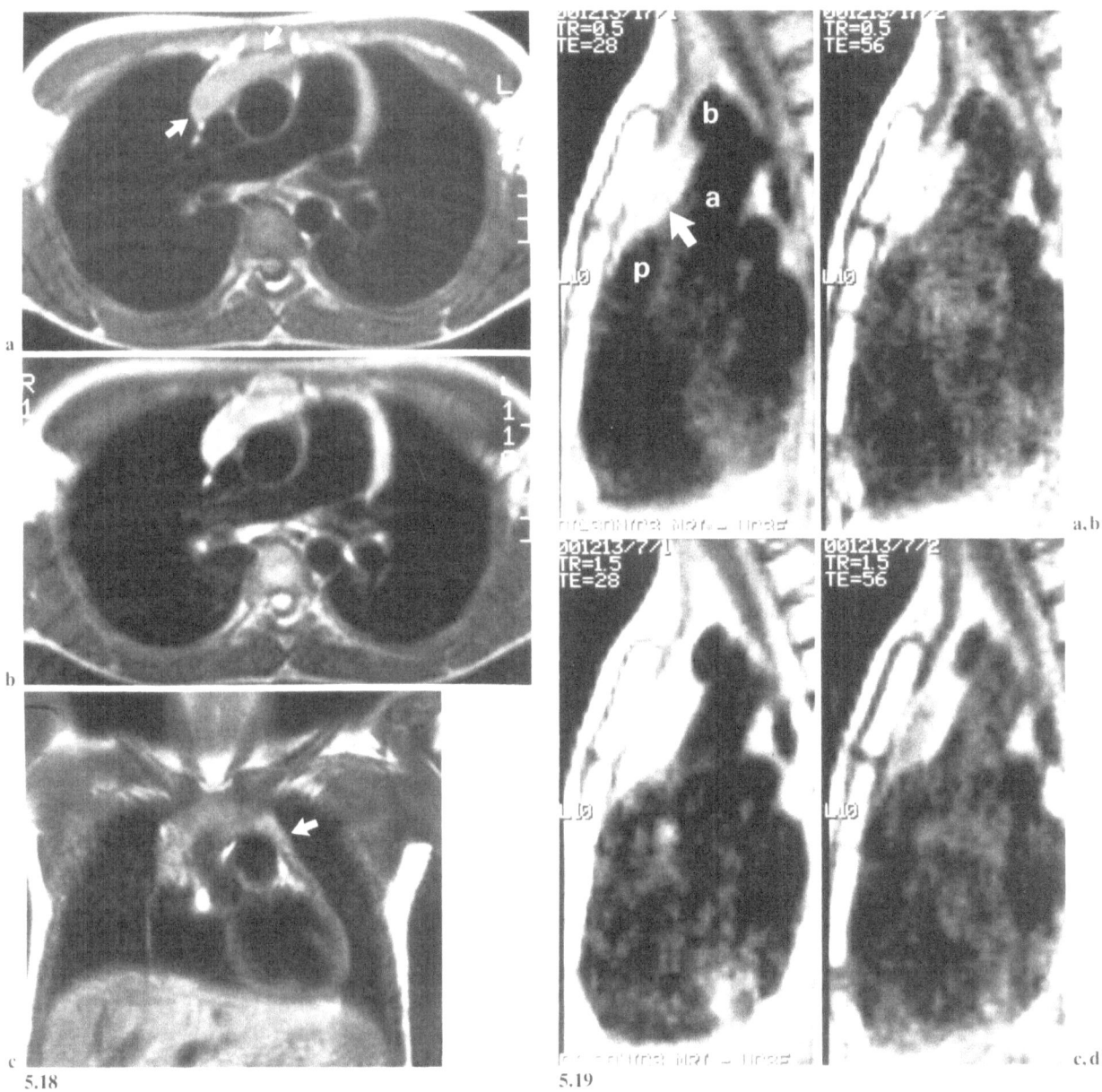

Fig. 5.18 a–c. Normal thymus in a 12-year-old boy. **a** A T1-weighted transaxial image (TR/TE = 750/20 ms) of the mediastinum shows homogeneous intensity of the thymus *(arrows)* anterior to the great vessels. The right mediastinal pleura is convex laterally. In this patient, the right lobe predominates. **b** A T2-weighted transaxial image (TR/TE = 2250/70 ms) shows an increase in intensity of the thymus, as compared with mediastinal fat. **c** A T1-weighted image (TR/TE = 750/20 ms) in the coronal plane shows the thymus occupying most of the superior mediastinum, extending inferiorly to the level of the right atrium. In this plane, the left thymic lobe *(arrow)* is also visible

Fig. 5.19 a–d. Normal thymus in a 14-year-old. The thymus *(arrow)* can be seen anterior to the ascending aorta *(a)*, below the level of the left brachiocephalic vein *(b)*, and above the pulmonary artery *(p)*. On most of the sequences, the thymus appears lower in intensity than surrounding mediastinal fat

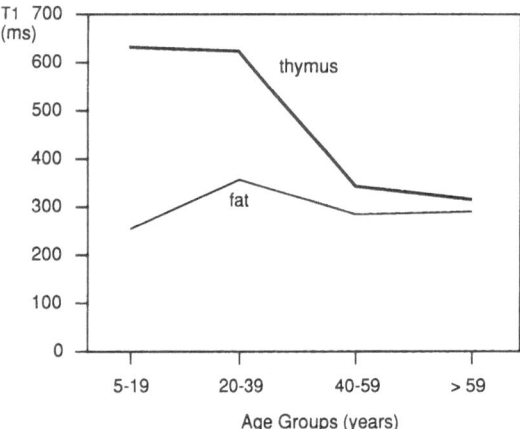

Fig. 5.20. Relative T1 values of thymus and fat in different age groups. T1 of thymus decreases in older patients because of fatty replacement. The T1 of fat remains constant

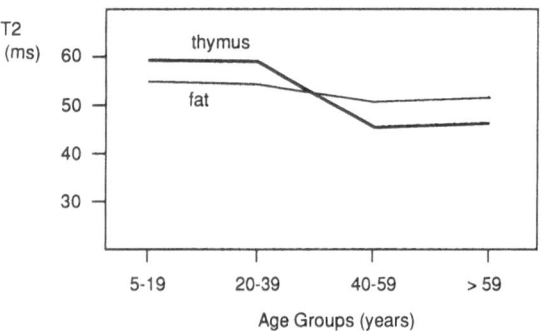

Fig. 5.21. Relative T2 values of thymus and fat in different age groups. There is a slight decrease in the T2 of thymus in adults, but this is much less than the changes in T1 which occur

Table 5.1. Thymic dimensions as measured using MRI at different ages (modified from SIEGEL et al. 1989 and DE GEER et al. 1986)

Age (years)	Right lobe		Left lobe	
	Width (cm)	Thickness (cm)	Width (cm)	Thickness (cm)
0–1	2.7	1.5	3.0	1.6
2–5	2.7	1.5	3.0	1.5
6–10	2.6	1.0	3.4	1.6
1–15	3.1	1.1	3.6	1.5
6–19	2.5	1.5	2.8	1.4
20–39			3.2	2.0
>40			2.5	1.8

Both the width and the thickness of the thymic lobes can be measured on transaxial images (Fig. 5.30). In more than half of children under 5 years of age, the right and left thymic lobes appear equal in thickness (approximately 1.5 cm) on MR images (SIEGEL et al. 1989). When the thymic lobes appear to be of different thicknesses, either may be larger, but it is more common for the left to be so. In children older than 5 years, there is a tendency for the left thymic lobe to be the thickest and widest (DE GEER et al. 1986; BATRA et al. 1987; SIEGEL et al. 1989) (Table 5.1). The left thymic lobe characteristically appears elliptical in shape, and parallels the lateral wall of the aortic arch.

On T1-weighted MR images, the thymus appears homogeneous, being lower in intensity than surrounding mediastinal fat and slightly more intense than chest wall muscle (Figs. 5.18, 5.19) (DE GEER et al. 1986; BATRA et al. 1987; SIEGEL et

al. 1989). In general, the intensity difference between fat and thymus is greatest for young children, and decreases with age. On T2-weighted images, the thymus increases in intensity relative to fat and muscle. It is typically more intense than muscle, and slightly less or equal in intensity to fat.

The greater contrast between thymus and mediastinal fat on T1-weighted images indicates a difference between thymus and fat in their T1 values. Indeed, in subjects 5–19 years of age whom we studied (DE GEER et al. 1986), the T1 of the thymus measured more than 600 ms. Furthermore, the T1 value of thymus decreases with age. In the 5-year-old we studied, we recorded a T1 value of 1028 ms. In comparison, in our study the T1 values of fat measured 280 ± 47.1 ms and did not vary with age (Fig. 5.20).

The T2 of the thymus in the same group of children had a mean value of 62.3 ± 14.6 ms, with no significant differences with age. The T2 of fat in this group was 52.3 ± 3.7 ms (Fig. 5.21). We also found a lower hydrogen density in thymus as compared to fat.

5.4.2 Adults

Proportionately, the thymus appears much smaller in adults than in children, and may be largely replaced by fat (Fig. 5.22). It usually appears more triangular than in children. In adults, as in children, the thymus appears homogeneous on MR images.

The characteristic changes of thymic involution and fatty replacement, which occur with increasing patient age, can be identified using MRI (DE GEER et al. 1986). Thus, in patients older than 40 years, the T1 values measured from thymus significantly decrease as compared to their childhood values, and become nearly equal to those of surrounding

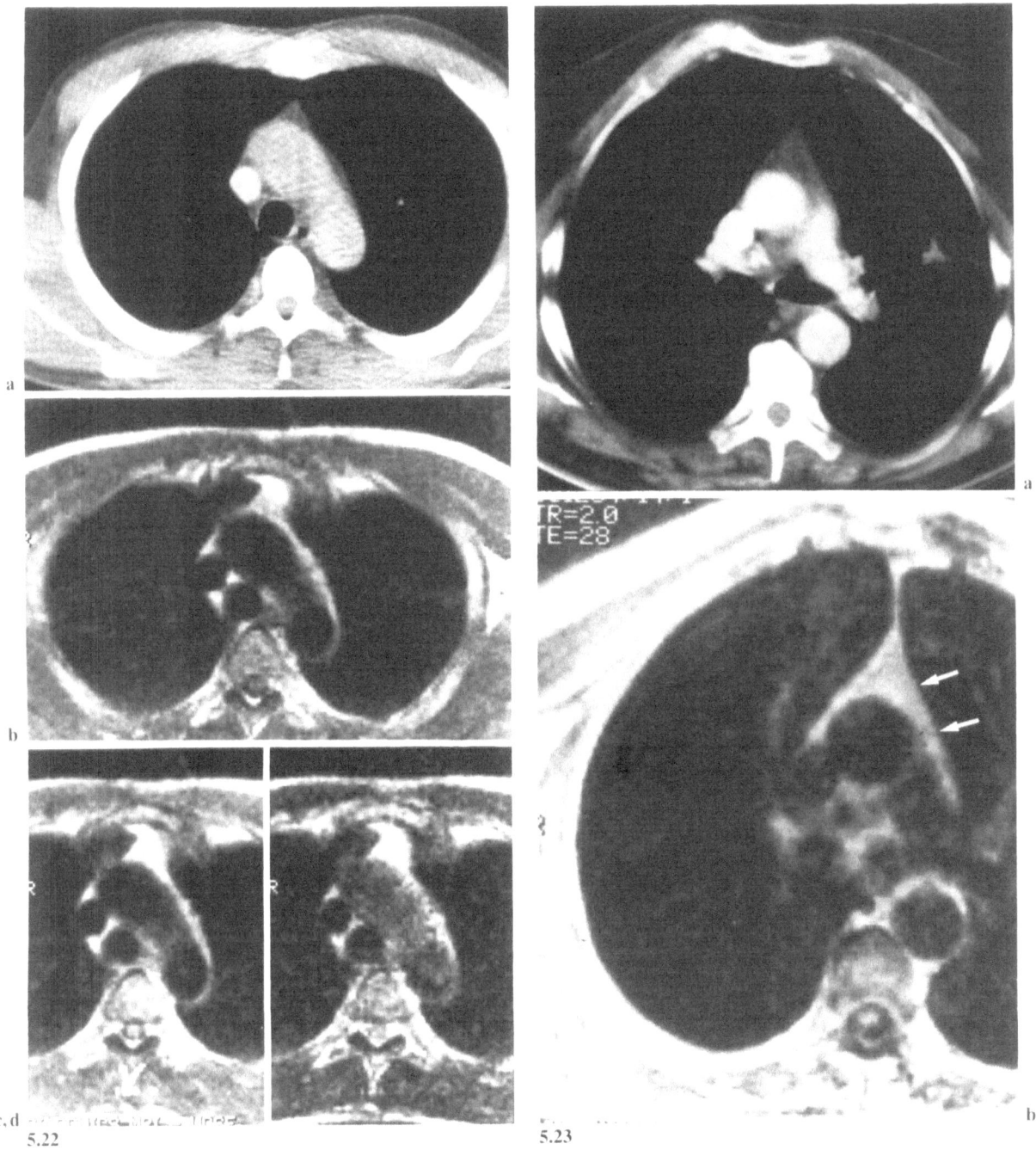

Fig. 5.22 a–d. Normal thymus in an adult. **a** CT shows a small amount of thymic soft tissue in the anterior mediastinum. **b** A T1-weighted image shows the thymus to be lower in intensity than surrounding fat. Note that the thymus appears somewhat different in shape than on the CT scan because of lower lung volume. With a longer TR (**c**) and on a T2-weighted image (**d**), the thymus is more difficult to contrast with adjacent fat

Fig. 5.23 a, b. Normal thymus in an adult. **a** CT primarily shows fat density in the anterior mediastinum. **b** On MRI, the left thymic lobe *(arrows)*, lateral to the aorta and left pulmonary artery, is predominant

mediastinal fat (Figs. 5.20, 5.22). In patients less than 30 years of age, the T1 of thymus averaged about 700 ms (703 ± 287 ms); in older patients, it averaged slightly more than 300 ms (311 ± 72 ms) (DE GEER et al. 1986). In the same group, the T1 value of mediastinal fat was quite constant regardless of age (297 ± 109 ms). Because of this, the thymus is less easily seen on MRI in adults than it is in children on T1-weighted images, but usually remains visible as a distinct structure. Its visibility likely reflects its lower hydrogen density (DE GEER et al. 1986). The ratio of hydrogen density of thymus to fat measured approximately 0.6, regardless of patient age (DE GEER et al. 1986).

The T2 value of thymus decreased slightly with age, but to a much lesser degree than the T1 value (Fig. 5.21). In patients less than 30, the mean T2 was 62 ± 16 ms; in those older than 30 it was 45 ± 6 ms. T2 measured from fat was 53 ± 6 ms and did not change significantly with age.

In adults, the left lobe of the thymus is the largest, typically being visible anterior and lateral to the lateral wall of the aortic arch on transaxial views (Fig. 5.23). The right thymic lobe may be inconspicuous and difficult to see.

In the sagittal plane, the thymus appears elliptical in shape, and 5–7 cm long. It is visible anterior to the ascending aorta and anteromedial to the superior vena cava, and is usually best seen in the midline.

5.5 Invasive Procedures (Pneumomediastinography, Arteriography, Phlebography)

E. WALTER

Since the thymus cannot be visualized in adults by means of conventional procedures, invasive techniques used to be necessary; chief among them was pneumomediastinography. With this technique the normal thymus appears bilobate and finger-shaped, though the size and configuration are variable. The surface is usually smooth. The length of the thymus has been reported as 5–15 cm, and the thickness of each lobe as 0.2–2.1 cm (SONE et al. 1980) (Fig. 5.24).

Selective arteriography of the thymus was performed via a catheter inserted into the internal thoracic artery, with ca. 10 ml of contrast medium being administered for visualization of the organ. Under normal conditions, phlebography, which entailed retrograde injection of the thymic veins, revealed a harmoniously organized venous network in the right and left thymic lobes; this technique, too, is no longer used.

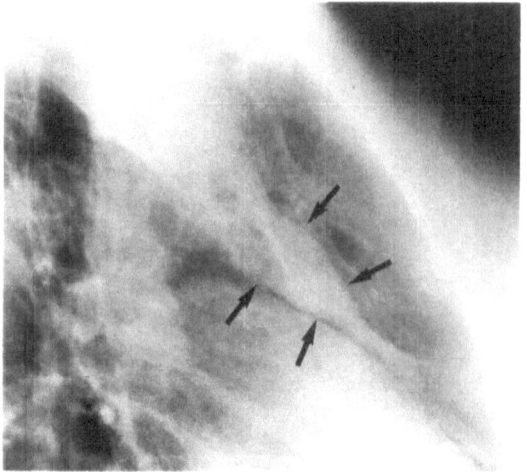

Fig. 5.24. Pneumomediastinography in a 27-year-old female patient. Demonstration of a normal thymus *(arrows)*. Spot film, oblique view

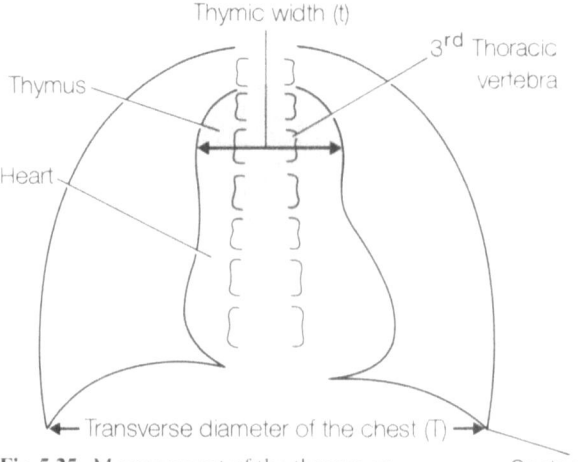

Fig. 5.25. Measurement of the thymus on radiographs (GEWOLB et al. 1979)

5.6 Measurement of the Size of the Thymus

E. Willich

5.6.1 Radiographic Method

Chest radiographs are produced with a focus-film distance of 1.2 m, while the patient is lying down (Gewolb et al. 1979). The width of the thymus is measured at the level of the carina and the third thoracic vertebral body and is related to the transverse diameter of the thorax at the level of the costophrenic angle. The quotient obtained from the width of the thymus and the transverse diameter of the thorax (i.e., the "cardiothymic index") forms the basis for the assessment of thymic size in scientific studies, e.g., the thymic reaction in the premature infant after the mother has received steroid therapy (Fig. 5.25). The mean value is generally 0.35 according to Gewolb et al. (1979) and 0.34 according to Mangelmann (1981) (see Sect. 6.3).

5.6.2 Computed Tomography

Using CT the size of the thymus can be exactly determined by measuring the craniocaudal extension (height) the maximum sagittal diameter (depth = thickness), and the maximum transverse diameter (width). Such measurements of the thymus were performed by: Baron et al. (1982: 154 patients, 6–64 years of age), Francis et al. (1985: 309 patients, 6 weeks to 81 years of age), Heiberg et al. (1982: 34 patients, 2 days to 20 years of age), and Amour et al. (1987: 25 children with thymic diseases and a control group of 71 healthy children).

According to the method of Baron et al., if the organ consists of two lobes, the thickness (T) and the width (W) are measured as shown in Fig. 5.26 a. If the two lobes come together in the form of an arrowhead, the thymus is divided along the line X–X^1 beginning at the top (Fig. 5.26 b). The other parameters remain as in Fig. 5.26 a. The normal values of these measurements are shown in Table 5.2.

Francis et al. (1985) measure the width in the real transverse diameter (frontal scan), the thickness in the same way as Baron et al., and the depth (X–X^2) in the sagittal diameter, including the lobe borders (Fig. 5.27). Thus two of these parameters differ from those employed by Baron et al. The normal values (thickness, sagittal diameter, transverse diameter, and height) obtained in this way in 82 patients aged 6 weeks to 60 years are shown in Table 5.3.

Due to the different parameters employed, the data reported by Baron et al. and Francis et al. can be compared only in respect of thymic thickness. The findings in respect of thickness showed a close similarity.

Francis et al. regard the logarithm of the product of thymic width and thickness as being more useful for differentiation against pathologically altered thymus glands than the thickness of the thymus alone.

Heiberg et al. (1982) obtained different results to Baron et al. in respect of thymic thickness (0.7 cm thicker ± 0.7 cm SD) and therefore doubted whether the thymic thickness is of any dif-

Fig. 5.26 a, b. Measurement of the thymus on CT-scans after Baron et al. (1982). **a** Bilobate organ. **b** In arrowtip forms, the thymus is divided by the line X–X^1. T, thickness; W, width

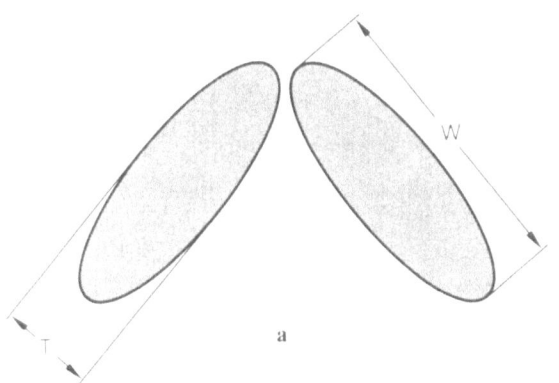
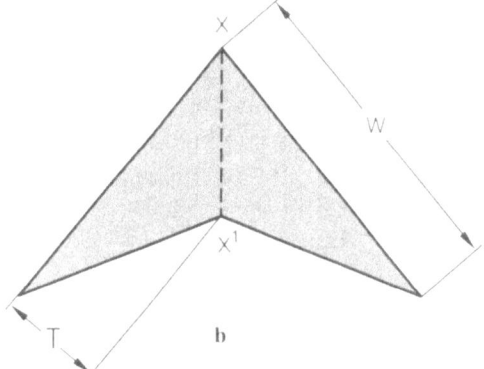

Table 5.2. Width and thickness of the thymus seen on transverse CT scans (after BARON et al. 1982)

Age group	No. of cases	Mean width in cm (SD)		Mean thickness in cm (SD)	
		Right lobe	Left lobe	Right lobe	Left lobe
6–19	11	2.0 (0.55)	3.3 (1.1)	1.0 (0.39)	1.1 (0.40)
20–29	11	1.9 (0.83)	2.3 (1.0)	0.7 (0.24)	0.8 (0.14)
30–39	13	1.3 (0.51)	2.0 (0.95)	0.5 (0.14)	0.7 (0.21)
40–49	14	1.4 (0.66)	1.9 (0.76)	0.6 (0.23)	0.6 (0.20)
> 49	16	1.4 (0.90)	1.4 (0.59)	0.5 (0.15)	0.5 (0.27)

Table 5.3. Thymic measurements in patients ($n = 82$) with normal glands (FRANCIS et al. 1985)

Age group (years)	No. of patients	Mean dimensions in cm (SD)			
		Thickness	Anteroposterior	Craniocaudal	Transverse
0–9	23	1.50 (0.46)	2.52 (0.82)	3.53 (0.99)	3.13 (0.85)
10–19	31	1.05 (0.36)	2.56 (0.88)	4.99 (1.25)	3.05 (1.17)
20–29	13	0.89 (0.16)	2.38 (0.72)	5.38 (1.80)	2.87 (0.86)
30–39	8	0.99 (0.34)	2.48 (0.86)	5.00 (1.12)	3.38 (1.37)
40–49	3	0.93 (0.58)	2.23 (0.93)	6.67 (2.08)	3.17 (0.76)
50–60	4	0.58 (0.33)	0.58 (0.33)	2.00 (1.15)	1.43 (0.48)

Table 5.4. Dimensions of the normal thymus in centimeters (AMOUR et al. 1987)

Age group (years)	No. of cases	Antero-posterior (SD)	Transverse (SD)	Right lobe (SD)		Left lobe (SD)	
				W	T	W	T
0–5	14	1.6 (0.5)	4.5 (0.6)	2.7 (0.7)	0.9 (0.3)	3.6 (0.9)	1.4 (0.5)
6–10	12	1.5 (0.6)	4.2 (1.0)	2.5 (0.7)	1.0 (0.5)	3.9 (1.2)	1.0 (0.4)
11–15	22	2.0 (0.8)	4.4 (0.5)	2.7 (0.7)	0.8 (0.3)	4.5 (0.7)	1.0 (0.5)
16–19	23	1.9 (0.6)	3.9 (0.8)	2.5 (0.7)	0.7 (0.2)	4.2 (0.9)	0.8 (0.4)
Mean (SD)		1.8 (0.6)	4.2 (0.7)	2.6 (0.7)	0.9 (0.3)	4.2 (0.9)	1.1 (0.4)

W, width; T, thickness

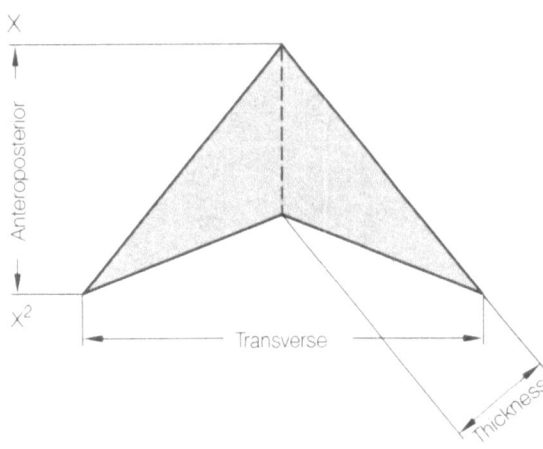

Fig. 5.27. Measurement of the thymus on CT scans after FRANCIS et al. (1985)

ferential diagnostic value with regard to pathologically altered thymus glands.

AMOUR et al. (1987) calculated six diameters for each thymus: anteroposterior diameter, transverse diameter, and the width and thickness of each lobe, whereby the "thickness" was taken as largest dimension perpendicular to the long axis of the lobe, the same definition as was used by BARON et al. (1982). In this way the measurements of BARON et al. (1982) and FRANCIS et al. (1985) are combined. The anteroposterior diameter corresponds to the distance $X–X^1$, which was not measured by BARON et al. (Table 5.4; Figs. 5.28, 5.29).

BODE and SCHEIDT (1988) reduced the measurements in 108 CT examinations to the dorsal transverse diameter of the thymus at the aortic arch level.

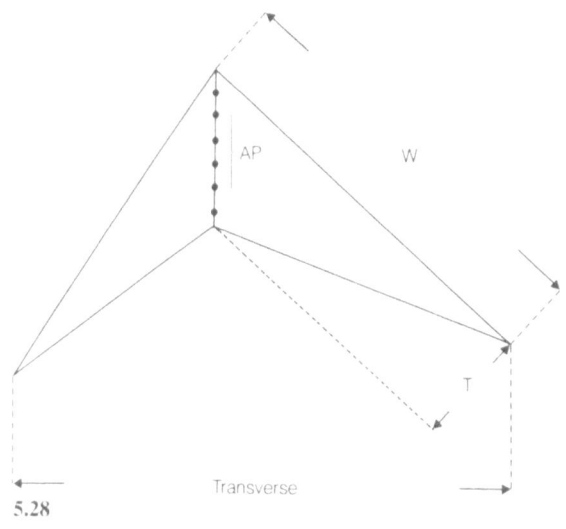

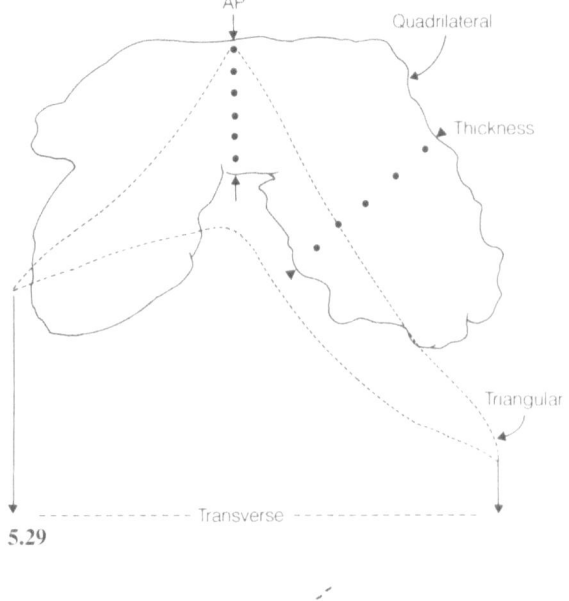

Fig. 5.28. Measurement of the thymus on CT scans after AMOUR et al. (1987). Six measurements were obtained for each thymus: the anteroposterior (*AP*) dimension, the transverse dimension, and the width (*W*) and thickness (*T*) for each lobe. The thickness is defined as the largest dimension perpendicular to the long axis of the lobe

Fig. 5.29. Measuring of the thymus on CT scans after AMOUR et al. (1987). The triangular *(dotted line)* and quadrilateral *(solid line)* glands are illustrated. With increasing age there is a gradual evolution in shape from the immature quadrilateral thymus with an isthmus of tissue connecting the two lobes to the triangular or arrowhead configuration

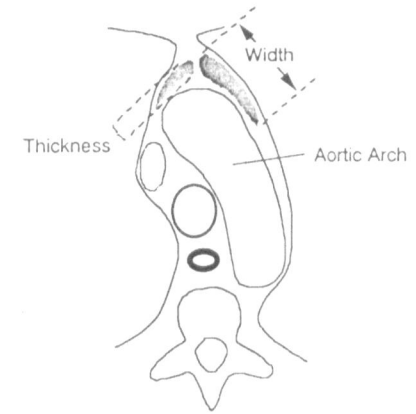

Fig. 5.30. Measurement of thymic dimensions on MRI

5.6.3 Magnetic Resonance Imaging

W. R. WEBB and G. DE GEER

The method of measuring thymic width and thickness by means of MRI is shown in Fig. 5.30. Generally speaking, the thymus appears thicker on MRI than it does on CT (DE GEER et al. 1986; BATRA et al. 1987; SIEGEL et al. 1989) (Table 5.5). This probably reflects two factors. First, lung volumes are lower on MR images made during quiet respiration than on CT performed at full inspiration. Thus, on MR images, the mediastinum characteristically appears wider than it does on CT.

Secondly, however, MRI also appears to better demonstrate true thymic size, particularly in adults (DE GEER et al. 1986; SIEGEL et al. 1989). On CT, in adult patients with thymic involution and fatty replacement, fat within the thymus cannot be clearly distinguished from surrounding mediastinal fat,

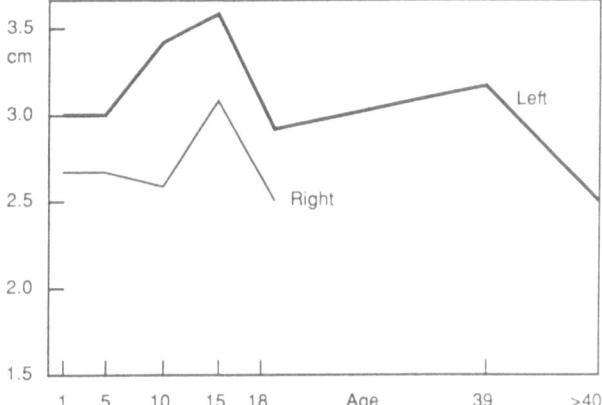

Fig. 5.31. Width of the thymic lobes measured using MRI in patients of different ages (from DE GEER et al. 1986; SIEGEL et al. 1989). These curves closely parallel plots of thymic weight versus age

Table 5.5. Thickness of left thymic lobe (cm) as measured using CT and MRI (modified from SIEGEL et al. 1989 and DE GEER et al. 1986)

Age (years)	CT	MRI
0–5	1.2	1.5
6–19	0.9	1.5
20–39	1.0	2.0
40–59	0.9	1.6
>59	0.9	2.0

and the thymus appears to be thinner and of decreased width, as compared to the thymus in children. In other words, on CT, only the residual glandular elements of the thymus are clearly seen, and the thymic thickness is underestimated. On MR in these patients, because of its better soft tissue contrast resolution, the entire thymus is usually visible, and it therefore appears thicker and wider. In one study of MRI of the thymus (DE GEER et al. 1986), thymus glands were similar in width and thickness, in patients of all ages. It is also of interest that a plot of the width of the left thymic lobe as seen on MRI closely approximates a plot of thymic weight versus age (Fig. 5.31).

It is of note that in children there is less difference between CT and MRI measurements than in adults.

References

Amann L (1962) Der Thymus beim Säugling und Kleinkind aus heutiger Sicht. Pädiatr Prax 1: 385

Amour TES, Siegel MJ, Glazer HS, Nadel SN (1987) CT appearance of the normal and abnormal thymus in childhood. J Comput Assist Tomogr 11: 645

Baron RL, Lee JKT, Sagel SS, Peterson RR (1982) Computed tomography of the normal thymus. Radiology 142: 121

Batra P, Hermann C Jr, Mulder D (1987) Mediastinal imaging in myasthenia gravis: correlation of chest radiography, CT, MR, and surgical findings. AJR 148: 515

Bode U, Scheidt W (1988) Change of thymic size during and following cytotoxic therapy in young patients. Pediatr Radiol 18: 20

de Geer G, Webb WR, Gamsu G (1986) Normal thymus: assessment with MR and CT. Radiology 158: 313

Dixon AK, Hilton CJ, Williams GT (1981) Computed tomography and histological correlation of the thymic remnant. Clin Radiol 32: 255

Ebel K-D (1980) Zur Röntgendiagnostik des Thymus im Kindesalter. Radiologe 20: 379

Francis IR, Glazer GM, Bookstein FL, Gross BH (1985) The thymus: reexamination of age-related changes in size and shape. AJR 145: 249

Gefferth K (1955) Thymus? Mediastinalpleuritis? Ein Beitrag zum diagnostischen Wert der interlobären Haarlinie. Fortschr Röntgenol 82: 462

Gewolb JH, Lebowitz RL, Taeusch HW (1979) Thymus size and its relationship to the respiratory distress syndrome. J Pediatr 95: 108

Goske Rudick M, Wood BP (1980) The use of ultrasound in the diagnosis of a large thymic cyst. Pediatr Radiol 10: 113

Haller JO, Schneider M, Kassner EG, Friedman AP, Waldroup LD (1980) Sonographic evaluation of the chest in infants and children. AJR 134: 1019

Heiberg E, Wolverson MK, Sundaram M, Nouri S (1982) Normal thymus: CT characteristics in subjects under age 20. AJR 138: 491

Helzel M (1985) Sonographische Topographie des oberen vorderen Mediastinums. Ultraschall Med 6: 101

Hoeffel JC, Fourchy E, Marchal AL, Pernot C (1984) Aspects radiologiques de l'hypotrophic thymique chez le nourrisson. Radiologie J CEPUR 4: 209

Kemp FH (1950) Factors influencing the mediastinal shadow in young children. Br J Radiol 23: 703

Kim Han B, Babcock DS, Oestreich AE (1989) Normal thymus in infancy: sonographic characteristics. Radiology 170: 471

Lack EE (1981) Thymic hyperplasia with massive enlargement. J Thorac Cardiovasc Surg 81: 741

Lanning R, Heikkinen E (1980) Thymus simulating left upper lobe atelectasis. Pediatr Radiol 9: 177

Lemaitre L, Marconi V, Avni F, Remy J (1987) The sonographic evaluation of normal thymus in infants and children. Eur J Radiol 7: 130

Mangelmann M (1981) Die Thymusreaktion im Neugeborenenalter. Klinisch-radiologische Untersuchung bei Frühgeborenen mit und ohne Steroidmedikation der Mütter. Thesis, Heidelberg

Miller JH (ed) (1985) Imaging in pediatric oncology. Williams and Wilkins, Baltimore, p 152

Moore AV, Korobkin M, Olanow W, Heaston DK, Ram PC, Dunnick NR, Silverman PM (1983) Age-related changes in the thymus gland: CT-pathologic correlation. AJR 141: 241

Moseley JE (1960) Loculated pneumomediastinum in the newborn, a thymic spinnaker sail sign. Radiology 75: 778

Mulvey RB (1963) The thymic wave sign. Radiology 81: 834

Oliva L (1973) Erkrankungen des Mediastinums. In: Schinz HR, Baensch WE, Frommhold W, Glauner R, Uehlinger E, Wellauer J (eds) Lehrbuch der Röntgendiagnostik, vol IV/2, 6. Pleura, Mediastinum und Lunge. Thieme, Stuttgart

Otlani T (1958) Thymusvergrößerung bei Kindern. Monatsschr Kinderheilkd 106: 143

Parker LA, Gaisie G, Scatliff JH (1985) Computerized tomography and ultrasonic findings in massive thymic hyperplasia. Clin Pediatr (Phila) 24: 90

Reither M (1984) Thoraxsonographie im Kindesalter. Röntgenpraxis 10: 375

Salonen OLM, Kivisaari ML, Somer JK (1984) Computed tomography of the thymus of children under 10 years. Pediatr Radiol 14: 373

Schnell VY (1975) Probleme der Thymusdiagnostik bei atypischer Lage und seltenen Begleitumständen. Thesis, Cologne

Siegel MJ, Glazer HS, Wiener JI, Molina PL (1989) Normal and abnormal thymus in childhood: MR imaging. Radiology 172: 367

Sone S, Higashihara T, Morimoto S et al. (1980) Normal anatomy of thymus and anterior mediastinum by pneumomediastinography. AJR 134: 81

Steinmann GG (1986) Changes in human thymus during aging. In: Müller-Hermenlink HK (ed) Current topics in pathology. The human thymus. Histophysiology and pathology. Springer, Berlin Heidelberg New York, p 43

Stern VN, Popow JA (1977) Der Einfluß des Thymus auf das Röntgenbild des Mediastinalschattens bei Kindern. Radiol Diagn (Berl) 18: 775

Swischuk LE (1980) Radiology of the newborn and young infant, 2nd edn. Williams and Wilkins, Baltimore, p 27

Tausend ME, Stern WZ (1965) Thymic pattern in the newborn. AJR 95: 125

von Lengerke HJ, Schmidt H (1988) Mediastinalsonographie im Kindesalter. Ergebnisse bei 310 Untersuchungen. Radiologe 28: 460

Walter E (1988) Erkrankungen und Tumoren des Thymus im Erwachsenenalter. In: Diethelm L, Heuck F, Olsson O, Strnad F, Vieten H, Zuppinger A (eds) Röntgendiagnostik der oberen Speise- und Atemwege und des Mediastinums. Springer, Berlin Heidelberg New York (Handbuch der medizinischen Radiologie, vol IX, 5c)

Weitzel D, Dinkel E, Dittrich M, Peters H (eds) (1984) Pädiatrische Ultraschalldiagnostik. Springer, Berlin Heidelberg New York, p 43

Wernecke K, Peters PR, Galanski M (1986) Mediastinal tumors: evaluation with suprasternal sonography. Radiology 159: 405

Willich E (1988) Bildgebende Diagnostik des Thymus vom Wachstums- bis ins Erwachsenenalter. In: Diethelm L, Heuck F, Olsson O, Strnad F, Vieten H, Zuppinger A (eds) Röntgendiagnostik der oberen Speise- und Atemwege und des Mediastinums. Springer, Berlin Heidelberg New York (Handbuch der medizinischen Radiologie, vol IX, 5c)

Zsebök Z (1958) Röntgenanatomie der Neugeborenen- und Säuglingslunge. Thieme, Stuttgart, p 118

6 Acute and Stress-Induced Involution of the Thymus

E. WILLICH

Age-related, physiologic involution of the thymus, which commences in puberty, stands in juxtaposition to acute, stress-related involution, which is of diagnostic and therapeutic significance especially during childhood and adolescence. The latter represents an endogenous (e.g. illness-related) or exogenous (e.g. drug-related) very rapid acceleration of physiologic, age-related involution, and is brought about by endogenous steroid release. This release induces lysis of lymphocytes and blocks their mitosis, resulting in a rapid reduction in the weight and size of the thymus which can be seen radiologically only a few days after the onset of the stress situation (e.g., after the beginning of an illness). Just as stress situations lead to atrophy of the thymus, so their termination (e.g., in convalescence or after exogenous induction) allows renewed growth of the thymus in the form of so-called regenerative hyperplasia (rebound phenomenon) (see Sect. 7.4.6).

6.1 Acute Endogenous Involution of the Thymus

Endogenously induced diminution of the thymic shadow accompanies numerous illnesses but can also occur following natural stress situations, such as a normal birth. Therefore, the thymic shadow is often absent in premature infants, but also in newborns (Fig. 6.1), and appears only in the first few days or weeks of life. On the other hand some babies are born with a large or even huge thymic shadow (Fig. 5.2 a).

In debilitating illnesses, e. g., sepsis, tuberculosis, and bronchopneumonia, or after operations, during childhood the thymus usually temporarily becomes smaller or even disappears totally (HARRIS et al. 1980).

Congenital cyanotic heart diseases represent "a chronic anoxic stress situation" for the affected child. Additionally, the nutritional status and general condition of health are usually worsened in such children. Therefore, the atrophic thymus cannot be seen by radiographic means.

RIZK et al. (1972) were able to demonstrate this in 40 children with transposition of the great vessels, in whom 80 operations were performed (mostly Mustard operations). In 1988, HOEFFEL et al. reported the same finding in eight children among whom there were cases of Fallot's tetralogy, ventricular septum defect, and coarctation of the aorta combined with ventricular septum defect, as well as the aforementioned cardiac abnormality. The postoperative appearance of a thymic shadow (in some cases there was thymic hyperplasia) was accompanied by a clinical improvement in these young patients which prevented misdiagnoses such as tumor, hematoma, or abscess.

6.2 Exogenous Involution of the Thymus: the Steroid Test

Thymic atrophy can be caused by exogenous influences, e.g., by heat injuries (GELFAND et al. 1972) or administration of lysozyme, an enzyme with a bacteriolytic effect to be found in saliva, tears, and other body fluids (LEVY et al. 1971). Alternatively, the reduction in the size of the thymus is sometimes caused for diagnostic or therapeutic reasons.

Irradiation of the hyperplastic thymus in newborns and infants in order to reduce the size of the organ was standard therapy until the end of the 1950s. Surface doses of 3–3.6 Gy, and later 1.2–2.4 Gy, were applied (COCCHI 1959). Usually one to three exposures were sufficient to bring about a reduction in the size of the thymus within 2 weeks: such a reduction was achieved in 60% of the children. This irradiation was discontinued only after numerous reports of late sequelae among these children, in the form of an increased incidence of leukemia and malignant tumors, especially thyroid carcinoma.

Out of 1722 infants irradiated between 1926 and 1951 in the United States, seven developed leukemia and 15 malignant tumors 3–26 years after exposure (SIMPSON and HAMPELMAN 1957, cited by COCCHI 1959).

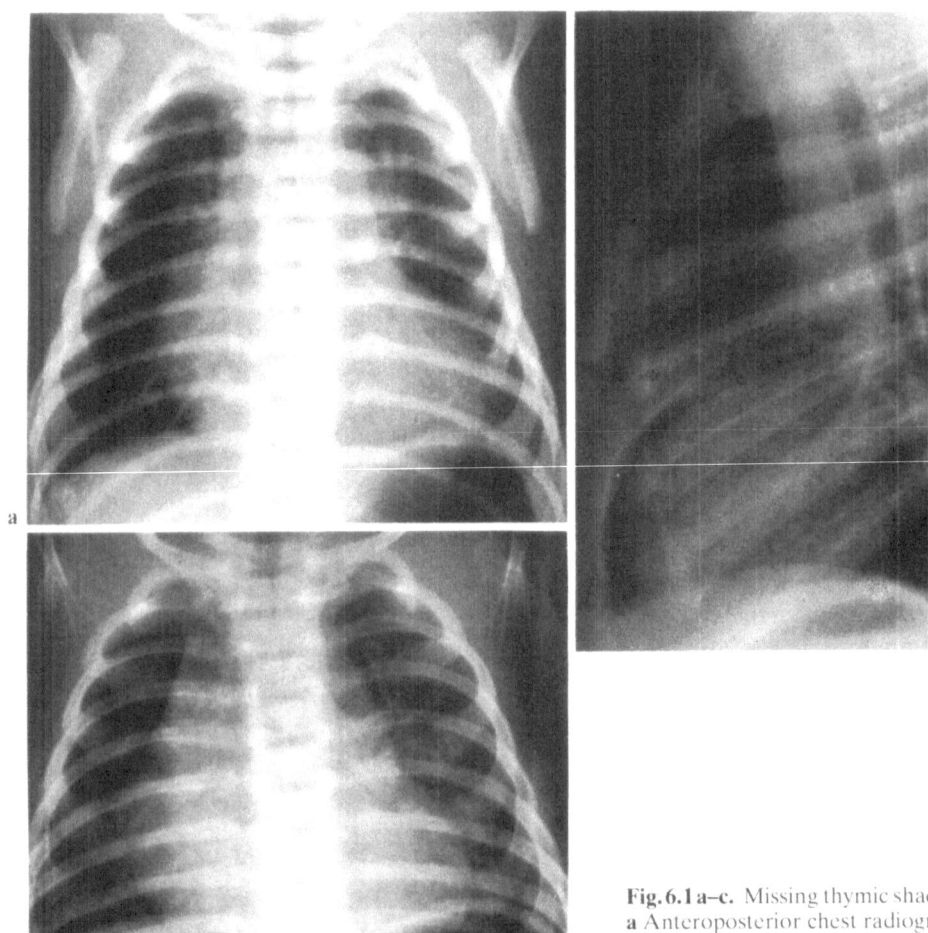

Fig. 6.1 a–c. Missing thymic shadow in a 5-day-old newborn. **a** Anteroposterior chest radiograph. **b** After 2 months presentation of a sail-like thymus. **c** Lateral view: thymus lying ventrally

Knowledge of the reason for endogenous thymic atrophy, namely the increased steroid production, led to use of the *steroid test.*

As early as 1959/60 CAFFEY and co-workers recognized the value of steroid medication in cases of dystopic or questionable thymus, a finding reiterated by GRIFFITH et al. (1961) shortly thereafter.

In these cases, 1 mg/kg ACTH or cortisone was given for 5 days and the condition of the thymus was controlled radiologically 3 or 4 days later. A large thymus was found to have diminished or disappeared totally in 80%–90% of cases, subsequently reaching or even exceeding its earlier size after approximately 2 weeks (artificial regenerative hyperplasia, see Sect. 7.4.6).

It was recognized, however, that not every thymus responds to steroids (a so-called steroid-refractory thymus exists in 5%–10% of cases according to CAFFEY and SILBEY 1960), and also that the test is not specific because lymphoid tissue can react similarly. Consequently thymic hyperplasia was frequently mistaken for non-Hodgkin's lymphoma, and vice versa, because in both cases ACTH treatment and cytostatics lead to a reduction in the solid mass (SCHNELL 1975; HASZE 1968).

The opponents of the steroid test, especially pediatric oncologists and pediatric surgeons (RINKE and OSCHATZ 1973; WILLNOW and TISCHER 1973; HASZE 1968), argue against it not only because of its unreliability but also because it delays any necessary tumor operation by at least 7 days (in the published case of HASZE the delay lasted 3 years, by which time the tumor was inoperable).

Nevertheless numerous authors are still in favor of the test under strict indications, especially if an operation can be avoided thereby. An analysis of the cases listed in tables 7.2–7.4 (see Sect. 7.4) shows that the results of the steroid test were positive in 19 and negative in 12.

When there is difficulty in differentiating congenital heart disease from thymic hyperplasia, invasive cardiac investigations can be avoided by applying the test (Fig. 5.2 b; see Sect. 7.4.7). Verification of the rare cases of stridor caused by a large thymus in infants can be achieved by the test, too (KEUTH 1978; see Sect. 7.4.8).

Even the suspicion of an ectopic thymus, for example in the posterior mediastinum, justifies use of the test (Fig. 7.4; SHACKELFORD and MCALISTER 1974). The objection regarding false-positive results, as in cases of malignant lymphoma, is to some extent countered by pointing out that such tumors rarely appear in the first year of life and are usually not localized in the posterior mediastinum (see Sect. 7.2.3).

On the other hand negative test results (absence of thymic atrophy) do not exclude pathologic processes of any kind, as BAUDAIN et al. thought in 1980.

In children undergoing tumor treatment (e. g., Wilms' tumors, rhabdomyosarcoma, acute lymphatic leukemia, osteosarcoma, and malignant lymphoma; see Sect. 7.4, table 7.4), mediastinal enlargement can result from 6 months until 5 years after the onset of treatment, during or following chemotherapy. Diagnosis of thymic enlargement can then be difficult, even if there are no other clinical or radiologic pathologic symptoms. In cases of doubt, the steroid test can be helpful and sometimes a surgical procedure can be avoided (COHEN et al. 1980; FORD et al. 1987).

COHEN suggests that, after leukemia and lymphoma are excluded, prednisolone 60 mg/m² be given daily for 7 days. On the 7th day chest x-ray is performed in order to assess the thymic reaction. If no such reaction has occurred, the medication is given for another 7 days and the situation is then again controlled by chest x-ray.

Positive experiences with the steroid test have also been reported by AMANN (1962), GUBBAWY and HOFMANN (1974), POELL et al. (1979), BAR-ZIV et al. (1984), DANILEWICZ-WYTRYCHOWSKA (1981), and HALLER et al. (1980), and by KOBAYASHI et al. in one of three cases (1986).

In cases of compression of the airways by a hyperplastic thymus, steroids should not be used as long-term therapy because of their short-term thymolytic effects.

With the use of ultrasound and computed tomography the steroid test has become less important.

The effects of *chemotherapeutic drugs* (cytostatics) on the thymus are similar to those of steroids.

Atrophy was recognized in larger patient groups aged 2–35 years by means of computed tomography (BODE and SCHEIDT 1988; CHOYKE et al. 1987). These were patients with malignant tumors or systemic diseases in whom the thymus decreased under therapy to as little as 43% of its original size, depending on the therapeutic cycle. A rebound of up to

>50% above the initial size was seen during therapy-free intervals. Such secondary hyperplasia takes place in about 25%–50% of the patients. The phenomenon can recur during subsequent therapeutic cycles, especially during relapses.

Similar effects of chemotherapeutic drugs have been recognized in cases of metastasizing non-seminomatous testicular carcinoma (HENDRICKX and DÖHRING 1989; ABILDGAARD et al. 1989) and in malignant metastasizing testicular tumors (KISSIN et al. 1987).

Again the follow-up was done by CT scans, with thymic measurements in 120 patients from 16 to 50 years old. Under treatment thymic atrophy was not seen; the subsequent rebound enlargement culminated 3–14 months after beginning of therapy in 14 (11.6%) patients (KISSIN et al. 1987). The subsequent involution phase lasted approximately 2 years. Metastasis-free patients who did not receive chemotherapy did not display any change in thymic size.

These investigations aim to show the incidence of thymic enlargement after chemotherapy, thereby helping to avoid misdiagnoses such as mediastinal lymphadenopathies and unnecessary "explorative" thoracotomies.

6.3 Transplacental Influence of Steroids on the Premature Infant's Thymus

Nowadays, gravidas are treated with steroids in the 30th–36th week of pregnancy in many gynecological hospitals in order to accelerate the fetus's pulmonary maturity and thus avoid postnatal respiratory distress syndrome in the premature infant. Because the thymus reacts very sensitively to steroids, it can be used as an indicator of the drugs' efficacy and can also be analyzed radiologically. This thymic reaction was verified and the thymic size measured in our own investigative series. The value of steroids in avoiding respiratory distress syndrome was investigated simultaneously.

Under standard conditions 103 premature infants from six gynecological hospitals were screened with a chest x-ray on the 1st day of life. The x-rays were analyzed and measured according to Gewolb's method, whereby a quotient is derived from the width of the thymus and the transverse diameter of the thorax. The thymus was measured at the level of the carina, and the thorax at the level of the costodiaphragmatic angle (Fig. 5.25). Group I comprised 52 premature infants, whose mothers had received steroids between the 30th and 36th week of pregnancy. Group II, consisting of 51 premature infants whose

Table 6.1. Results of thymic measurement in 103 premature infants (quotient: thymic width/transverse diameter of the chest; mean quotient = 0.34) (MANGELMANN 1981)

| RDS | No. | Quotient | Steroids | | | | | |
| | | | With | | | Without | | |
			No.	Quotient	SD ±	No.	Quotient	SD ±
With	38	0.35	17	0.35	0.09	21	0.34	0.15
Without	65	0.33	35	0.32	0.12	30	0.34	0.09
Total	103		52	0.33	0.13	51	0.34	0.16

RDS, respiratory distress syndrome

mothers had not received steroid therapy, served as the control group. Additionally all stress factors in both the mother and child (approximately 15 in each case) which might influence the thymic size had to be documented. Statistical analyses were performed quantitatively using the Wilcoxon-Frank sum test and the Krushal-Wallis test, and qualitatively using the Irwin-Snedecor test and the Fisher test. Statistically only the respiratory distress syndrome was recognized as a uniform stress factor in premature infants.

Table 6.1 shows the results (MANGELMANN 1981). No statistically significant differences in the thymic size were found between the two groups. No relation was found between the thymic size and either prenatal steroid treatment of the mother or the occurrence of respiratory distress syndrome. Furthermore no relation was found between the thymic size and gestational age or between the frequency of respiratory distress syndrome and any specific gestational age, not taking into account steroid medication. The thymic size did not depend on the time of the mother's last steroid intake or on the steroid dosage.

However, respiratory distress syndrome was observed to be less frequent in premature infants born in the 30th–31st week of pregnancy to mothers who had received prenatal steroid medication, as compared with similar infants born to untreated mothers (Fig. 6.2).

The average thymic quotient of 0.34 was almost identical to that reported by GEWOLB et al. (0.35).

The influence of numerous further maternal and infant stress factors, whose effect on the thymus cannot be differentiated from those of steroids, may explain the above results. Irrespective of this, the favorable effect of prenatal steroid medication on the frequency of respiratory distress syndrome in the premature infant has been proven and fetal steroid insufficiency represents one of the pathogenetic factors in respiratory distress syndrome. Therefore, a postnatally large thymus in the premature infant can serve as a radiologic indication for the early diagnosis of respiratory distress syndrome (FLETCHER et al. 1979).

References

Abildgaard A, Lien HH, Fossa SD, Høie J, Langholm R (1989) Enlargement of the thymus following chemotherapy for non-seminomatous testicular cancer. Acta Radiol 30: 259–262

Amann L (1962) Der Thymus beim Säugling und Kleinkind aus heutiger Sicht. Pädiatr Prax 1: 385–392

Bar-Ziv J, Barki Y, Itzschak Y, Mares AJ (1984) Posterior mediastinal accessory thymus. Pediatr Radiol 14: 165–167

Baudain P, Terraube P, Crouzet A (1980) Une tumeur peu banale du médiastin postérieur chez l'enfant. Arch Fr Pédiatr 37: 609–611

Bode U, Scheidt W (1988) Change of thymic size during and following cytotoxic therapy in young patients. Pediatr Radiol 18: 20–23

Caffey J, Di Liberti (1959) Acute atrophy of thymus induced adrenocorticosteroids observed roentgenologically. AJR 82: 530–540

Caffey J, Silbey R (1960) Regrowth and overgrowth of the thymus after atrophy induced by the oral administration of adrenocorticosteroids to human infants. Pediatrics 26: 762–770

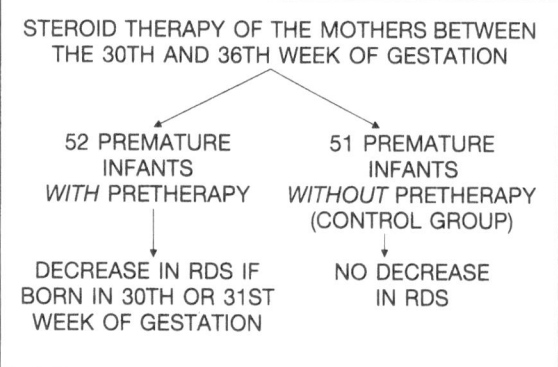

STEROID THERAPY OF THE MOTHERS BETWEEN THE 30TH AND 36TH WEEK OF GESTATION

52 PREMATURE INFANTS *WITH* PRETHERAPY

51 PREMATURE INFANTS *WITHOUT* PRETHERAPY (CONTROL GROUP)

DECREASE IN RDS IF BORN IN 30TH OR 31ST WEEK OF GESTATION

NO DECREASE IN RDS

Fig. 6.2. Reaction of the thymus in 103 premature infants. *RDS*, respiratory distress syndrome

Choyke PL, Zeman RK, Gootenberg JE, Greenberg JN, Hoffer F, Frank JA (1987) Thymic atrophy and regrowth in response to chemotherapy: CT evaluation. AJR 149: 269–272

Cocchi U (1959) Röntgendiagnostik und Strahlentherapie des Thymus. Strahlentherapie (Sonderbd) 109: 426–440

Cohen M, Hill CA, Cangir A, Sullivan MP (1980) Thymic rebound after treatment of childhood tumors. AJR 135: 151–156

Danilewicz-Wytrychowska T (1981) Zur Röntgendiagnostik und Differentialdiagnose der Thymuserkrankungen im Kindesalter. Radiologe 21: 542–546

Fletcher BD, Masson M, Lisbona A, Riggs T, Papageorgiou AN (1979) Thymic response to endogenous and exogenous steroids in premature newborn infants. J Pediatr 95: 111–114

Ford EG, Lockhardt SK, Sullivan MP, Andrassy RJ (1987) Mediastinal mass following chemotherapeutic treatment of Hodgkin's disease: recurrent tumor or thymic hyperplasia? J Pediatr Surg 22: 1155–1159

Gelfand DM, Goldman AS, Law EJ (1972) Thymic hyperplasia in children recovering from thermal burns. J Trauma 12: 813–817

Gewolb JH, Lebowitz RL, Taeusch HW (1979) Thymus size and its relationship to the respiratory distress syndrome. J Pediatr 95: 108–111

Griffith SP, Levine QR, Kaber DH, Blumenthal S (1961) Evaluation of enlarged cardiothymic image in infancy: thymolytic effect of steroid administration. Am J Cardiol 8: 311–318

Gubbawy H, Hofmann A (1974) Der Thymus im Säuglings- und Kindesalter. Prax Pneumol 28: 615–628

Haller JO, Schneider M, Kassner EG, Friedman AP, Waldroup LD (1980) Sonographic evaluation of the chest in infants and children. AJR 134: 1019–1027

Harris VJ, Ramilo J, White H (1980) The thymic mass as a mediastinal dilemma. Clin Radiol 31: 263–269

Hasze W (1968) Die Geschwülste des Mediastinum im Kindesalter. Langenbecks Arch Chir 322: 1236–1243

Hendrickx P, Döhring W (1989) Thymic atrophy and rebound enlargement following chemotherapy for testicular cancer. Acta Radiol 30: 263–268

Hoeffel JC, Pernot C, Worms AM, Bretagne MC, Bernard C (1988) L'hypertrophie thymique post-opératoire dans les cardiopathies congénitales graves. Ann Pédiatr (Paris) 35: 440–444

Keuth U (1974) Thymushyperplasie. Pädiatr Prax 14: 447–448

Kissin CM, Husband JE, Nicholas E, Eversman W (1987) Benign thymic enlargement in adults after chemotherapy: CT demonstration. Radiology 163: 67–70

Kobayashi T, Hirabayashi Y, Kobayashi Y (1986) Diagnostic value of plain chest roentgenogram and CT-findings in four cases of massive thymic hyperplasia. Pediatr Radiol 16: 452–455

Lévy JM, Stoll C, Francfort JJ (1971) L'hypertrophie thymique du nourrisson: effect du lysozyme. Ann Pédiatr (Paris) 18: 138–145

Mangelmann M (1981) Die Thymusreaktion im Neugeborenenalter. Klinisch-radiologische Untersuchung bei Frühgeborenen mit und ohne Steroidmedikation der Mutter. Thesis, Heidelberg

Poell J, Stanisic M, Morger R (1979) Beitrag zum akzessorischen Thymus. Z Kinderchir 26: 62–66

Rinke W, Oschatz R (1973) Neurogene Mediastinaltumoren im Kindesalter. Zentralbl Chir 98: 590–598

Rizk Gh, Cueto L, Amplatz K (1972) Rebound enlargement of the thymus after successful corrective surgery for transposition of the great vessels. AJR 116: 528–530

Schnell VY (1975) Probleme der Thymusdiagnostik bei atypischer Lage und seltenen Begleitumständen. Thesis, Cologne

Shackelford GD, McAlister WH (1974) The aberrantly positioned thymus. A cause of mediastinal or neck masses in children. AJR 120: 291–296

Willnow U, Tischer W (1973) Thymusgeschwülste im Kindesalter. Zentralbl Chir 98: 581–589

7 Developmental Abnormalities of the Thymus

E. WILLICH, E. WALTER, H. F. OTTO, and W. J. HOFMANN

7.1 Aplasia, Hypoplasia, and Dysplasia

E. WILLICH and E. WALTER

Absence or hypoplasia of the thymus is usually caused by immunodeficiency diseases or syndromes (Table 7.1).

In all cases a lateral chest x-ray or a CT scan is necessary to determine absence or dysplasia (thinness) of the thymus.

Clinically it is of great importance that malignant tumors of the hematopoietic system, especially malignant lymphoma, occur 100 times more frequently in children with primary immunodeficiency than in those with a healthy immune system. In addition to the usual immunodeficiency diseases, Wiskott-Aldrich syndrome and Louis-Bar syndrome can be responsible for such tumors.

Since 1959, 231 cases of DiGeorge syndrome (involving congenital absence or hypoplasia of the thymus associated with hypoparathyroidism, heart defects, and vessel anomalies) have been reported (BELOHRADSKY 1985).

7.2 Dystopia

Thymic ectopia is very rare; cases have been reported by FINCH and GOUGH (1972), TOVI and MARES (1978), EBEL (1980), COHEN et al. (1983), BAR-ZIV et al. (1984), and GOEBEL (1985), among others.

The ectopia is caused by interrupted migration of the thymus from the right and left pharyngeal pouch into the anterior superior mediastinum. Furthermore, tissue can split off from the caudally

Table 7.1. Immunodeficiency diseases with thymic alterations (after DAY and GEDGAUDAS 1984)

Syndrome	Thymus	Humoral immunity	Cellular immunity	Immuno-globulins	Lympho-cytes	Heredity	Additional findings
DiGeorge syndrome	Absent	Normal	Deficient	Normal	Normal/ low	–	Absence of parathyroid; anomalies of heart and great vessels
Nezelof syndrome (congenital thymic dysplasia)	Hypo-plasia	Normal or slightly deficient	Deficient	Normal or slightly deficient	Reduced	Autosomal recessive	–
Reticular dysgenesis	Hypo-plasia	Deficient	Deficient	Deficient	Reduced	–	Leukopenia
Agammaglobulin-emia (Swiss type)	Hypo-plasia	Severely deficient	Absent or deficient	Deficient	Markedly reduced	Autosomal recessive	Dyschondroplasia, ulcerative colitis
Thymic alymphoplasia	Hypo-plasia	Deficient	Absent or deficient	Deficient	Reduced	Sex-linked recessive, only male	–
Louis-Bar syn-drome (ataxia telangiectasia)	Hypo-plasia	Slightly deficient	Deficient	Normal or slight IgA deficiency	Variable	Autosomal recessive	Cerebellar ataxia, telangi-ectasia, lymphoma, dys-chondroplasia, endocrine anomalies, neutropenia
Agammaglobu-linemia with thymoma	Spindle cell tumor	Deficient	Deficient	Deficient	Reduced	–	–

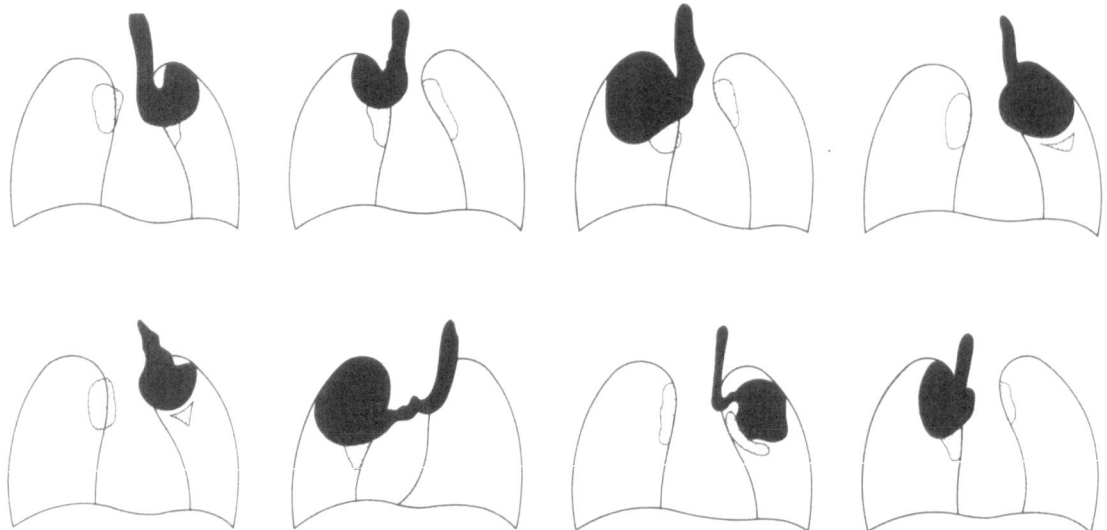

Fig. 7.1. Forms of ectopic accessory thymic lobes (schematic drawing after KABELKA et al. 1977). Punctated areas, orthotopic thymus; *black areas,* accessory lobes

Fig. 7.2 a, b. Sonographic identification of a cervical thymus (5-month-old infant). Clinically there was bulging in the jugular fossa, which was intensified by crying and pressing. **a** Longitudinal scan above the jugular fossa. A part of the thymus reaches into the cervical soft tissue. The other part is normally located in the anterior superior mediastinum. **b** Schematic drawing. (Courtesy of Dr. W. Uhlig, University Children's Hospital of Tübingen, FRG)

moving organ; sometimes, however, this is accessory thymic tissue that has originated from the fourth visceral cleft (OTTO 1984). Therefore, in most of the studied cases a double-lobed thymus exists in the normal location in addition to the ectopic thymus (Fig. 7.1; SAADE et at. 1976; EBEL 1980).

Ectopic thymic tissue usually does not cause any clinical symptoms. If there are any such symptoms, they are usually determined by the location of the ectopic tissue and therefore vary enormously.

In 20% of pathoanatomically investigated patients, aberrant thymic islands are also found (GIL-MOUR 1941). However, because of their microscopic growth these islands cannot be equated with

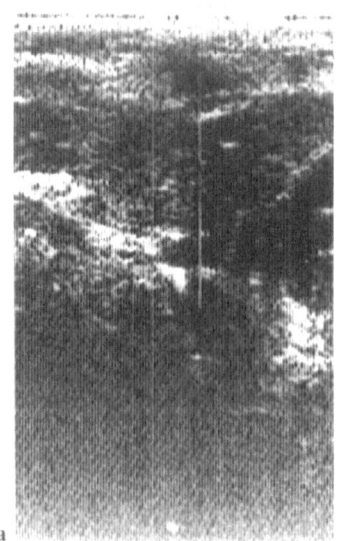

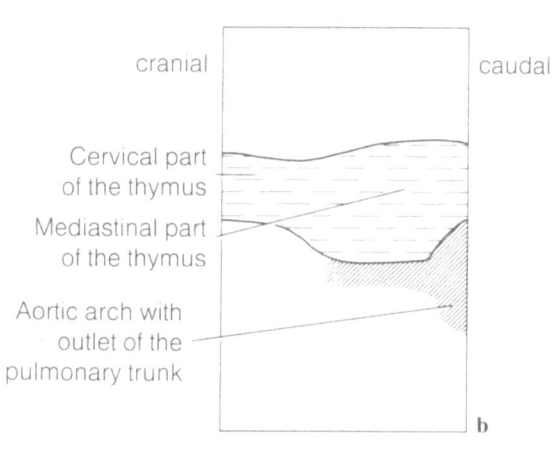

cranial   caudal

Cervical part
of the thymus

Mediastinal part
of the thymus

Aortic arch with
outlet of the
pulmonary trunk

ectopic thymus glands. Usually they are found accidentally during surgery and are only important in patients with myasthenia gravis (because of the question of thymectomy).

7.2.1 Cervical and Superior Mediastinum

Embryologically the cervical thymus results from a failure of descent from the mandibular angle into the anterior mediastinum and therefore entails the persistence of a thymopharyngeal duct.

In cases cervical thymus, too, there is either a gland accessory to the normaly situated thymus or a real ectopic thymus on the anterolateral neck side in the absence of a normally situated thymus. The former presentation is also called cervico-mediastinal or "pseudocervical" thymus: The normal thymus is lengthened cranially and reaches the anterolateral neck in the superior mediastinum. The thymus will become visible and palpable when there is increased intrathoracic pressure, e.g., during severe screaming by infants and small children and during Valsalva's maneuver (KABELKA and HORAK 1976; HURLEY 1977). Further reports on solid thymic tissue in the lateral cervical triangle in infants and small children have been provided by THORRENS et al. (1969), FINCH and GOUGH (1972), and DOMARUS and von BLAHA (1987, including a literature review).

The most important literature review of cases of cervical thymus is that by TOVI and MARES (1978), who reported on 68 cases. Thirty of these had histologically proven normal thymic tissue. SPIGLAND et al. (1990) have reported three more cases and supplied a literature review.

The cervical thymus usually does not show *clinical symptomes*. When there is bulging on the anterior neck in children, differential diagnosis involves many possibilities: branchial cysts, thyroglossal cysts, cervical fistulas, dermoid cysts, cartilaginous deposits, parotid cysts, lymphangiomas, lymphadenomas, cystic hygromas, hemangiomas, and, rarely, lymph node metastases.

In the past operative treatment was the only means of reliable diagnosis. Now, *ultrasonography* can narrow or even secure the diagnosis (GRUMBACH et al. 1985) (Fig. 7.2). Solid thymic tissue is displayed as a homogenous hypoechoic structure outside the thyroid gland. Although the echo texture alone is insufficient evidence for a diagnosis of cervical thymus, the diagnosis can be made on the basis of cranial displacement of thymic tissue on real-time imaging during screaming or pressing

and ultrasonographic proof of a connection of the cervical portion with the mediastinal orthotopic thymus (UHLILG, personal communication, 1986; RYPENS et al. 1989). Cystic tissue, e.g., in thymic cysts, can be differentiated easily.

Today, *computed tomography* (CT) allows reduction of the number of differential diagnostic possibilities. The ectopic thymus can be differentiated from cystic processes. Pathognomonic CT findings, however, are not known; uncharacteristic absorption values can only lead to suspicion of the diagnosis.

Often the cervical thymus is situated in a close topographic relationship to the thyroid gland (GILMOUR 1941; BATSAKIS 1974). Thymic islands have even been found inside the thyroid and parathyroid, as reported by TESSERAUX (1953) in his extensive literature review. TOVI and MARES (1978) described a case in which parathyroid-located thymic tissue was accidentally removed during a nodular goiter operation.

Cystic degeneration is supposed to occur more often in cervical thymus glands than in normally located glands (ROSAI and LEVINE 1976). This theory is supported, for example, by the 40 thymic cysts found among 43 cervical tumors in the review of BARRICK and O'KELL (1969). Other authors, however, do not agree (see Sect. 9.1).

Although the cervical thymus is usually found by accident, it sometimes narrows the trachea and esophagus, leading to clinical compression symptoms: POELL et al. (1979) described a submandibular swelling in 2-month-old female which caused inspiratory stridor and was operated on under the tentative diagnosis of a lymphangioma or parotid cyst. The mandarin-sized tumor was revealed histologically to be the cervical portion of a normal intrathoracic thymus. In 1985, BISTRITZER et al. reported the case of a 5-month-old boy who suffered from a cervical thymus with severe respiratory insufficiency and dysphagia. The cervical thymus weighed 75 g and 4 days after the operation all symptoms had disappeared. Stridor and chronically recurrent infections of the upper respiratory tract were also found in one of two cases described by RYPENS et al. (1989).

Radiologically tracheal displacement may be observed without pathologic findings being present on the esophagogram (MICHELSON and SENDER 1956). With a retrotracheal position of the thymus a tracheal impression may be found (SHACKELFORD and MC ALISTER 1974; MARTIN 1975; KABELKA and HORAK 1976; KABELKA et al. 1977). According to BARON et al. (1982) an ectopic cervical thymus can

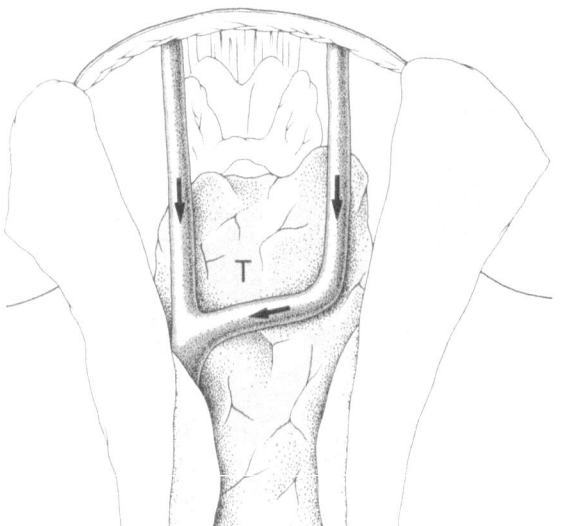

Fig. 7.3. Retrovenous thymus. The hypertrophic thymus is situated in the middle mediastinum behind the great veins. *T*, thymus; *arrows*, internal jugular vein, brachiocephalic vein, superior vena cava. (After Lucien et al. In: Testut-La-target 1966)

only be suspected on the basis of CT because it does not show any characteristic signs in comparison to the other anatomic structures in the neck.

Like Ebel (1980), Tovi and Mares (1978) and Goebel (1985) described cases with persistence of the thymus in the upper thoracic aperture near the jugulum. Because of the narrow topographic relations of the thymus to the esophagus and trachea, clinical symptoms of dysphagia and dyspnea were very striking in a 16-year-old girl described by Goebel (1985) and also in patients described by Tovi and Mares (1978). Conventional tomography of the trachea, tracheobronchography, or esophagography can show pathologic impression signs in such cases. On CT scans the thymus appears as a structure of soft tissue density with uncharacteristic absorption values between 40 and 50 H (Goebel 1985), as also are observed in the orthotopic thymus. For definite histologic proof of the mass, fine needle biopsy or even an operation is nevertheless necessary (Goebel 1985).

By reference to six patients between 4 and 14 years old, Cory et al. (1987) highlighted possible confusion between the thymus situated in the superior mediastinum and adenopathies. All six patients suffered from malignant disease. The suspicious "nodes" were situated above the left brachiocephalic vein. These mediastinal eminences could be identified as the thymus by CT scans and in one instance by biopsy.

It must be noted that the cervical thymus can develop into a tumorous mass: thymomas, thymic teratomas, and thymic lipomas may occur. In their review of the literature, Barrick and O'Kell (1969) found only three cases of solid, undescended thymic tissue among 43 cervical thymic tumors.

Finally, with regard to therapy Rypens et al. (1989), unlike most other authors, are of the opinion that the cervical thymus regresses by physiologic involution synchronously with the accompanying orthotopic thymus, thereby rendering surgery or any other form of therapy unnecessary.

7.2.2 Middle Mediastinum

A dystopic thymus in the middle mediastinum was first described in the radiologic literature by No-back in 1926, and later by Castellanos et al. (1971), Schnell (1975), and others.

In such cases the thymus is situated between the ascending aorta or the aortic arch and the upper vena cava or between the great vessels and the trachea but behind the left anonymeous vein. Therefore, Lucien (1966) distinguishes this "retrovenous thymus" from the so-called prevenous thymus (Fig. 7.3).

Retrovenous thymus occurs very seldom and will only be detected if it causes symptoms, as, for example, in the case of the 4-month-old infant described by Shackelford and Mc Alister in 1974. Because of compression and displacement of one main bronchus, it was not diagnosed radiologically to be thymic tissue; rather the diagnosis was made through extirpation. In another case reported by the same authors, the thymus was situated laterally to the upper vena cava; it displaces the trachea ventrally and the esophagus to the left.

7.2.3 Posterior Mediastinum

Normal thymic tissue can extend into the posterior mediastinum. However, the thymus is seldom missing from its normal position. More often there is an ectopic, accessory thymus that may be either connected to the orthotopic gland by a parenchymatous bridge (Bar-Ziv et al. 1984; Saade et al. 1976; Cohen et al. 1983; Koecher 1959; Ebel 1980; Faure 1978) or totally divided from it. A connection between the ectopic thymus and the orthotopic gland is observed six times more often than a disconnected ectopic thymus (Ebel 1980).

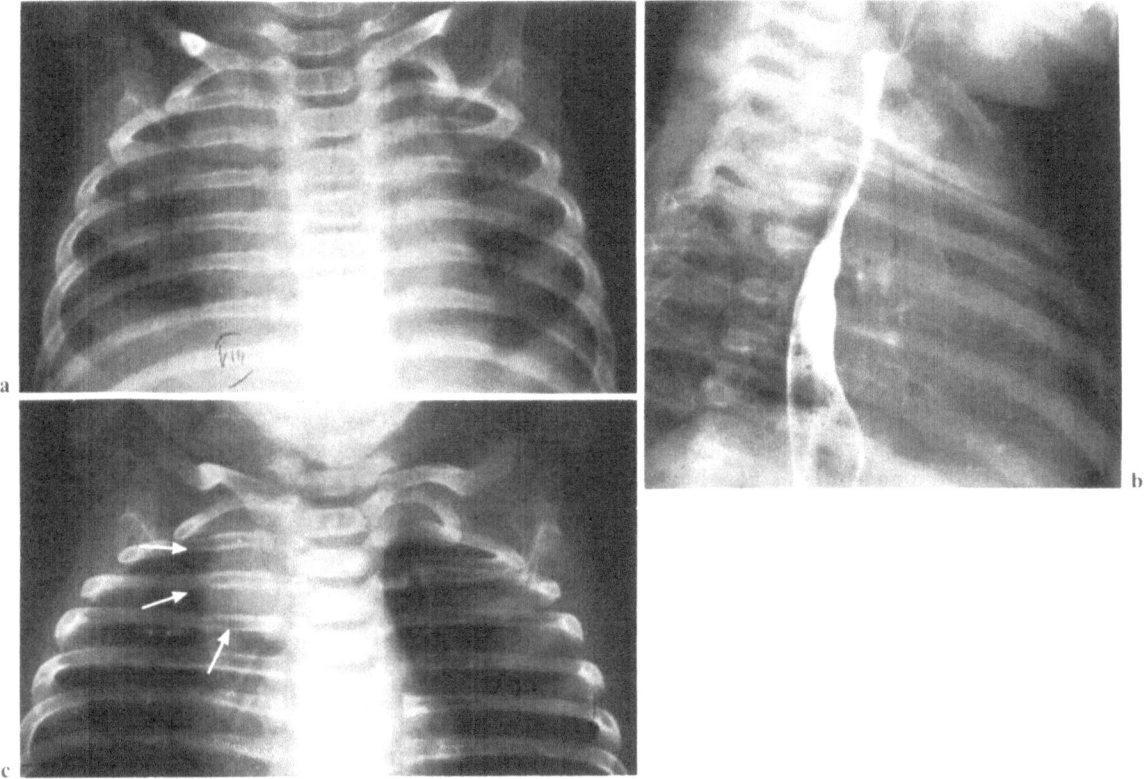

Fig. 7.4 a–c. Accessory thymus in the posterior mediastinum ($3^1/_2$-month-old infant without clinical symptoms). **a** Large thymic shadow, symmetrically adjacent to the cardiac shadow. Within the right lobe there is a rounded shadow of higher density. **b** Spot film with esophagography; lateral view. There is displacement of the esophagus ventrally by an oval mass in the posterior mediastinum with a sharp border caudally. **c** Steroid test; control radiograph 7 days later. The normally situated part of the thymus is clearly diminished and is overlapped by the mass in the posterior mediastinum, the size of which has remained unchanged *(arrows)*. Operation because of suspicion of tumor: spherical thymic tissue with a tissue bridge to the orthotopic thymus. Histology: normal thymic tissue. (Courtesy of Prof. Dr. EBEL, Department of Radiology, Children's Hospital, Cologne-Riehl, FRG)

Clinically such normal variations usually do not cause any symptoms. Thus the ectopic thymus will typically be discovered accidentally on chest x-rays (COWART 1980; EBEL 1980; SAADE et al. 1976). Nevertheless, posteriorly situated thymus glands have also been described that have caused unspecific symptoms such as stridor (BAR-ZIV et al. 1984), chronic coughing or dyspnea (COHEN et al. 1983), and compression effects on the neighboring trachea and lung parts (see also Sect. 7.4.3.2).

Whereas conventional radiologic methodes usually fail when there is ectopic thymus place-ment in the neck region (EBEL 1980), if the thymus is situated in the posterior mediastinum chest x-rays in two planes show a sharply outlined, smooth "tumor," paravertebrally situated and without signs of calcification (KOECHER 1959; SAADE et al. 1976; EBEL 1980; COHEN et al. 1983).

On sagittal chest x-rays, two overlapping tumorous opacities may be seen; during barium swallow the esophagus is displaced ventrally (Fig. 7.4.). A substernal thymus can best be discovered on lateral radiographs.

Differential diagnosis includes esophageal cysts, mediastinal abscesses, intrathoracic meningoceles, bronchoesophageal cysts, lymphomas and aneurysms of the thoracic aorta, thoracic duct cysts, spinal masses, mesenchymal tumors, and especially neuroblastomas, which develop in the same age group, namely during early childhood. *Ultrasound diagnosis* nowadays plays an important role in differential diagnosis (CLAUS and COPPENS 1984; BAR-ZIV et al. 1984). Good results have also been obtained with *computed tomography* (PARKER et al. 1985). COHEN et al. (1983) described the ectopic thymus as a smoothly contoured tumor of soft tissue density without calcifications erosion of the neighboring bony structures. Cystic processes such as bronchogenic cysts, but also abscesses, can be differentiated on the basis of their absorption values with normal CT. Differentiation of aneurysms on CT requires the use of water-soluble contrast media.

Although the use of CT has rendered the diagnosis more reliable, all the cases reported in recent years nevertheless underwent thoracotomy, in part because of severe symptoms (BAR-ZIV et al. 1984; MALONE and FITZGERALD 1987) and in part because a malignant tumor could not be definitely excluded.

Magnetic resonance imaging (MRI) seems to make possible reliable diagnosis of ectopic thymus in the posterior mediastinum. MRI can be valuable in diagnosing ectopic thymus in children who are thought to have a mediastinal mass because of a plain radiographic abnormality. In one recent case (ROLLINS and CURRARINO 1988), extension of the right lobe of the thymus into the middle and posterior mediastinum was detected using MRI. Furthermore, in a recent study (SIEGEL et al. 1989) of 47 children who underwent MRI for the diagnosis of congenital heart disease, thymus was seen extending into the posterior mediastinum in four. This posterior extension is typically continuous with the normally positioned thymus in the anterior mediastinum, allowing it to be correctly diagnosed, and has an MRI signal intensity identical to that of the remainder of the thymus. The posterior extension of the right thymic lobe typically passes between the superior vena cava and the trachea.

In summary, the diagnosis of thymus in the posterior mediastinum has become more reliable by means of MRI because of:

1. The possibility of visualizing a connection between the orthotopic thymus and a solid mass situated in the posterior mediastinum
2. The identical signals from the anterior and posterior thymic parts
3. The typical homogeneous signal intensity of thymic tissue, which is higher than that of muscle tissue and less than that of fat tissue on T1- and to a moderate extent also on T2-weighted images
4. The characteristic dorsal extension of the thymus between the upper vena cava and the trachea

In the experience of JOHNSON et al. (1978), 67 gallium citrate *scintigraphy* can be used for tissue typing, although the mechanism of isotope concentration in the thymus is still unclear. EBEL (1980) and also ALT and HOCHMAN (1982) could not verify this

activity uptake in thymic hyperplasia; therefore nuclear tissue typing does not allow reliable conclusions.

The *steroid test* recommended by CAFFEY and DI LIBERTI (1959) can be tried, especially if this will enable an operation to be avoided through steroid reduction of the thymus, as in the case reported by BAUDAIN et al. (1980). Other authors point out, however, that thymus glands situated in the posterior mediastinum react less to steroids than does a normal thymus, or, indeed, do not react at all (SAADE et al. 1976; KABELKA et al. 1977; COHEN et al. 1983). EBEL (1980) observed one case in which the normally situated thymus reacted to steroids while the accessory posterior part did not (Fig. 7.4 c).

Finally it must be pointed out that hyperplastic thymus glands can extend from the anterior into the posterior mediastinum (Fig. 7.14).

7.2.4 Miscellaneous

The Annular thymus (thymus anularis) can wind itself around the upper vena cava; the vessel may thereby be congested and a chylothorax or chyloabdomen may even develop. Such a case was reported by JUZBASIC and PASINI (1965) in a small child.

In addition ectopic thymus glands can occur in the region of the tympanic cavity, together with severe malformations of the ears (HAGENS 1932) and the pharynx (EPSTEIN and LOEB 1955). Excessive caudal displacement of the thymus with pediculation is also known (TESSERAUX 1953). In "thymoptosis" the thymus reaches to the diaphragm.

An extremely rare ectopic *intratracheal thymus* has been described in two cases, a subglottic submucous mass being present in the trachea (FALK 1936; MARTIN and MC ALISTER 1987).

Combined malformations occur more often. The dystopia described by GOEBEL in 1985 was combined with a malformation of the petrosal bones.

References

Alt W, Hochman HI (1982) Thyrotoxicosis and myasthenia gravis. Clin Pediatr (Phila) 21: 749

Baron RL, Lee JKT, Sagel SS, Peterson RR (1982) Computed tomography of the normal thymus. Radiology 142: 121

Barrick B, O'Kell RT (1969) Thymic cysts and remnant cervical thymus. J Pediatr Surg 4: 355

Bar-Ziv J, Barki Y, Itzchak Y, Mares AJ (1984) Posterior mediastinal accessory thymus. Pediatr Radiol 14: 165

Batsakis JG (1974) Tumors of the head and neck: clinical and pathological considerations. Williams and Wilkins, Baltimore, p 233

Baudain P, Terraube P, Crouzet A (1980) Une tumeur peu banale du médiastin postérieur chez l'enfant. Arch Fr Pédiatr 37: 609

Belohradsky BH (1985) Thymusaplasie und -hypoplasie mit Hypoparathyreoidismus, Herz- und Gefäßmißbildungen (Di-George-Syndrom). Ergeb Inn Med Kinderheilkd 54: 35

Bistritzer T, Tamir A, Oland J, Varsano D, Manor A, Gall A, Aladjem M (1985) Severe dyspnea and dysphagia resulting from an aberrant cervical thymus. Eur J Pediatr 144: 86

Caffey J, Di Liberti (1959) Acute atrophy of thymus induced adrenocorticosteroids observed roentgenologically. AJR 82: 530

Castellanos A, Peireiras R, Garcia O (1971) Angiocardiography in huge hypertrophy of the thymus. AJR 112: 40

Claus D, Coppens JP (1984) Sonography of mediastinal masses in infants and children. Ann Radiol (Paris) 27: 150

Cohen MD, Weber TR, Sequeira FW, Vane DW, King H (1983) The diagnostic dilemma of the posterior mediastinal thymus. CT manifestations. Radiology 146: 691

Cory DA, Cohen MD, Smith JA (1987) Thymus in the superior mediastinum simulating adenopathy: appearance on CT. Radiology 162: 457

Cowart MA (1980) Radiologic seminar CCVII: ectopic thymus. J Miss State Med Assoc 21: 217

Day DL, Gedgaudas E (1984) The Thymus. Radiol Clin North Am 22: 519

Domarus H, von Blaha J (1987) Ectopic thymus in the neck; a case report and review of the literature. Br J Plast Surg 40: 532

Ebel KD (1980) Zur Röntgendiagnostik des Thymus im Kindesalter. Radiologe 20: 379

Epstein HC, Loeb WJ (1955) Thymic tumor of the pharynx. J Pediatr 47: 105

Falk P (1936) Über ortsfremde gutartige Gewebsbildungen, Thymus und Thyreoidea-gewebe im Kehlkopf. Arch Ohren-, Nasen-, Kehlkopfkrankh 141: 118

Fauré C (1978) Le thymus. In: Lefèbvre J et al. (eds) Traité de radiodiagnostic: Radiopédiatrie, vol 19. Masson, Paris, p 53

Finch DRA, Gough MH (1972) Ectopic thymic tissue presenting as a lateral cervical swelling. Br J Surg 59: 885

Gilmour JR (1941) Some developmental abnormalities of thymus and parathyroids. J Pathol Bacteriol 52: 213

Goebel N (1985) Lokalisation des Thymus im unteren Halsbereich. Digitale Bilddiagn 5: 8

Grumbach S, Uhlig W, Schöning M (1985) Weichteilschwellung im Kopf-Halsbereich – sonographische Diagnostik Vortr 81. Tag Dtsch Gesellsch Kinderheilkd. Frankfurt (M)

Hagens EW (1932) Malformation of the auditory apparatus in the newborn, associated with ectopic thymus. Arch Otolaryngol 15: 671

Hurley MF (1977) Cervicomediastinal thymic cyst: cyst puncture and contrast radiographic demonstration. Br J Radiol 50: 676

Johnson PM, Berdon WE, Baker DH, Fawwaz RA (1978) Thymic uptake of gallium-67 citrate in a healthy 4 year-old boy. Pediatr Radiol 7: 243

Juzbasič D, Pasini M (1965) Thymus anularis. Dtsch Med Wochenschr 90: 1050

Kabelka M, Horák J (1976) Pneumomediastinography in the diagnosis of ectopic lobe of the thymus in respiratory obstruction. J Pediatr Surg 11: 265

Kabelka M, Sintáková B, Zitková M (1977) Dysontogenetic accessory lobe of the thymus. A new clinical entity? Z Kinderchir 20: 116

Koecher PH (1959) Fehldiagnose eines Tumors im hinteren oberen Mediastinum durch ungewöhnlich gelegene Thymusdrüse. ROFO 90: 515

Lucien et al (1966) see Testut-Latarget A (1966)

Malone PS, Fitzgerald RJ (1987) Aberrant thymus: a misleading mediastinal mass. J Pediatr Surg 22: 130

Martin DJ (1975) Experiences with acute surgical conditions. Radiol Clin North Am 8: 297

Martin KW, McAlister WH (1987) Intratracheal thymus: a rare cause of airway obstruction. AJR 149: 1217

Michelson H, Sender B (1956) Cervical thymus: report of a case. Arch Surg 72: 275

Noback NG (1926) Thymus in newborn and early infancy. Radiology 7: 416

Otto HF (1984) Pathologie des Thymus. In: Doerr W, Seifert G (eds) Spezielle pathologische Anatomie, vol 17. Springer, Berlin Heidelberg New York Tokyo

Parker LA, Gaisie G, Scatliff JH (1985) Computerited tomography and ultrasonographic findings in massive thymic hyperplasia. Clin Pediatr 24: 90

Poell J, Stanisic M, Morger R (1979) Beitrag zum akzessorischen Thymus. Z Kinderchir 26: 62

Rollins NK, Currarino G (1988) MR imaging of posterior mediastinal thymus. J Comput Assist Tomogr 12: 518

Rosai J, Levine GD (1976) Tumors of the thymus. In: Atlas of tumor pathology, 2nd ser, fasc. 13. Armed Forces Institute of Pathology, Washington DC

Rypens F, Avni F, Müller F, Buran D, von Struy J (1989) Thymus ectopique cervical. J Radiol 70: 721

Saade M, Whitten DN, Necheles TF, Leape L, Darling D (1976) Posterior mediastinal accessory thymus. J Pediatr 88: 71

Schnell VY (1975) probleme der Thymusdiagnostik bei atypischer Lage und seltenen Begleitumständen. Thesis, Cologne

Shackelford GD, McAlister WH (1974) The aberrantly positioned thymus. A cause of mediastinal or neck masses in children. AJR 120: 291

Siegel MJ, Glazer HS, Wiener JI, Molina PL (1989) Normal and abnormal thymus in childhood: MR imaging. Radiology 172: 367

Spigland N, Bensoussan AL, Blanchard H, Russo P (1990) Aberrant cervical thymus in children: three case reports and review of the literature. J Pediatr Surg 25: 1196

Tesseraux H (1953) Physiologie und Pathologie des Thymus unter besonderer Berücksichtigung der pathologischen Morphologie. Barth, Leipzig

Testut-Latarget A (1966) Tratado de Anatomia Humana, 9th edn. Salvat Editors, SA, Barcelona, p 940

Thorrens SJ, Pantzer JG, Bennett JE (1969) Cervical thymus gland. Plast Reconstr Surg 44: 86

Tovi F, Mares AJ (1978) The aberrant cervical thymus. Embryology, pathology, and clinical implications. Am J Surg 136: 631

7.3 Persistent Thymus

E. WILLICH

7.3.1 Introduction

The apparently paradoxical expression "persistent" derives from radiologic observations of a deceleration in, or even absence of, the relative diminution of the thymus in comparison to the growing mediastinum that usually occurs after the 2nd year of life. In such cases the thymus consequently exceeds the age-dependent physiologic size. This is reflected in the appearance of the organ on CT scans, and on chest radiographs in two planes it overlaps the mediastinal borders. Since the size of the thymus in any case varies markedly up to the age of 6 years (it is therefore sometimes still visible until the 5th year of life), it is at school age and in adulthood that its persistence can be of importance, causing misinterpretation including suspicion of a tumor.

Pathoanatomically and clinically the persistent thymus is generally without significance and does not require therapy, especially surgery. Cases of myasthenia gravis pseudoparalytica represent an exception; this disorder is combined with incomplete regression of the thymus, and therefore with persistence of this organ, in 15% of cases (see also Chap. 11).

The typical structure of the thymus, with cortex, medulla, and Hassall's corpuscles, is also found in cases of persistent thymus.

7.3.2 Pathophysiologic Causes

A persistent thymus can be caused by prevention of involution of the organ as a result of delayed "lipomatous atrophy" (STEINMANN 1984).

For the diagnosis of persistent thymus to be made, it is necessary to exclude a preceding stress-related illness or steroid treatment as these can lead to a certain rebound phenomenon, even if the thymus was not previously visible.

7.3.3 Clinical Features

Normally, the persistent thymus will be asymptomatic and detected by chance. Rarely, however, clinical symptoms are present, as in thymic hyperplasia.

7.3.4 Imaging Methods

On conventional radiography (sagittal view) a persistent thymus appears as a bilateral or sometimes unilateral enlargement of the mediastinum. The enlargement does not correspond to normal glands after the 1st year of life (BARON et al. 1982). The extent of the enlargement varies, sometimes reaching the size of hyperplasia. The retrosternal localization must be confirmed by the lateral radiograph. On fluoroscopy the size of the thymus typically depends on respiration (PARKER et al. 1985). Conventional tomography, and also the former technique of pneumomediastinography, does not allow differential diagnosis from thymic enlargement of other causes. (LISSNER 1963; POHLENZ 1968; SONE et al. 1980) (Fig. 7.5).

The most frequent radiologic sign in late infancy and at school age is a "prominent pulmonary segment" or an "effaced heart waist," a thymus "tip" (or "residue") in the pulmonary concavity which can suggest a congenital heart disease in children (Fig. 7.6). This persisting thymus tip is sometimes visible after traumatic pneumomediastinum. By means of CT it is usually possible to identify the retrosternal – and/or paratracheal-situated enlarged organ, which in most cases has a clearly defined contour (Fig. 7.7). The solid, homogeneous, dense tissue parts show absorption values equivalent to those of normal thymus (WALTER and HÜBENER 1980; BARON et al. 1982); however, fatty infiltration can give rise to heterogeneous absorption values. Therefore it is easier to identify the thymic tissue by means of MRI (Fig. 7.8).

7.3.5 Differential Diagnosis

Persistent thymus sometimes cannot be distinguished from hyperplasia or a solid tumor (LACK 1981). KOOK SANG OH et al. reported in 1971 that three patients aged 10–15 years with persistent thy-

---

Fig. 7.5 a–f. Persistent thymus in a 3-year-old. **a** Enlargement of mediastinal shadow in frontal chest radiograph which had remained constant over several months and was suspected to be a tumor. **b** Lateral view: A dense shadow is seen in the anterior part of the superior mediastinum, with a blurred lower border. The density exceeds that of the heart shadow. **c,d** Tomograms, 5 and 8 cm: Bronchial diameters are normal; ventrally there is a well-defined contour that is convex-arched to the right. No surgery; clinically asymptomatic. **e,f** Control radiograph in two planes 5 months later: Diminution of the thymus in the frontal view; laterally the retrosternal shadow is diminished

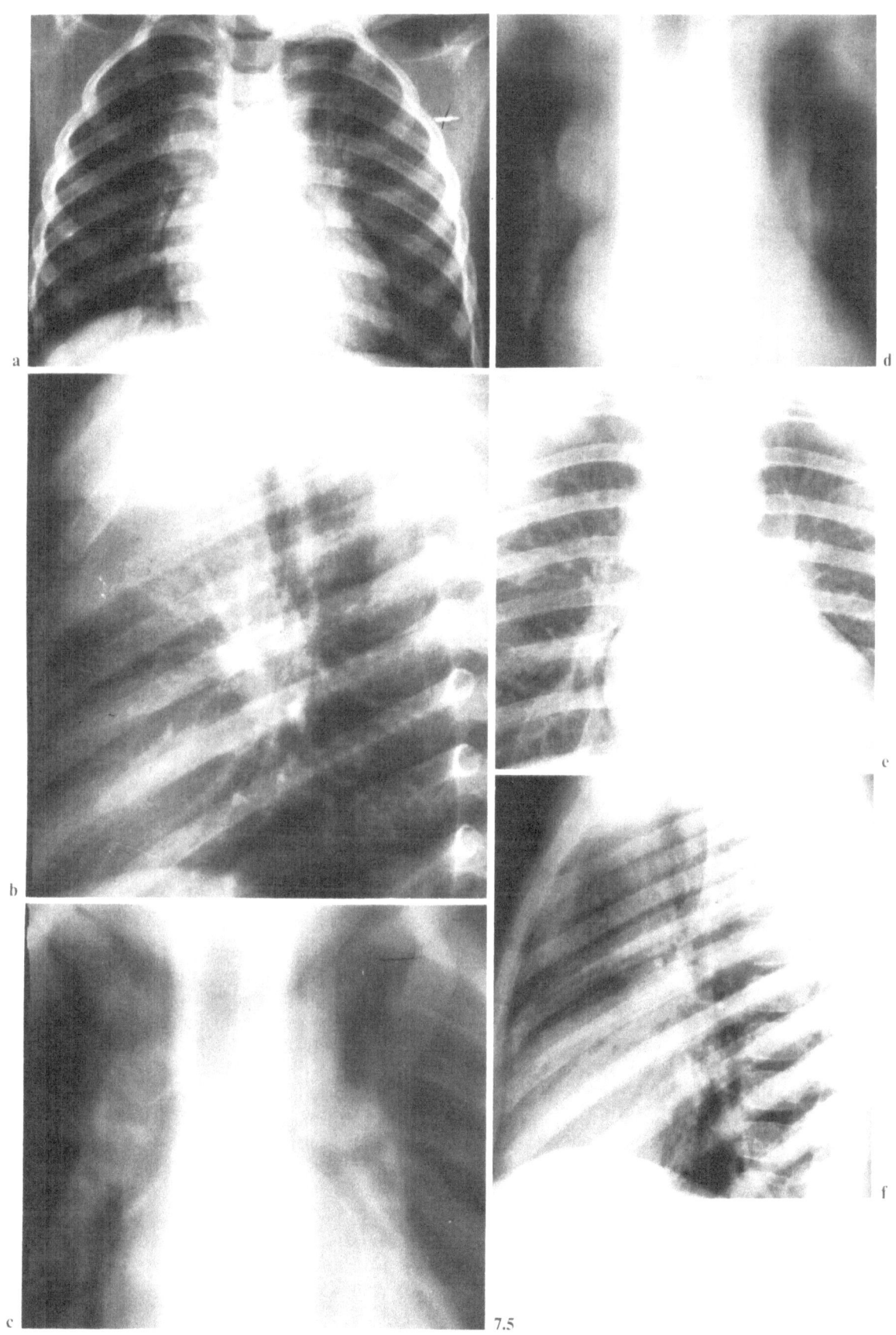

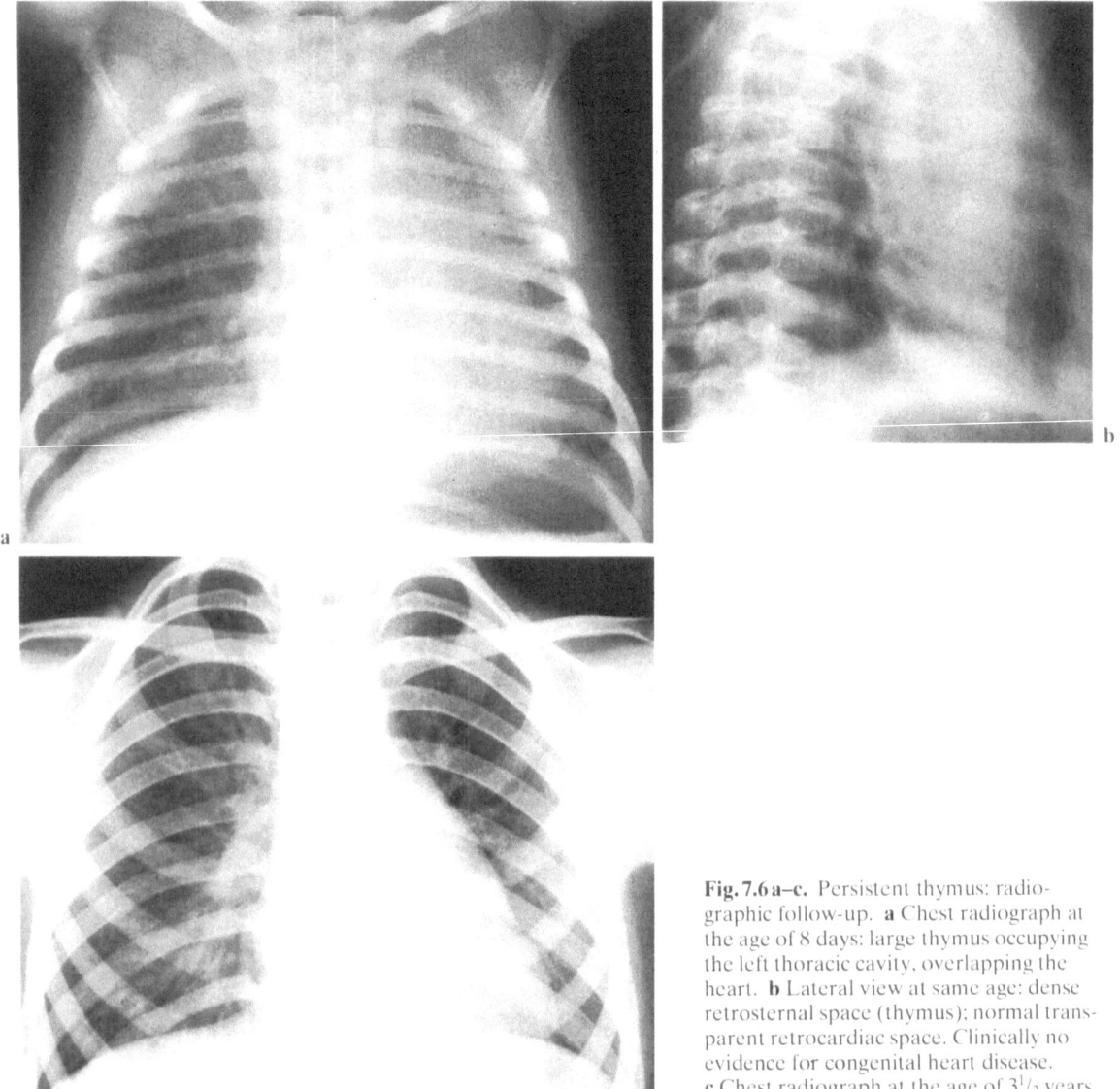

Fig. 7.6 a–c. Persistent thymus: radiographic follow-up. **a** Chest radiograph at the age of 8 days: large thymus occupying the left thoracic cavity, overlapping the heart. **b** Lateral view at same age: dense retrosternal space (thymus); normal transparent retrocardiac space. Clinically no evidence for congenital heart disease. **c** Chest radiograph at the age of 3½ years shows a persistent thymus tip as the symptom of an "effaced heart waist"

mus underwent thoracotomy either because it was assumed a solid tumor was present, or in order to exclude such a tumor. Narrowing of the trachea tends to suggest a pathologic mass, e.g., a thymic tumor, because persistent or hyperplastic thymus usually does not compress the neighboring organs or structures. In particular it does not affect the trachea and the great vessels although very rarely tracheal impressions have been reported in the presence of a persistent thymus (EBEL 1980). In cases of myasthenia gravis pseudoparalytica the enlargement of the organ can be so slight that there is no difference from delayed involution. In

our own case material and in the report of BARON et al. (1982), a pathologic process was not visible on normal chest x-rays in 50%–60% of patients with myasthenia gravis pseudoparalytica although thymic hyperplasia or persistent thymus was found on thoracotomy.

A systemic lymphatic disease is often suspected, especially in children, and sometimes thoracotomy or extirpation of the thymus is erroneously performed.

Congenital heart disease or cardiomegaly can resemble a normal or persistent thymus in all age groups (Fig. 7.9). Nowadays, pathologic cardiac

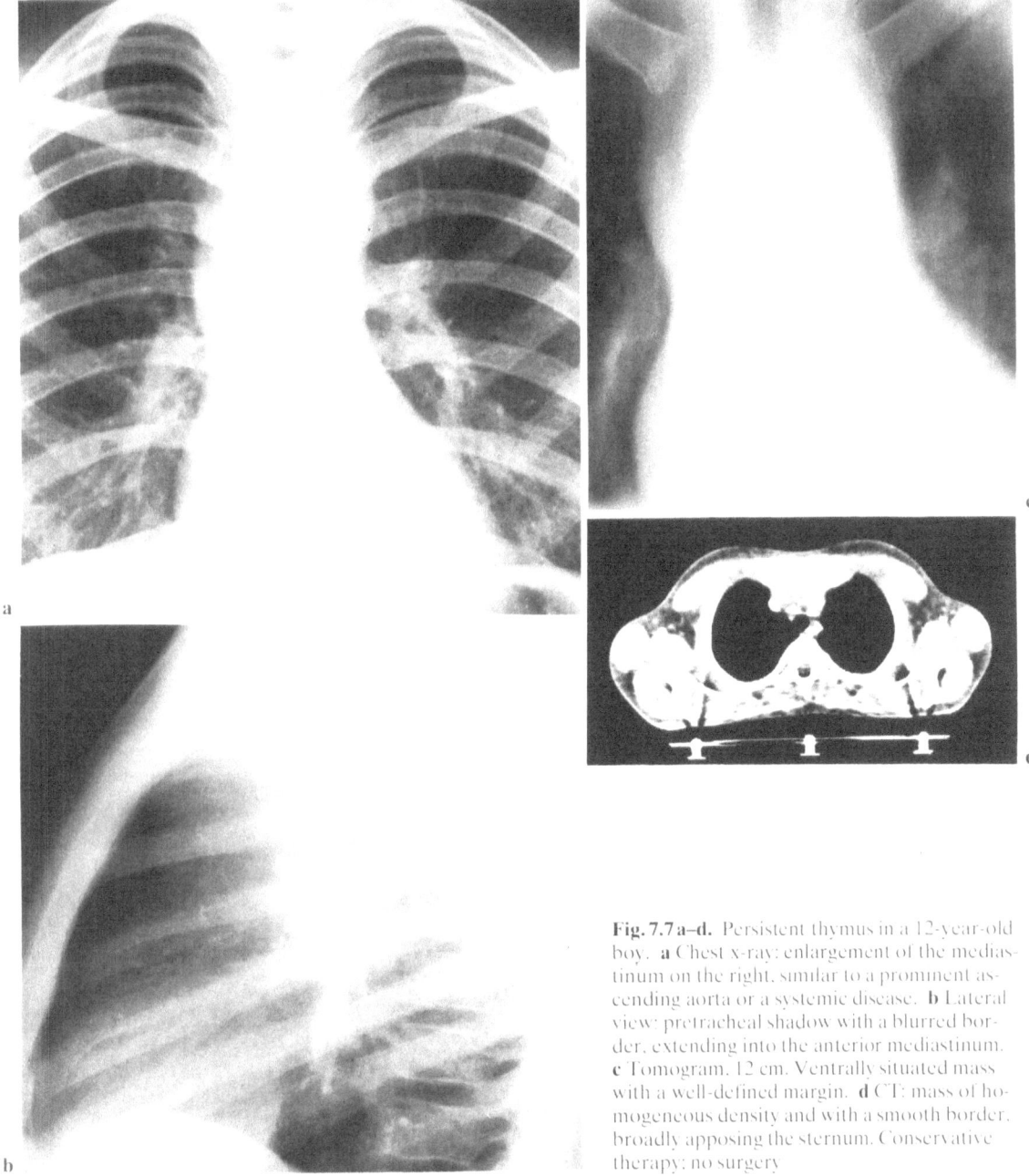

Fig. 7.7 a–d. Persistent thymus in a 12-year-old boy. **a** Chest x-ray: enlargement of the mediastinum on the right, similar to a prominent ascending aorta or a systemic disease. **b** Lateral view: pretracheal shadow with a blurred border, extending into the anterior mediastinum. **c** Tomogram, 12 cm. Ventrally situated mass with a well-defined margin. **d** CT: mass of homogeneous density and with a smooth border, broadly apposing the sternum. Conservative therapy; no surgery

symptoms can be excluded more easily on the basis of clinical, electrocardiographic, and echocardiographic parameters. The normally sized retrocardiac space seen in the lateral view or during fluoroscopy in an oblique projection with barium swallow can also be of considerable help. The formerly used technique of angiocardiography, which entailed the intravenous introduction of contrast material (CASTELLANOS et al. 1971), has been largely replaced by CT.

The previously mentioned radiologic visualization of a persistent thymic lobe in the form of a so-called effaced heart waist or a prominent pulmonary segment (Figs. 5.2d, 7.6c) occurs at an age (late infancy and school age) when a thymus does not generally spring to mind as a possible cause. The left thymic lobe overlaps the main branch of the pulmonary artery in a way which can resemble an enlarged pulmonary artery (Fig. 7.11; POHLENZ 1968; STRAUBE and RAUTENBURG 1974).

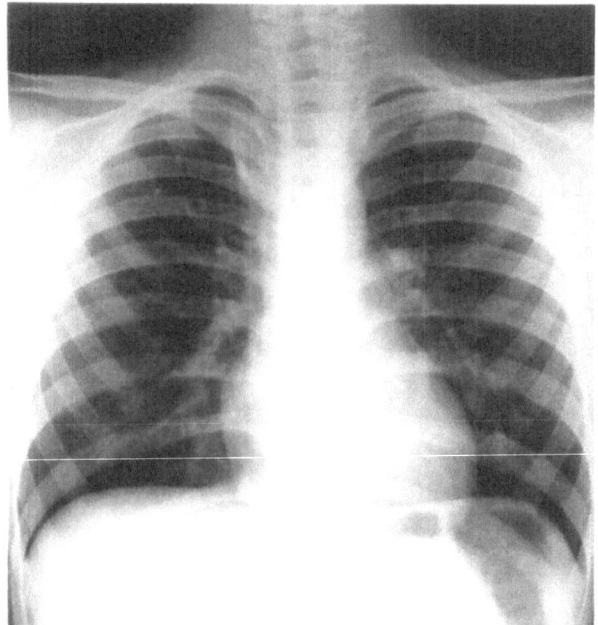

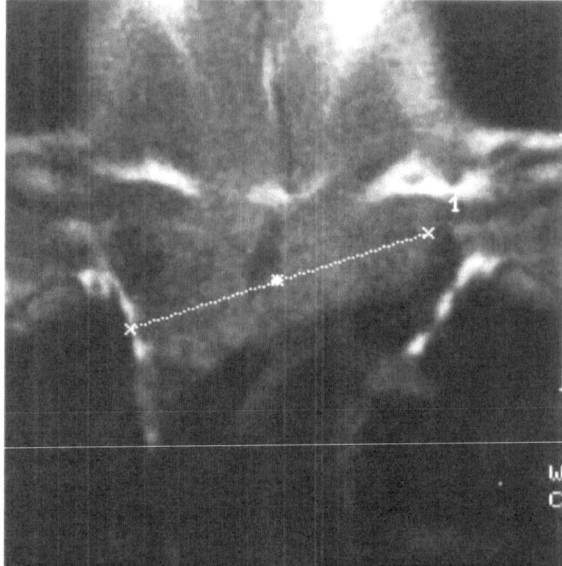

a

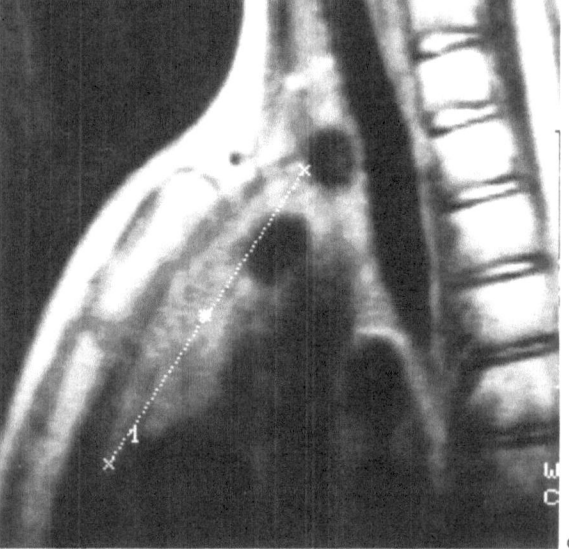

Fig. 7.8 a–c. Persistent thymus in a 10-year-old boy. **a** Plain chest radiograph, routine examination: Enlargement of the mediastinum is seen on the right in the upper part (slightly rotated). On the left there is a triangular shadow of low density in the hilar region. Secondary finding: lobus venae azygos. (Lateral view: no findings.) **b,c** MRI in two planes: A retrosternal thymic shadow is present, embracing the trachea. The mass is of low signal intensity and homogeneous; it is not suggestive of a tumor. (Courtesy of Prof. Dr. G. BENZ-BOHM, Pediatric Department of the Radiology Institute, University of Cologne, FRG)

Fig. 7.9 a, b. Simulation of cardiomegaly by a persistent thymus in a 1-year-old boy. Chest radiograph: bilaterally "enlarged heart," smooth borders, small mediastinal shadow at the level of the thymus. Transparent marginal zones! **b** Lateral view: free retrocardiac space. Homogeneous shadowing of the anterior mediastinum by the thymus. Clinically no evidence for congenital heart disease

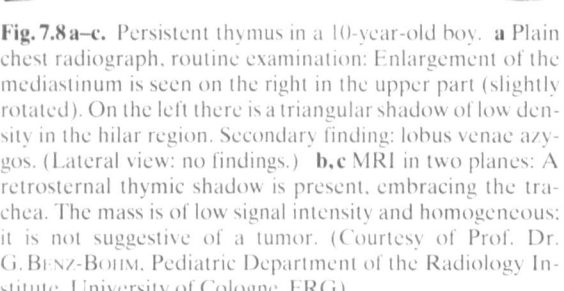

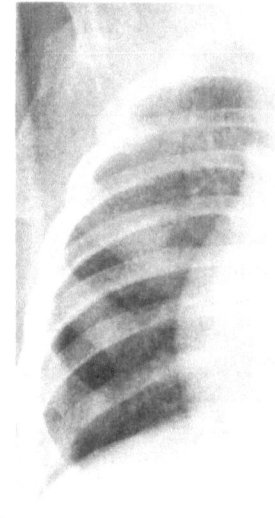

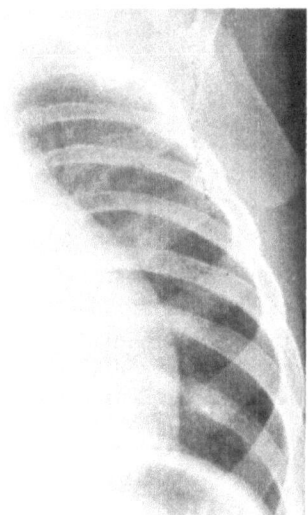

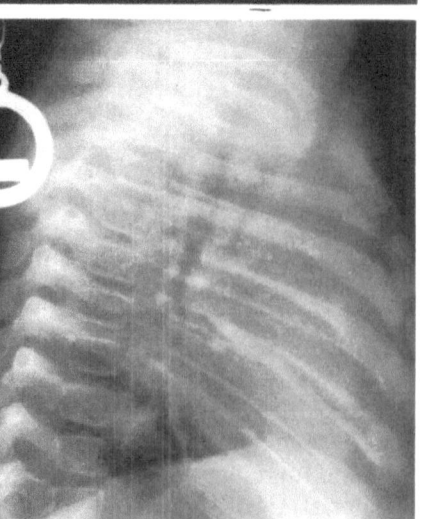

a   b

Fig. 7.10. Definition of the basis point to which the left pulmonary artery can extend if there is a "prominent pulmonary segment." Normal finding in a 6-year-old boy. (Courtesy of Prof. Dr. F. BALL, Dept. of Pediatric Radiology, University Children's Hospital, Frankfurt/M, FRG)

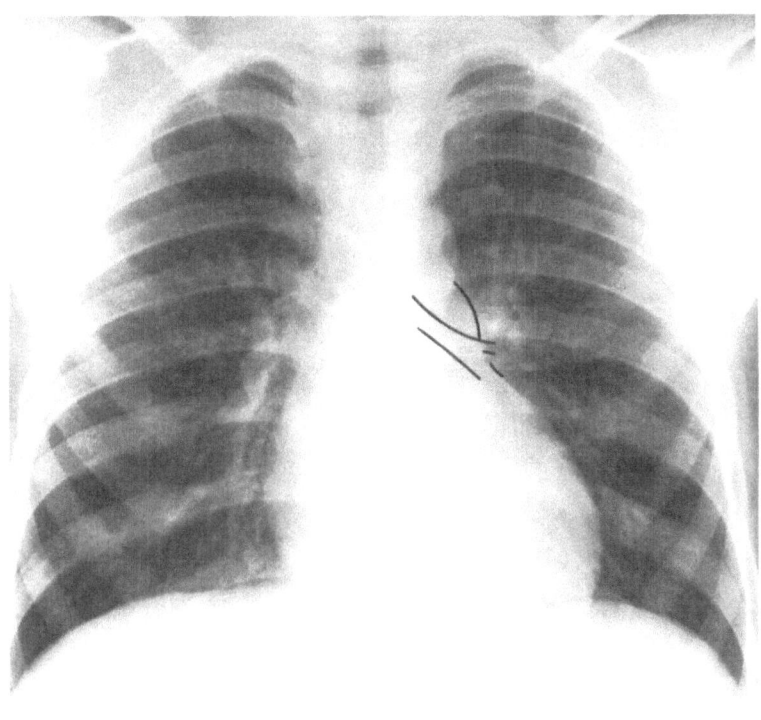

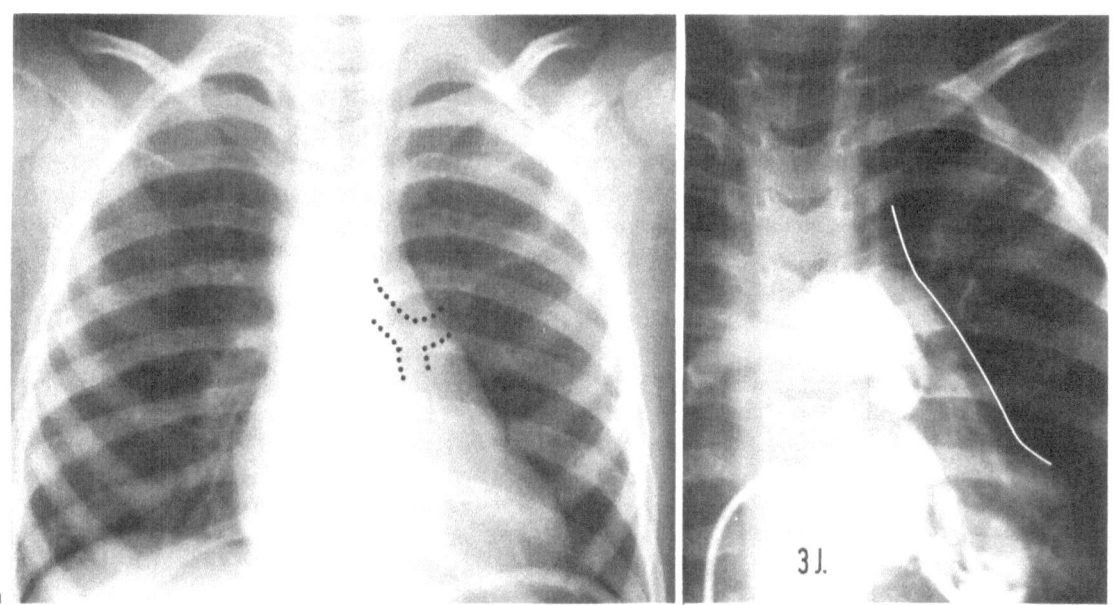

Fig. 7.11 a, b. Prominent pulmonary segment due to persistent thymus in a 3-year-old girl with Fallot's tetralogy. **a** Chest radiograph: slight prominence of the pulmonary segment. The thymus widely overlaps the lower border of the left upper lobe bronchus and the basis line, prolonged by the transverse diameter of this bronchus. **b** Angiocardiography: the left thymic border (see *line*) overlaps the contrast-filled pulmonary artery by 1 cm laterally and 2.5 cm caudally (see also Fig. 5.6 of the same child at the age of 1 year). (Courtesy of Prof. Dr. F. BALL, Dept. of Pediatric Radiology, University Children's Hospital, Frankfurt/M, FRG).

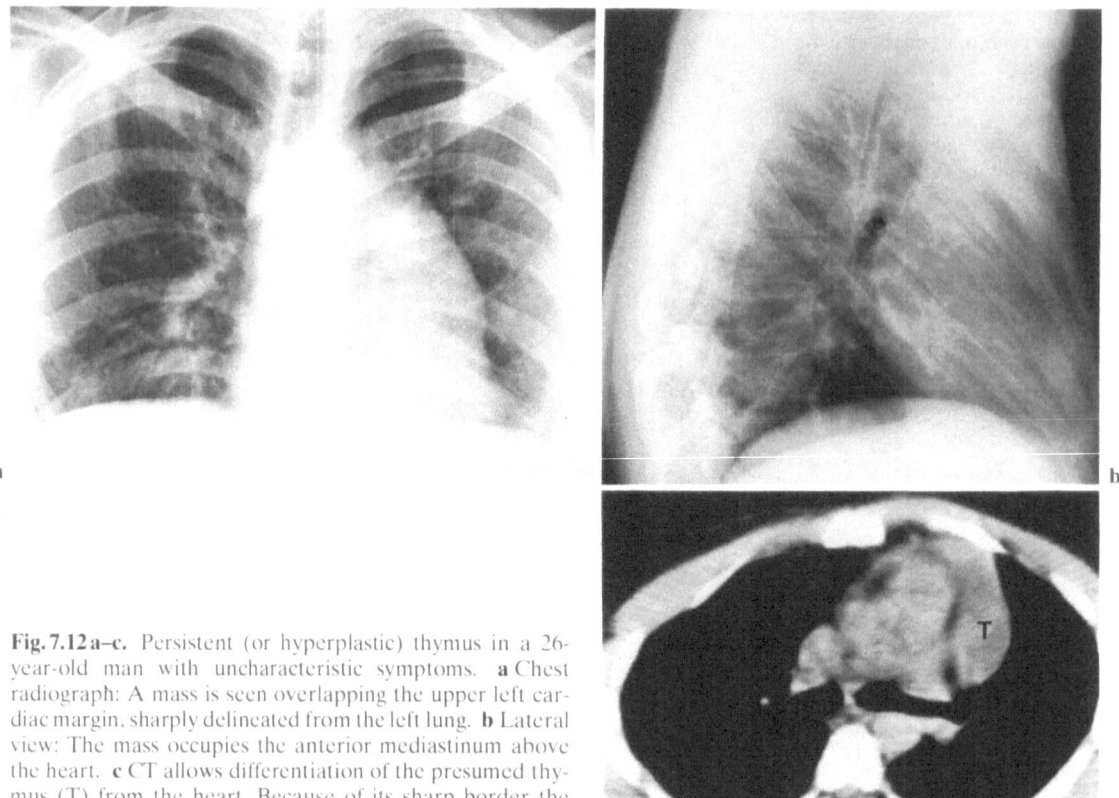

Fig. 7.12 a–c. Persistent (or hyperplastic) thymus in a 26-year-old man with uncharacteristic symptoms. **a** Chest radiograph: A mass is seen overlapping the upper left cardiac margin, sharply delineated from the left lung. **b** Lateral view: The mass occupies the anterior mediastinum above the heart. **c** CT allows differentiation of the presumed thymus (T) from the heart. Because of its sharp border the mass was supposed to be benign

STÖVER et al. (1975) and BALL et al. (1982) have described a simple and relatively reliable discriminatory radiodiagnostic sign on the basis of angiocardiography in children with suspicion of a heart defect or with an isolated valvular pulmonary stenosis: On plain chest x-rays a pulmonary segment formed by the pulmonary trunk is seen at the lower border of the left upper lobe bronchus directly after its outlet from the cardiac margin. However, this pulmonary segment is never situated more caudally than double the transverse diameter of the upper lobe bronchus. If such an eminence in the pulmonary artery region overlaps the left heart silhouette caudally, it is usually the left-sided outline of the thymus (Fig. 7.10). If a prominent pulmonary segment enlarges, as occurs, for example, in cases of pulmonary artery stenosis or left to right shunt, it usually elongates cranially. To this extent a persistent thymus in the pulmonary concavity can also be differentiated in children with congenital heart disease by means of plain chest x-rays (Fig. 7.11).

In cases of doubt, the enhancement seen on CT enables the heart and great vessels to be distinguished from the thymus (Fig. 7.14 e, f; SIEGEL et al. 1982). In a 9-month-old boy who showed "cardiomegaly" on radiographs HEIBERG et al. (1982) were able to identify a "soft tissue lobe" adjoining the heart as the thymus by means of CT, after cardiac catheterization and angiography had previously shown normal findings.

The problem of differential diagnosis between persistent thymus, cardiomegaly, and hyperplastic thymus is illustrated by Fig. 7.12. The patient had uncharacteristic clinical symptoms. The enlarged mediastinum above the upper left cardiac margin simulates cardiomegaly; in the lateral view the "mass" is retrosternally situated and suspected of being a hyperplastic or tumorous thymus. CT allows differentiation from the heart and a preliminary diagnosis of a persistent thymus.

References

Ball F, Stöver B, Vettermann HE, Müller U (1982) Zum Aussagewert der Thoraxaufnahmen bei isolierter valvulärer Pulmonalstenose. Monatsschr. Kinderheilkd. 130: 41

Baron RL, Lee JKT, Sagel SS, Peterson RR (1982) Computed tomography of the normal thymus. Radiology 142: 121

Castellanos A, Pereiras R, Garcia O (1971) Angiocardiography in huge hypertrophy of the thymus. AJR 112: 40

Ebel KD (1980) Zur Röntgendiagnostik des Thymus im Kindesalter. Radiologe 20: 379

Heiberg E, Wolverson MK, Sundaram M, Nouri S (1982) Normal thymus: CT characteristics in subjects under age 20. AJR 138: 491

Kook Sang Oh, Weber AL, Borden SP (1971) Normal mediastinal mass in late childhood. Radiology 101: 625

Lack EE (1981) Thymic hyperplasia with massive enlargement. J Thorac Cardiovasc Surg 81: 741

Lissner J (1963) Die röntgenologische Diagnostik der Thymustumoren. Radiologe 1: 31

Parker LA, Gaisie G, Scatliff JH (1985) Computed tomography and ultrasonographic findings in massive thymic hyperplasia. Clin Pediatr (Phila) 24: 90

Pohlenz O (1968) Röntgenologische Thymusdiagnostik. Med Klin 63: 1255

Siegel MJ, Sagel SS, Reed K (1982) The value of computed tomography in the diagnosis and management of pediatric mediastinal abnormalities. Radiology 142: 149

Sone S, Higashihara T, Morimoto S et al. (1980) Normal anatomy of the thymus and anterior mediastinum by pneumomediastinography. AJR 134: 81

Steinmann GG (1984) Altersveränderungen des menschlichen Thymus. Thesis, Medical Faculty, University of Kiel

Stöver B, Ball F, Müller U (1975) Die radiologische Differenzierung eines prominenten Pulmonalsegmentes. Vortrag 12. Jahrestagung, Ges für Pädiatr Radiol, Vienna

Straube EM, Rautenburg HW (1974) Der prominente Pulmonalisbogen im Säuglings- und Kindesalter. Klin Pädiatr 186: 107

Walter E, Hubener K-H (1980) Computertomographische Charakteristika raumfordernder Prozesse im vorderen Mediastinum und ihre Differentialdiagnose. ROFO 133: 391

7.4 Hyperplasia

7.4.1 Introduction

The term "hyperplasia of the thymus" is used in two different ways. The first usage refers to abnormal enlargement of the thymus (e.g., "gross hyperplasia") and is an imaging finding. It is histologically normal (LEVINE and ROSAI 1978). This type of hyperplasia is often difficult to define because thymic size varies widely in the normal population and is also dependent on age. The second usage refers to the presence of thymic lymphoid germinal centers, as revealed by histopathologic investiga-

tion. This type does not clearly relate either to thymic size or to the degree of fatty involution (MOORE et al. 1983) (see. Sect. 7.4.2).

The thymus is an essential organ for the development and maintenance of cell-mediated immunity, and it can be the site of origin of numerous pathologic conditions, including developmental abnormalities, hyperplasia, and tumors (ROSAI and LEVINE 1976; JANOSSY et al. 1980, 1986; HOFMANN et al. 1984, 1985; OTTO 1984; MÜLLER-HERMELINK 1986). Numerous experimental and clinicopathologic investigations have demonstrated that the immunologic functions of the thymus are closely dependent on the presence of normal thymic structures (GOLDSTEIN and MACKAY 1969; ALPERT et al. 1981; Ciba Foundation 1981). Past experience has shown that a number of autoimmune diseases – including myasthenia gravis – coincides with structural changes of the thymus. One of those changes is thymic hyperplasia.

Hyperplasia is an increase in volume in a tissue or organ by the formation of new cellular elements in a normal microscopic arrangement. Thymic hyperplasia is one of numerous conditions which present themselves clinically and/or roentgenologically as mediastinal masses. Therefore, the diagnosis of a mediastinal mass represents a challenging diagnostic and management problem (HALLER et al. 1969; SAEGESSER and ZOUPANOS 1970; WYCHULIS et al. 1971; BLASIMANN et al. 1977; BOWER and KIESEWETTER 1977; BARCIA and NELSON 1979; FILLER et al. 1979; SILVERMAN and SABISTON 1980; HOFMANN et al. 1987, 1990). Currently on the basis of morphologic criteria, two types of thymic hyperplasia are recognized (LEVINE and ROSAI 1978; OTTO 1984): (a) true hyperplasia; and (b) lymphofollicular hyperplasia defined by the presence of lymph follicles with germinal centers, regardless of the size or weight of the thymus (CASTLEMAN and NORRIS 1949). This is the type classically associated with myasthenia gravis (SLOAN 1943).

Using imaging techniques, no clearly defined border exists between a "large thymus" and hyperplasia. The age-dependent enlargement can be illustrated by the fact that the normal thymus in young infants is to be classified as pathologically enlarged just 2 years later.

From the clinicoradiologic point of view, hyperplasia must be assumed if the thymus occupies markedly more than half of a hemithorax (even the entire hemithorax may be filled) (Fig. 5.2 a). Consequently a radiologically large thymus in young infants does not necessarily justify the diagnosis of true hyperplasia: a large thymus is indeed visible in half of all children under 9 months old although these infants are healthy and eutrophic. Therefore the enlargement does not represent pathologic hypertrophy but a relative physiologic growth which relates to the immune system of the child and is indicative of a good constitution and good immune reactivity of the organism. Thus such enlargement is without diagnostic or therapeutic consequences (COCCHI 1959; TISCHER 1967).

The incidence of hyperplasia during childhood is the subject of controversy, varying according to the literature between 0.12% and 63% (SZAKALL 1973). This variation can be explained by the different definitions of hyperplasia that are employed.

As regards the classification of hyperplasia, a distinction is drawn between true or "idiopathic" hyperplasia and a regenerative form that occurs following stress situations, debilitating illness, chemotherapy, steroid administration, etc. Thymic hyperplasia occurring in association with other diseases constitutes a third type (see Sect. 7.4.4).

7.4.2 Pathologic Features

W. J. HOFMANN and H. F. OTTO

7.4.2.1 True Thymic Hyperplasia

True hyperplasia is characterized by an increase in both the size and the weight of the thymus, with a normal microscopic appearance appropriate for the patient's age. True thymic hyperplasia is rare. The three clinicopathologic subtypes of this form of hyperplasia are:

1. Thymic hyperplasia with massive enlargement of the gland (massive thymic hyperplasia)
2. Thymic rebound in childhood and adolescence
3. Rare instances of thymic hyperplasia which are associated with other diseases, endocrinopathies being of major importance here

7.4.2.2 Thymic Hyperplasia with Massive Enlargement of the Gland

There are very few well-documented examples of thymic hyperplasia with massive enlargement, and these are summarized in Table 7.2. In our review of the literature we found only 14 cases of this con-

dition. The cause and functional significance of giant thymic hyperplasia (thymomegaly) are unclear.

"Enlargement of the thymus" is a common observation in infancy. HALLER et al. (1969) reported a series of 80 children who were seen for "mediastinal masses" at the Johns Hopkins Hospital, Baltimore, between July 1933 and Juli 1968; there were eight "hyperplastic thymus glands" in four newborn infants and four children 3 months to 5 years old. In a review of 16 cases of thymic hyperplasia by BLASIMANN et al. (1977), nine were found in infants in their 1st year of life. BARCIA and NELSON (1979) reported a series of 11 children, 1–13 years of age, who underwent thymectomy for an undiagnosed thymic enlargement. The weight of the resected masses was 47–92 g. On histologic examination, one proved to be an anaplastic thymic malignancy; the other ten were shown to be histologically normal thymuses without germinal center formation.

Clinical symptoms in this type of thymic hyperplasia range from none at all to respiratory distress (Table 7.2). Four of the cases in Table 7.2 (cases 4, 5, 6, and 13) were asymptomatic and mediastinal widening was discovered by chance on a routine chest radiograph. If the mediastinal mass is symptomatic, most of the symptoms are local ones and due to the irritation of mediastinal structures. Respiratory symptoms, i.e., mild dyspnea, nonproductive cough, bronchopneumonia, or acute respiratory distress, occurred in four of the 14 cases (cases 3, 7, 9, and 11). However, some of them might have been unrelated to the mediastinal mass which was then detected during the routine diagnostic procedure for an upper respiratory infection, for example. Other, nonlocal symptoms which have been reported are a moderate and disseminated lymphadenopathy in one of the 14 cases (case 10) and hepatomegaly with questionable splenomegaly which disappeared 6 months after thymectomy in another case (case 2). It is tempting to correlate the lymphadenopathy with the thymic hyperplasia although there was only a peripheral leukocytosis, but without lymphocytosis. The hepatomegaly, on the other hand, might be correlated with the thymic hyperplasia since the patient also had an increase in the number of peripheral T cells and a disturbance of the architecture of a mediastinal lymph node, owing to an expansion of the thymus-dependent lymph node area (see also Sect. 7.4.3).

Table 7.2. Clinicopathologic features of thymic hyperplasia with massive enlargement, but normal, age-related histology. Summary of 14 well-documented cases, compiled by W. J. HOFMANN and H. F. OTTO (see Table 7.3 for details on the clinico-radiologic features of 27 further cases)

Case no.	Age/sex	Clinical and laboratory findings	Treatment	Weight and size of thymus	Reference
1	8 mo, –	Decreased breathing sounds. Large extra-pulmonary mass in the right lower two-thirds of the hemithorax, obliterating right cardiac margin and right hemidiaphragm	Thoracotomy	– 9 × 8 × 5 cm	BARTH et al. 1976
2	7 mo, m	Hepatomegaly. Peripheral blood and bone marrow lymphocytosis. "Large soft tissue density in the right hemithorax." Two years after thymectomy: reduced serum IgG	Thymectomy	224 g 9 × 8 × 6 cm	KATZ et al. 1977
3	12 mo, m	Respiratory distress. "Large anterior me-diastinal mass . . . (decreased in size after steroid therapy, but quickly enlarged again)." Peripheral blood lymphocytosis, 92 % T lymphocytes[a]	Corticosteroids Thymectomy	420 g	O'SHEA et al. 1978
4	4 yr, f	Asymptomatic. Moderate peripheral lym-phocytosis[b]. Median opacity occupying almost entirely both lung fields	Thymectomy	800 g	RASORE-QUARTINO et al. 1979
5	14 yr, m	"Anterior mediastinal mass . . . (discovered in routine chest roentgenogram)"	Thymectomy	490 g	LACK 1981[c]
6	11 yr, m	"Right anterior mediastinal mass . . . (dis-covered on routine chest roentgenogram)"	Thymectomy	324 g 15.2 cm in diam.	LACK 1981[c]
7	7 mo, f	Large liver cyst. Respiratory distress syn-drome ("by displacement and compression of the bronchopulmonary system"). "Huge" mediastinal mass	Corticosteroids (for 3 weeks)[d] Thymectomy	230 g 18 × 11 × 8.5 cm	LAMESCH 1983
8	15 mo, m	"Pneumonia" without response to therapy. Density of the left hemithorax, mass in the anterior and middle mediastinum	Thoracotomy	200 g	PARKER et al. 1985
9	10 yr, f	Cough. A regularly outlined x-ray shadow in the anterior mediastinum	Thymectomy	93 g	NEZELOF and NORMAND 1986
10	5 yr, f	Slighly asthenic. Moderate and disseminat-ed lymphadenopathy. Leukocytosis with-out lymphocytosis[e]. Abnormal mediastinal shadow	Biopsy	–	NEZELOF and NORMAND 1986
11	11 yr, f	Mild, nonproductive cough, localized bron-chitis, bronchopneumonia. Homogeneous mass occupying the thymic region	Biopsy	–	NEZELOF and NORMAND 1986
12	12 yr, m	Respiratory distress, dysphagia. Large an-terior mediastinal mass	Thymectomy	245 g 13 × 8 × 3.5 cm	JUDD 1987
13	15 yr, m	Multiple childhood viral infections. Chronic persistent hepatitis 2 years before the detec-tion of a large anterior mediastinal mass	Thymectomy	680 g 17 × 16 × 6 cm	ARLISS et al. 1988
14	14 yr, m	Shortness of breath. Huge anterior medias-tinal mass with a smooth margin enveloping normal mediastinal structures	Thymectomy	1950 g	GRAHAM et al. 1990

[a] Lymphocytosis disappeared after total thymectomy. Phytohemagglutinin blastogenesis was normal in peripheral blood lymphocytes but diminished in the thymic cells. The etiology of lymphocytosis is unknown. The authors postulated that a disorder in T suppressor activity may have been a factor in their case

[b] Disappeared after thymectomy

[c] In both instances the hyperplasia was demonstrated by morphometric studies using the point-counting method

[d] Steroid therapy without effect on the mediastinal mass

[e] Normal number of peripheral T lymphocytes and normal lymphocyte proliferation assays

Pathologic laboratory findings may also be absent, but, if present, they mostly concern the peripheral leukocyte blood count. Seven of the 14 cases in Table 7.2 (cases 5, 6, 7, 9, 11, 12, and 13) did not reveal any abnormal results of routine laboratory tests. The remaining four cases presented with leukocytosis (case 10) or lymphocytosis (cases 2, 3, 4) with (cases 2, 3) or without (case 4) and increase in the number of peripheral T lymphocytes. Hypogammaglobulinemia was detected in one case (case 2) 6 months after thymectomy. The authors postulate that the thymic hyperplasia might have induced hypogammaglobulinemia through an imbalance of the T–B cell ratio in the peripheral lymphoid organs (a mediastinal lymph node with an expanded T cell zone was examined) and blood. This hypothesis, however, could not be proven and congenital or acquired hypogammaglobulinemia could not be ruled out.

The morphology in many instances is not well illustrated or defined and it is conceivable that many cases of "thymic hyperplasia" (borderline enlargement) are examples of lymphofollicular hyperplasia. This might be true not only for those cases without histologic examination, but also for those in which only a small biopsy obtained through mediastinoscopy or only one random section of the thymectomy specimen is examined. The number of lymph follicles in lymphofollicular hyperplasia of the thymus varies considerably from case to case and between different histologic slides from the same specimen (GRODY et al. 1986). Therefore, if only one random section of the specimen is examined, the correct diagnosis of lymphofollicular hyperplasia might be overlooked.

Thymectomy specimens of very well documented cases are macroscopically encapsulated. Histologic examination reveals a normal, lobular thymic architecture with a clear demarcation of the dark cortical and the lighter medullary areas. As usual the cortex contains many more lymphocytes than the medulla, were Hassall's corpuscles, normal in distribution and number, can be found. No lymph follicles with germinal centers occur within the specimen.

Etiology and pathogenesis of this rare lesion still remain to be elucidated. The most convenient explanation for its formation is thymic hyperfunction or dysfunction, which might be related to the endocrine activity of the thymic epithelial cells. This was suggested by LACK (1981), KATZ et al. (1977), and more recently NEZELOF and NORMAND (1986). The findings of lymphocytosis with high numbers of peripheral T cells in some of the reported cases, and the expansion of the thymus-dependent area in a lymph node near the resected thymus in another case, would argue for thymic hyperfunction with an effect on the peripheral lymphoid organs. Thymic dysfunction, on the other hand, with an arrest in T cell differentiation and an accumulation of immature T cells, could be postulated on the basis of the findings of NEZELOF and NORMAND (1986). They found that the number of mature T lymphocytes, estimated by the intracellular dot-like α-naphthyl acetate esterease activity, was markedly reduced in three cases of massive thymic hyperplasia in comparison with normal control thymus. Lastly, besides the functional disturbances a mechanical one has been discussed by LACK (1981), who found an increase in perivascular collagen in one of his two reported cases. Since the perivascular spaces are believed to be the pathway of lymphocyte emigration from the thymus (see Sect. 2.2), an increase of the perivascular collagen might inhibit the normal migration and lead to a local accumulation of T cells.

The fact that thymic hyperplasia with massive enlargement can simulate malignant mediastinal tumors and tumor-like lesions, however, is of greater practical concern (see also Sect. 7.4.7). Tumors of the anterior mediastinum to be considered in the differential diagnosis of thymic hyperplasia with massive enlargement are thymoma, carcinoid tumors of the thymus, thymolipoma, Hodgkin's disease or non-Hodgkin's lymphomas, neoplasms of germ cell origin, Castleman's disease, and cysts of various histogenesis. If a child with a newly recognized mass is thriving and if most of the alternative possibilities have been ruled out by appropriate clinical and laboratory evaluation, the patient can just be observed carefully. A trial of corticosteroid therapy, as proposed by CAFFEY and SILBEY (1960), should only be done if a corticosteroid-sensitive tumor can be ruled out. A brief course of corticosteroids will often shrink the hyperplastic thymus within a few days. However, this measure is not conclusive in all cases and also failed to be effective in one of two cases in Table 7.2 (see also Sect. 6.2). Therefore, diagnostic mediastinoscopy or, in the case of severe respiratory symptoms, a thoracotomy with resection of the mediastinal mass may be recessary. Thymic hyperplasia can then be easily diagnosed because it is histologically different from all the tumors mentioned here.

7.4.2.3 Thymic Rebound in Childhood and Adolescence (see also Sect. 7.4.6)

The phenomenon of rebound or regeneration of thymic tissue in children has been described in a number of conditions, including recovery from severe thermal burns (GELFAND et al. 1972; LEE et al. 1979) or cardiac surgery (RIZK et al. 1972), after ending oral administration of steroids (CAFFEY and SILBEY 1960), and following recovery from tuberculosis (BERTOYE et al. 1956).

This phenomenon of thymic rebound has also been reported after treatment for Hodgkin's disease (GRISSOM et al. 1983; SHIN and HO 1983; CARMOSINO et al. 1985; TARTAS et al. 1985). Furthermore, it has been described after treatment for other malignancies such as lymphoblastic leukemia, malignant lymphoma, poorly differentiated lymphocytic lymphoma, Wilms' tumor, osteosarcoma of the left distal femur, malignant abdominal teratoma (HILL and DODD 1970; COHEN et al. 1980), embryonal rhabdomyosarcoma of the left testicle (BELL et al. 1984), and germ cell tumors of the ovary and testicle (CARMOSINO et al. 1985; DÜE et al. 1988; DIECKMANN et al. 1988).

The histologic appearance of this type of thymic hyperplasia is the same as that of true thymic hyperplasia with massive enlargement of the gland as discussed in the previous section. It is merely the circumstances and the possible pathogenetic explanations of this type of thymic hyperplasia that differentiate the two. The microtopography and cellular composition of the enlarged thymus glands are the same as in normal thymus, as could be shown by immunohistologic examination of one case of thymic rebound hyperplasia (DÜE et al. 1988). After treatment of a malignant tumor, this form of thymic hyperplasia may simulate radiologically a recurrence or a metastasis.

Pathogenetically, different factors can be implicated as the cause of thymic hyperplasia in these patients. The reversal of greatly elevated endogeneous corticosteroid levels in patients with severe thermal burns (GELFAND et al. 1972), the withdrawal of exogenous corticosteroids and antimitotic drugs in patients with malignancies (HILL and DODD 1970; SHIN and HO 1983), or the stimulatory effects of the cellular-mediated immunity by viral infections (GRISSOM et al. 1983) might, alone or in combination, cause thymic hyperplasia under certain conditions. However, these factors can only cause thymic hyperplasia in a susceptible thymus. The age-dependent size of the thymus with thymic atrophy during ageing indicates a functionally active thymus in childhood and adolescence which might be suceptible to such effects. Indeed, most of the reported cases were 20-month- to 12-year-old children; only four patients were between 19 and 33 years old. The occurrence of thymic rebound hyperplasia in patients with malignant tumors has recently been reported to represent an immunologic rebound phenomenon that can be used clinically as a good prognostic indicator of successful control of Hodgkin's disease and other malignancies (COHEN et al. 1980).

7.4.2.4 True Thymic Hyperplasia in Association with Other Diseases (see also Sect. 7.4.4)

Rare instances of nonneoplastic enlargement of the thymus have also been described in patients with endocrine abnormalities, sarcoidosis (OH et al. 1971; PARDO-MINDAN et al. 1980), or the Beckwith-Wiedemann syndrome (BALCOM et al. 1985). This enlargement is due to a true thymic hyperplasia which again, on histologic grounds, cannot be distinguished from true thymic hyperplasia with massive enlargement or thymic rebound hyperplasia as discussed in the two previous sections. For instance, it has been found that in cases of thyrotoxicosis (the so-called thymic form of Graves' disease) and in children treated for hypothyroidism (NICHOLSON 1978; YULISH and OWENS 1980; ROSE and LAM 1982) an enlargement of the thymus occurred.

SCHEIFF et al. (1977) studied the influence of thyroid hormones on the size of the thymus in their experimental work on thymic hyperplasia. To our knowledge, this is the only experimental study on this subject. In their murine model of thymic hyperplasia induced by triiodothyronine administration, they demonstrated a twofold increase in the total number of epithelial cells in both the cortex and the medulla. However, whereas the number of epithelial cells per unit volume also increased in the medulla, this value decreased in the cortex, indicating that the volume of the thymic cortex was mainly increased by the nonepithelial component, i.e., the lymphocytes.

Thus, thymic hyperplasia induced by triidothyronine administration is caused by multiplication and proliferation of epithelial cells in both the cortex and the medulla on the one hand and by invasion or proliferation of lymphocytes in the cortex on the other hand. Thereby the cortical volume is increased twofold and the medullary volume about 1.6-fold. Since these data were obtained by delicate morphometric studies using semithin and ultrathin sections of the tissue, it is doubtful whether these criteria can be used in the differential diagnosis of thymic hyperplasia in normal histologic tissue sections.

Other conditions in which true thymic hyperplasia occurs include Addison's disease, acromegaly, congenital absence of the pituitary gland, and anencephaly (GOLDSTEIN and MACKAY 1969; POTTER and CRAIG 1975).

7.4.2.5 Lymphofollicular Hyperplasia of the Thymus

Lymphofollicular hyperplasia of the thymus has been described in autoimmune diseases such as myasthenia gravis, systemic lupus erythematosus, scleroderma, rheumatoid arthritis, periarteritis nodosa, Hashimoto's thyroiditis, autoimmune anemia, Behçet's disease, and Sjögren's syndrome (ROSAI and LEVINE 1976; LEVINE and ROSAI 1978; OTTO 1984; TRIDENTE 1985). The characteristic nonneoplastic lesion of the thymus in myasthenia gravis, for example, is lymphofollicular hyperplasia. Between 60% and 90% of myasthenia patients show such thymic changes (SLOAN 1943; CASTLEMAN and NORRIS 1949; KIRCHNER et al. 1986). Further thymic abnormalities include an increased number of B lymphocytes, T helper cells, myoid cells (JUDD 1987; SATO and TAMAOKI 1989), and epithelial cells containing detectable intracytoplasmic thymosin (DALAKAS et al. 1981; SCADDING et al. 1981; THOMAS et al. 1982; KORNSTEIN et al. 1984).

Lymphofollicular hyperplasia of the thymus can also be observed in patients with ulcerative colitis, multiple sclerosis, and hepatic cirrhosis and other liver diseases, in some endocrinopathies (Addison's disease, thyrotoxicosis, acromegaly, gonadal hypofunction, diabetes), and in chronic disseminated infections (toxoplasmosis). Lymphofollicular hyperplasia has also been found in epithelial thymic tumors and in the uninvolved portion of a thymus with a thymoma.

The size of the thymus in lymphofollicular hyperplasia lies within the normal range (CASTLEMAN and NORRIS 1949; ROSAI and LEVINE 1976; LEVINE and ROSAI 1978). Lymphofollicular hyperplasia of the thymus is defined by its histologic appearance (CASTLEMAN and NORRIS 1949; ROSAI and LEVINE 1976).

Histologically lymph follicles with germinal centers are found in the thymic medulla (Fig. 7.13).

Their number, however, varies considerably from case to case and even within one case (GRODY et al. 1986). Thus, if lymphofollicular hyperplasia of the thymus is suspected, sections from different regions of the organ should be examined in order to rule out the presence or absence of lymph follicles. The medullary area seems to be blown up by the presence of lymph follicles and the thymic cortex is arranged in the form of a cap covering this region. Thymuses with lymphofollicular hyperplasia may also present with fatty involution, depending on the patient's age.

The configuration, microtopography, cellular composition, ultrastructure, and immunohistologic findings of thymic germinal centers in lymphofollicular hyperplasia associated with myasthenia gravis are essentially the same as in those occurring in lymph nodes and in other lymphatic tissue. Ultrastructurally and immunohistologically the cellular population is composed of long branching dendritic reticulum cells, lymphocytes in various stages of transformation, and "starry sky" macrophages, and the marginal zone is populated by small lymphocytes.

Immunohistology with monoclonal antibodies against B cell differentiation antigens is a useful tool in those cases where the lymph follicles are rare or difficult to detect morphologically. Aggregates of the B cell population are clearly visible by the reaction of the cells with such antibodies. Furthermore, the relation of the lymph follicles in lymphofollicular hyperplasia to the different compartments of the thymus becomes evident when using immunohistologic methods.

Staining with antikeratin serum quite clearly reveals the borders between thymic and extrathymic compartments. Thus two statements about the localization of the lymph follicles in the lymphofollicular hyperplastic thymus can be made: (a) there is a very clear demarcation line between the lymph follicles and the thymic medulla, consisting of a continuous row of epithelial cells; and (b) the lymphofollicular hyperplastic tissue is connected with the surrounding fat and connective tissue of the interlobular septa.

These two facts suggest that the lymphofollicular hyperplastic tissue originates from the interlobular fibrous septa; as the connection to the fibrous septa has the shape of a stalk, it depends very much on the section level whether this connection is visible or not. Thus, for geometric reasons the most frequent picture to be seen is that of lymph follicles seeming to be embedded in the thymic medulla.

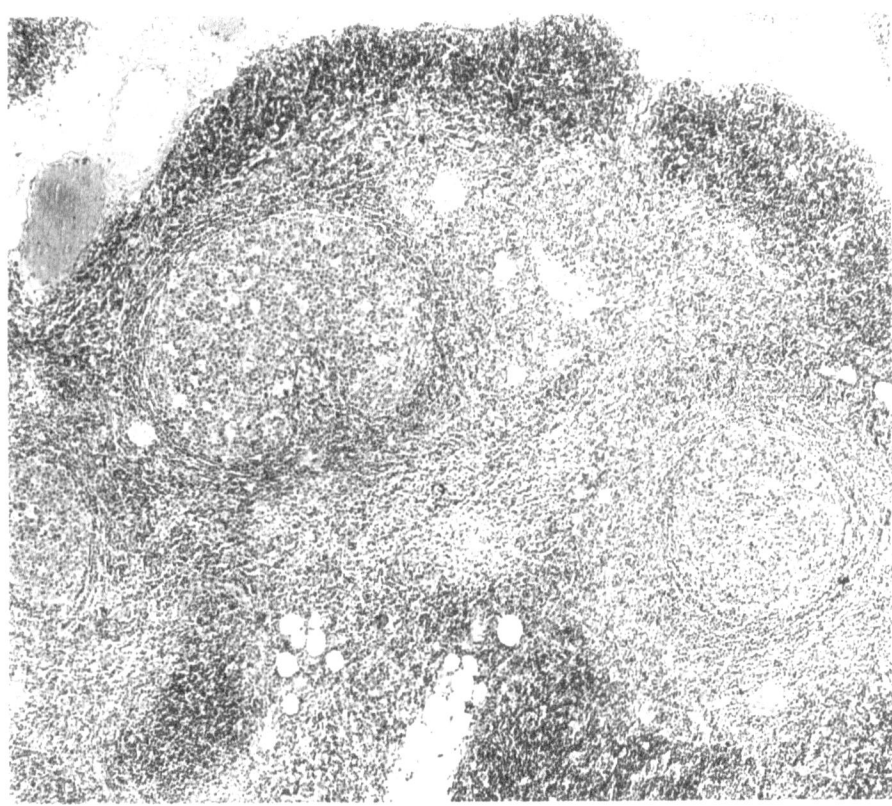

Fig. 7.13. Lymphofollicular hyperplasia of the thymus with active germinal centers. Three lymph follicles are seemingly situated within thymic medulla. Atrophic thymic cortex. Epithelial cells and Hassall's corpuscles are seen in the intervening zone. Female, 31 years old, myasthenia gravis, thymectomy specimen 80 g. (OTTO 1984) H&E, x80

During further development of the lesion this border between the extraparenchymal zone with the lymph follicles and the thymic medulla may be interrupted (BOFILL et al. 1985; KIRCHNER et al. 1986), thus facilitating the B lymphocytes infiltrating the thymic medulla, a situation which is also called "thymitis" (OTTO 1984; KIRCHNER et al. 1986). This infiltration of the thymic medulla by B lymphocytes in the course of lymphofollicular hyperplasia and myasthenia gravis, however, has to be distinguished from the previously reported physiologic occurrence of B lymphocytes within the thymic medulla (HOFMANN et al. 1988 a, b.).

Diagnosis of lymphofollicular hyperplasia of the thymus should not be difficult in those cases where a thymectomy is performed for myasthenia gravis when a thymus of normal weight is removed, showing the typical histologic picture of lymphofollicular hyperplasia. However, if a biopsy of an anterior mediastinal tumor shows thymic tissue with lymphofollicular hyperplasia this is most probably not the cause of the mediastinal widening, since a thymus with lymphofollicular hyperplasia is not greatly enlarged and its weight lies within normal limits. Thus, tumors of the anterior mediastinum which can be associated with lymphofollicular hyperplasia of the thymus, i.e., thymoma or metastasizing tumors, should be ruled out by a second biopsy.

Lesions which might be confused with lymphofollicular hyperplasia of the thymus because of their microscopic appearance are angiofollicular lymph node hyperplasia (giant lymph node hyperplasia, Castleman's disease) of the anterior mediastinum and follicular lymphomas. Both lesions, however, clinically present as mediastinal masses, a feature uncommon for lymphofollicular hyperplasia of the thymus. On histologic examination, the absence of thymic tissue, the hyalinization of the centers of lymphoid follicles in the hyaline–vascular type of giant lymph node hyperplasia, and the numerous plasma cells in the plasma cell type of giant lymph node hyperplasia help to distinguish this lesion from lymphofollicular hyperplasia of the thymus.

7.4.3 Clinical Features

E. WILLICH

The hyperplastic thymus is clinically important:
- If it causes clinical symptoms like stridor or dyspnea (TISCHER 1967; LAMESCH et al. 1974)
- If it limits the normal expansion of the lungs (PARKER et al. 1985): compression atelectasis of the lungs can lead to respiratory distress, chronic recurrent infections, and bronchopneumonia
- If it cannot be distinguished from tumor
- If it causes cardiac symptoms: an enlarged thymus can compress the heart and the great vessels in such a manner that the pulmonary blood circulation (input as well as output) is impaired.

7.4.3.1 Asymptomatic Thymic Hyperplasia

In half of the cases thymic hyperplasia is incidentaly detected on a routine chest radiograph (WHITTAKER and LYNN 1973). As long ago as 1934 CAPPER and SCHLESS correlated clinical symptoms with radiologically enlarged thymus glands in 1074 newborns and did not find any close relationships. CAFFEY (1950) also rejected the large thymus as a cause of clinical symptoms.

The asymptomatic thymus presents the physician with the question of appropriate therapeutic procedure (see Sect. 7.4.8).

7.4.3.2 Symptomatic Thymic Hyperplasia

The relationship between a large or hyperplastic thymus and clinical symptoms has been discussed since the beginning of the century (HOCHSINGER 1903; FRIEDJUNG 1910; BIRK 1918). Thymic hyperplasia, proven by autopsy, was held responsible for the sudden infant death syndrome ("mors thymica") by anatomists (PALTAUF 1910) and clinicians (WALDBOTT 1934). Furthermore, irradiation of the enlarged thymus was first suggested in 1907 (see Sect. 7.4.8), since its disappearance had been observed after radiation therapy. Stridor caused by hyperplastic thymus also disappeared (see below).

The findings in symptomatic thymic hyperplasia are mostly unspecific, and it is not always possible to establish clearly that the hyperplasia is responsible for these symptoms, as, for example, in the case of the four young infants reported by KOBOYASHI et al. (1986) (Table 7.3, cases 22–25), in whom an increase in the respiratory symptoms following compression of thoracic organs or narrowing of the airways had been assumed. Dyspnea, cyanosis, asthmoid coughing, dysphagia, and recurrent upper respiratory tract infection have been described, as has stridor (so-called stridor thymicus) in newborns.

In 1903 HOCHSINGER became the first to claim that so-called congenital stridor was due to the thymus. For decades this view was reiterated in journals (e.g., BRUCE and GRAVES 1922) and also in numerous pediatric textbooks (FRIEDJUNG 1910; FISCHL 1923; MITCHELL-NELSON 1945; PFAUNDLER 1948; GLANZMANN 1949). Radiation therapy of the thymus and operative intervention were the consequences. Doubt was subsequently cast on the existence of "thymogenic stridor," until numerous authors flatly rejected any possibility that a large thymus could influence respiration (CAFFEY and SILBEY 1960; AMANN 1962; HOPE et al. 1963; HALLER et al. 1969; THAL 1972).

On the other hand FISCHL in 1923 on 30 published cases of thymogenic stridor, and other authors subsequently reported cases which were either confirmed at operation and displayed disappearance of the stridor postoperatively (LEINISCH 1963; TISCHER 1967: six out of ten operated cases; POKORNY and SHERMAN 1974; EBEL 1980; LAMESCH 1983; see Table 7.2, case 7, and Table 7.3, cases 5–10, 14) or in which the stridor disappeared after steroid therapy, in conjunction with a reduction in the size of the thymus. After discontinuing the medication the thymus grew again, causing stridor, which, however, disappeared after steroid intake (BIERICH and SCHMIDT-GRIMMINGER 1966). When ste-

Fig. 7.14a–f. Hyperplastic thymus in a 6-month-old infant with "congenital stridor." **a** Chest radiograph – frontal view: Massive homogeneous shadowing of the left upper lung field. Mediastinal enlargement on the right side. **b** Lateral view: the "mass" occupies the whole middle and posterior mediastinum in the upper half. Stenosis of the trachea to 2 mm (arrows). **c₁** Transverse ultrasonographic scan: the thymus is demonstrated as a region of homogeneous echo texture with moderate echogenicity. **d₁** Longitudinal ultrasonographic scan (transducer positioned ventrally in the jugulum): extension of the thymus from ventral to dorsal (see **c₂, d₂**). **e,f** CT without and with enhancement: The extension of the thymus from substernal to the left posterior thoracic cavity is recognizable. There is a broad connection with the anterior thoracic wall. Density 60 HU. After contrast injection (**f**) the great vessels are not impressed by the adjacent thymus. Definite exclusion of a tumor was nevertheless not possible. Thoracotomy with partial extirpation. Histology: normal thymic tissue. (Courtesy of Priv. Doz. Dr. H. TSCHÄPPELER, Bern, Switzerland)

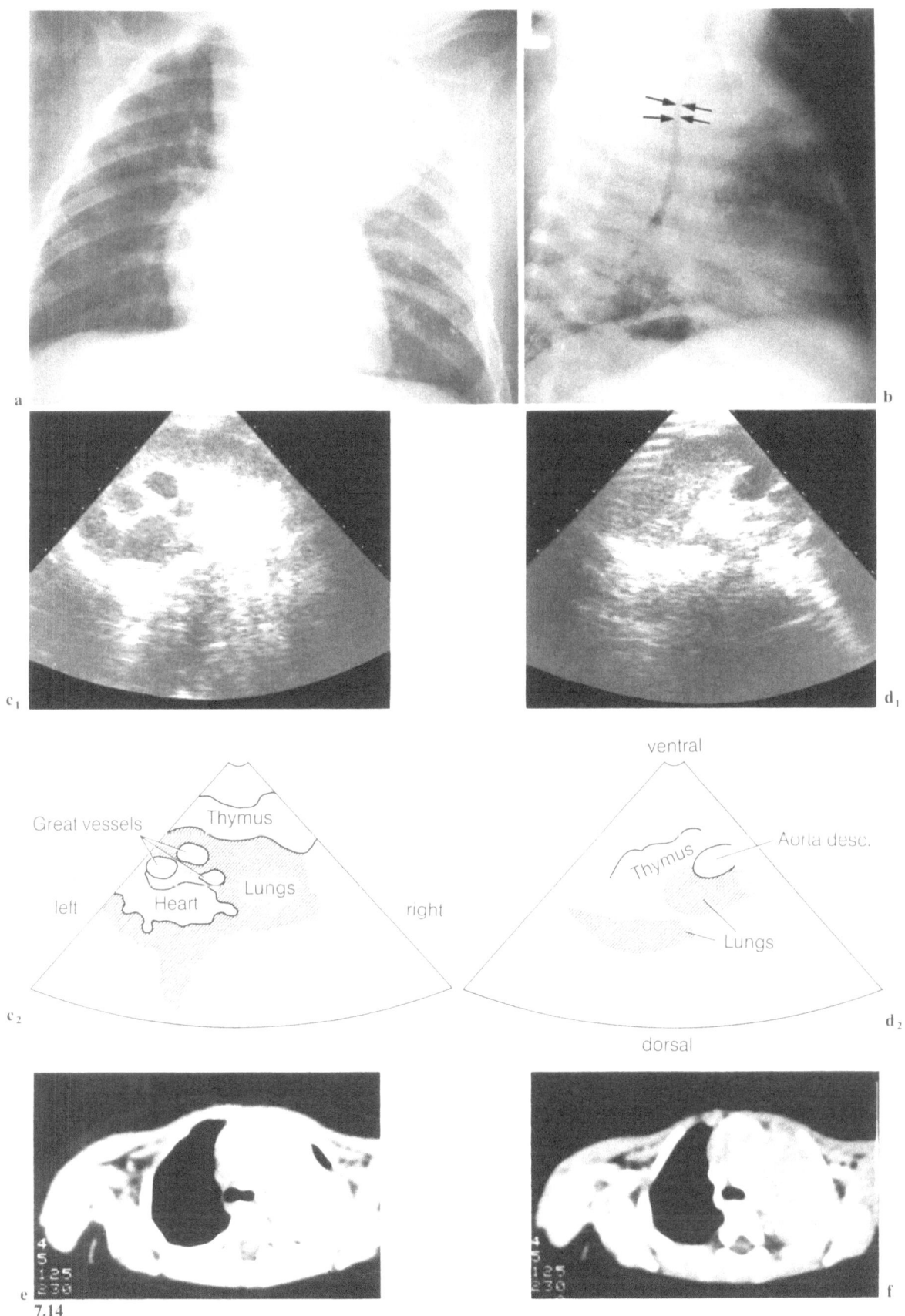

7.14

Table 7.3. Clinicoradiologic features of thymic hyperplasia with massive enlargement. Analysis of 27 cases since 1970, compiled by E. Willich (excludes the 14 cases detailed in Table 7.2)

Case no.	Age/sex	Clinical and radiologic findings	Imaging method	Treatment	Weight and size of the thymus	Follow-up	Reference
1	4 mo, m	Dyspnea, cyanosis, sub- and intercostal retraction, rapid deterioration. Massive shadow of the right hemithorax	Chest radiography	Extirpation	80 g	–	Kim et al. 1972
2	3 wk, f	Dyspnea, cyanosis, cervicofacial angioma, expiratory bulging substernally, wearingness. Rounded shadow in the anterior and superior mediastinum with compression of the trachea	Chest radiography	Substernal excision of two nodules. "Benign thymoma"?	–	–	Kim et al. 1972
3, 4	15 yr, m; age and sex not reported in other case	Suspected for mediastinal tumor. No clinical symptoms. Radiography: right mediastinal enlargement	Chest radiography. Fluoroscopy: mass observed to pulsate. Angiocardiography: normal. Esophagography: normal	Thoracotomy, excision	–	–	Whittaker and Lynn 1973
5–10	0–28 mo	Mild respiratory distress shortly after birth. Bronchoscopy was performed in three cases; two showed anterior-posterior compression of the trachea	Chest radiography	Thoracotomy in one case, conservative treatment in five	51.5 g, 4 × 6 cm (one case)	Postoperative course uneventful	Pokorny and Shermann 1974
11	5½ yr, f	Recurrent pharyngotonsillitis. Wolff-Parkinson-White syndrome. Routine examination: shadow in the left superior mediastinum. Steroid test positive	Chest radiography	Thoracotomy	36 g	Uneventful	Blasimann et al. 1977
12	9 mo, m	Pleural empyema at the age of 1 mo; 4 months later "shadow" in the upper third of the left hemithorax	Chest radiography	Surgical exploration	78 g	Uneventful	Blasimann et al. 1977
13	22 mo, f	Scalding 4 weeks previously. Large anterior mediastinal mass. No symptoms. Retraction of the substernal notch and intercostal muscles during respiration. Lung fields bilaterally specified. Prednisone test: no regression	Chest radiography. Ultrasonography: solid mass. Isotope angiography: nonvascular	Thoracotomy Excision	550 g 19 × 12 × 4.5 cm	Uneventful	Lee et al. 1979
14	4 mo, m	Stridor, inspiratory and expiratory. Suspected vitium cordis; bilateral tumorous shadows in the upper lung fields. Stenosis of the trachea. Steroid test positive	Chest radiography		–	Improvement, but stridor unchanged. Tracheal stenosis probably due to innominate artery	Ebel 1980
15	8 mo, f	Osteomyelitis of the right humerus at birth. Since the age of 2 months, massive shadow in the left upper hemithorax, with progression	Chest radiography, ultrasonography	Operation	–	Uneventful	Ebel 1980
16	7 mo	Since the 5th week of life, infections of the upper airways, compression of the right upper lobe bronchus. Mass in the right upper thorax	Chest radiography, tomography, bronchography	Exploratory thoracotomy	–	Gradual shrinkage of the thymus; reexpansion of the right upper lobe 2 years later	Harris et al. 1980

No.	Age, sex	Clinical findings	Diagnostic method	Treatment	Size/weight	Outcome	Reference
17	11 yr	No clinical symptoms. Mass in the anterior right mediastinum	Chest radiography, pneumomediastinography, tomography	None	–	–	HARRIS et al. 1980
18	"Infant"	"Cardiomegaly," severe sepsis. Apparent mediastinal mass; pulmonary congestion after shrinking thymus – regrowth!	Chest radiography, bronchography	Thoracotomy (excision)	–	–	HARRIS et al. 1980
19	3 yr, m	Suspected tumor of the lung. Respiratory and vascular insufficiency. Radiography: giant mass in the anterior mediastinum in both hemithoraces	Chest radiography	Probative irradiation: regression. Regrowth at 7 years of age: extirpation	–	Death 7 days after operation	DANILEWICZ-WYTRY-CHOWSKA 1981
20 (brother of no. 19)	4 yr 5 mo, m	For the previous 3 years, mass and enlargement of the mediastinum, initially without clinical symptoms. Status at 4 yr 5 mo: respiratory insufficiency, dyspnea, cyanosis, stridor, and fever. Giant mass over both lungs, occupying three-quarters of the thoracic volume	Chest radiography	Extirpation	80 % of the thoracic volume	Follow-up to 18 years of age. Healthy, radiography normal	DANILEWICZ-WYTRY-CHOWSKA 1981
21 (2nd brother of no. 19)	14 yr, m	Six months after birth, normal thymus without clinical findings. Observation with routine controls. Present status: Massive enlargement of the thymus into the left hemithorax at the thoracic wall. Calcifications in the mass. Laboratory findings: normal	Chest radiography	Corticosteroids: slight regression. Regrowth after 2 months. Conservative treatment with steroids	–	Without clinical symptoms	DANILEWICZ-WYTRY-CHOWSKA 1981
22	1 mo, m	Dyspnea, cough, wheezing, and cyanosis, without fever. Massive shadow in the right upper hemithorax. Steroid test negative	Chest radiography, CT	Intensive care	–	Well	KOBAYASHI et al. 1986
23	2 mo, m	Cough, dyspnea, nasal discharge, pneumonia shadow in both upper lobes and a mass in the right upper chest (anterior mediastinum). Steroid test positive	Chest radiography, CT	Intensive care	–	Well	KOBAYASHI et al. 1986
24	4 mo, m	Severe productive cough. Huge mass in the right middle and upper chest. Pneumonia shadow without fever. Steroid test negative	Chest radiography, CT	Symptomatic	–	Improvement	KOBAYASHI et al. 1986
25	2 wk, f	Cough, severe dyspnea, and tachypnea, without fever. Mass in the right upper hemithorax	Chest radiography? CT	–	–	–	KOBAYASHI et al. 1986
26	7 wk, m	Upper respiratory tract infections, bronchiolitis, anemia, tracheal stenosis, anterior mediastinal mass in the left hemithorax	Chest radiography, Perfusion and ventilation scintigraphy	Thoracotomy	72 g	Uneventful	THOMAS and GUPTA 1988
27	17 mo, f	Respiratory distress, anterior mediastinal mass, right upper lobe atelectasis. Huge mass in the entire right thoracic cavity	Chest radiography	Prednisolone. Open biopsy (mini-sternotomy). Endotracheal intubation, mechanical ventilation	–	8 months later, malignant mesenchymoma	ATTAR et al. 1988

roid therapy fails it is still unclear whether this is due to a nonresponsive thymus or to other causes, as has been suggested by EBEL (1980) in one case of tracheal stenosis due to innominate artery (see table 7.3, case 14).

With regard to differential diagnosis, in the presence of a large thymus, frequent causes of stridor should be excluded clinically and radiologically. Such causes include tracheomalacia, physiologic congenital stridor in the 1st year of life, aortic ring or other vessel anomalies, laryngeal malformations, congenital guiter, and foreign bodies (TISCHER 1967; STROBL 1985). Apart form chest radiography in two planes, functional examination of the trachea on 100 mm spot films, ultrasonography, and esophagography in two planes are indispensable.

Diagnosis of thymogenic stridor is only justified if:

- There is radiologic evidence of hyperplastic, dystopic, or accessory thymic tissue (Figs. 7.4, 7.14)
- There is bronchoscopic or operative evidence of stenosis in the respiratory system
- If, after thymectomy or steroid therapy, the thymus and the stenosis on the radiograph and also the clinical symptoms have disappeared and do not return.

On the basis of their own experience with a 6-week-old infant, BAR-ZIV et al. (1984) pointed out that thymus-related stridor is always expiratory and is caused by a pathologic organic process, i.e., that the trachea is compressed by a dystopic thymus or accessory thymic lobes in the posterior mediastinum without enlargement of the gland (cf. two young infants reported by SHACKELFORD and McALISTER (1974)], or that a thymic cyst or a thymic tumor compressed the trachea, causing stridor (cf. case 2, Table 7.3, reported by KIM et al. 1972).

Extirpation of the thymus is only indicated if the symptoms are definitely caused by the thymus and if steroid resistance, severe symptoms, or recurrence upon discontinuation of steroid medication are present (KIM et al. 1972) (see also Sect. 7.4.8).

Overall, thymogenic stridor remains a "rarity worthy of publication" (KEUTH 1974).

Respiratory or cardiovascular symptoms can be caused by the thymus compressing or displacing neighboring organs such as the lungs and great vessels. Numerous case reports have discribed severe symptoms in association with thymic hyperplasia, necessitating surgery. Such cases include: two

children with respiratory distress syndrome and tracheal stenosis (SEALY et al. 1965), a young infant with cyanosis and shortness of breath (KIM et al. 1972), two relatives with severe respiratory symptoms (DANILEWICZ-WYTRYCHOWSKA 1981), a 14-year-old girl (OH et al. 1971), one infant with compression of the upper lung lobe (HARRIS et al. 1980), and one infant with lung compression (PARKER et al. 1985) (see Table 7.2, case 8, and Table 7.3, cases 1, 2, 16, 19, and 20).

However, symptoms can arise as a result of thymic dystopia alone, i.e., without hyperplasia, as in the third case reported by SHACKELFORD and McALISTER (1974): a 4-month-old girl with stenosis and dislocation of the right main and intermediary bronchi causing obstructive emphysema of the middle and lower lung lobes. BISTRITZER et al. (1985) described a 5-month-old boy with dyspnea and dysphagia caused by a cervical thymus weighing 75 g. Another patient of our own with chronic recurrent infections is described in Fig. 7.20. He suffered from bronchial compression caused by a large thymus and upper lung lobe atelectasis.

Children with slight or mild respiratory problems should not be operated on. Such problems existed, for example, in five out of seven pediatric cases reported by POKORNY and SHERMAN (1974); bronchoscopy was performed in three of these children, revealing tracheal compression in one. A 3-year-old boy reported by DANILEWICZ-WYTRYCHOWSKA (1981) (Table 7.3, case 19) and four young infants reported by KOBAYASHI et al. (1986) (Table 7.3, cases 22–25) were also treated conservatively.

Esophageal compression with dysphagia as a result of a hyperplastic thymus is an absolute rarity. One such case was a 12-year-old boy with a thymic weight of 245 g (average for age: 34 ± 15 g, described by JUDD (1987) (Table 7.2, case 12).

Tables 7.2 and 7.3 reviews 41 case histories, detailing the clinicopathologic and clinicoradiologic features.

According to SILVERMAN (1985) 80 % of cases of thymic hyperplasia occur in males.

BIRK (1918), SLOWIKOWSKI (1968), and DANILEWICZ-WYTRYCHOWSKA (1981) have described a certain familial disposition toward thymic hyperplasia.

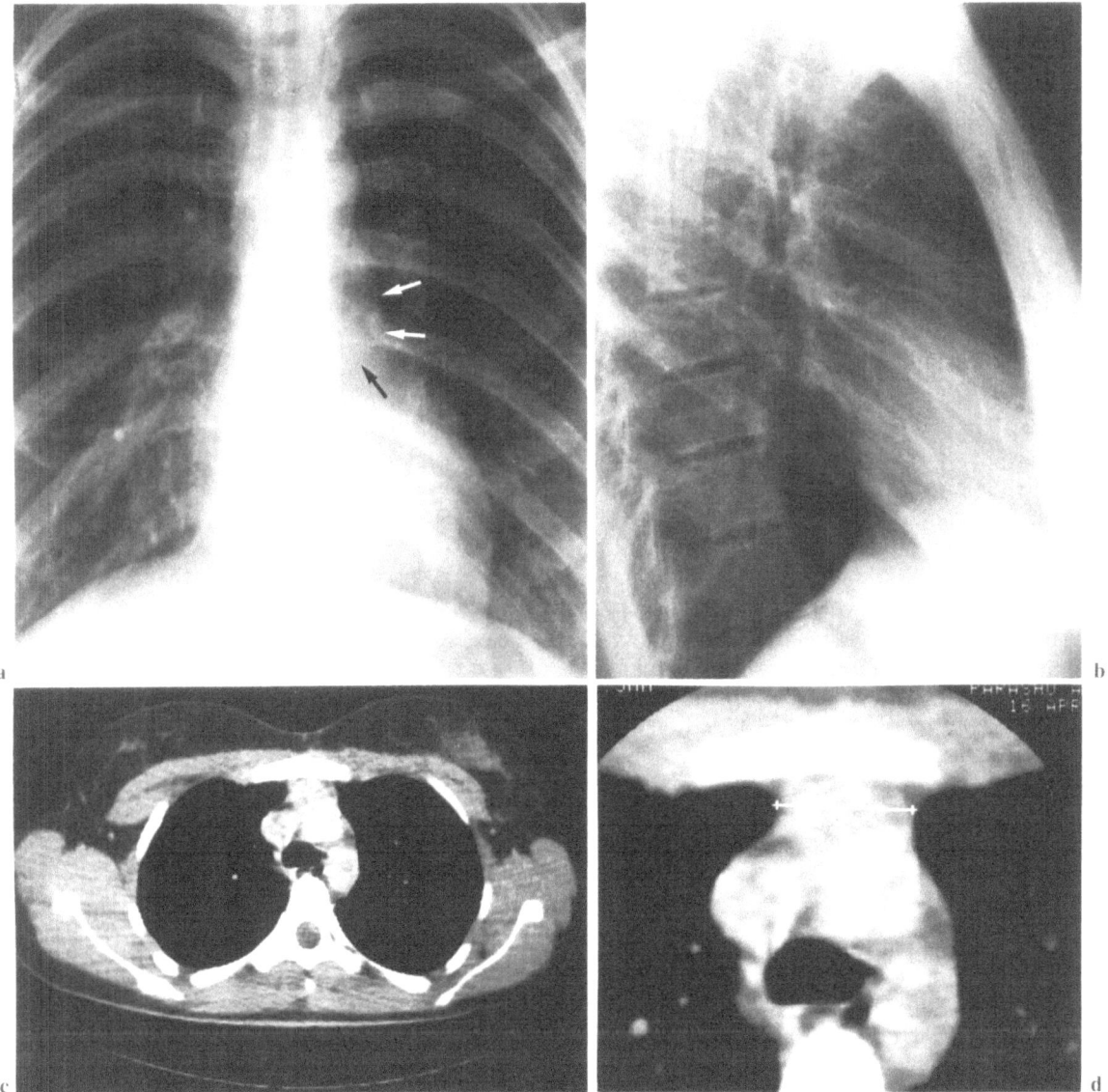

7.4.4 Associated Diseases (see also Sect. 7.4.2.4)

Myasthenia gravis pseudoparalytica is the fore-most disease associated with thymic hyperplasia (see Chap. II). In 65% of cases of myasthenia, thymic hyperplasia or persistence is found; in 25% there is a normal thymus and the other 10% relate to thymomas. However, there are three different forms of manifestation according to age group:

Thymic hyperplasia in the *newborn,* which is detected in 10%–15% of young infants of mothers with myasthenia, seems to represent a transient form. The *juvenile form* begins earlier than the 21st year of life, presenting with blepharoptosis, general weakness, shortness of breath, bulbar par-

Fig. 7.15a–d. Thymic hyperplasia associated with myasthenia gravis in a 15-year-old girl. **a** Chest radiograph: para-aortally situated and 3 cm long shadowing, laterally convexed *(arrows)* and overlapping the left upper border of the heart. **b** Lateral view: suspected pigeon egg-sized shadow above the upper heart border. No clear-cut pathologic finding. **c,d** CT at the aortic level. Total scan and magnification: 4 × 2 × 4 cm mass, suspicious for thymic tumor in the anterior mediastinum, reaching to the aortic arch. Surgery: extirpation of the tumor. Histology: lymphofollicular hyperplasia of the thymic parenchyma. (Courtesy of Prof. Dr. M. Georgi, Mannheim, FRG)

alysis, or ophthalmoplegia. The *adult form* only starts after the 21st year of life. This distinction is important because of the thymic histology: 10 %– 15 % of the adults suffer from thymomas, whereas they are very rarely found in the juvenile form. In contrast, thymic hyperplasia has been diagnosed in between 50 % (TORKALSRUD et al. 1970, cited by THURMOND and BRASCH 1978) and 75 % (THURMOND and BRASCH 1978) of juvenile cases (Fig. 7.15).

THURMOND and BRASCH reported in 1978 on 19 patients, 9–20 years old, 16 of whom were females. Nothing abnormal had been detected on 17 chest radiographs in two planes, but only 2 of the 19 patients had normal thymus glands histologically: the rest displayed hyperplasia and/or abnormal germinal centers inside the thymus. Computed tomography (CT) had been performed in one 16-year-old boy and did not reveal any pathology (nor was any evident histologically). In the age group up to 21 years, CT is only recommended following suspicious plain radiographs. Since the average weight of the ten extirpated thymus glands (26 g; range, 16–56 g) was within normal limits, CT seems to be insecure in the diagnosis of hyperplasia, as is also proved by the case illustrated in Fig. 7.15).

MOORE et al. (1982) reported on 2 of 23 thymectomized patients with myasthenia gravis, aged 13 and 22 years, in whom CT yielded a false-positive diagnosis of thymoma. While MOORE et al. (1983) discovered thymic hyperplasia microscopical in 15 (28.3 %) of 53 myasthenia patients, CASTLEMAN (1966) found this disorder in as many as 80 %. CT nevertheless revealed differences between thymic hyperplasia and normal fatty involution only in the four patients aged 11–22 years, because replacement by fatty tissue had not yet taken place. Put another way, in patients aged 20–40 years, with physiologic fatty involution, no such differences were revealed by CT. KIRKS and KOROBKIN (1980) also emphasized the insecurity of CT diagnosis of the thymus in children with myasthenia.

Thymic hyperplasia also occurs in association with thyroid function disorders, and in 5 % of patients in association with hyperthyroidism (VAN HERLE and CHOBRA 1971; NICHOLSON 1978; ROSE and LAM 1982; ALT and HOCHMAN 1982; FORD et al. 1987; SCHNYDER and CANDARDJIS 1987). The question of whether an enlarged thymus can lead to thyrotoxicosis, or conversely, whether thyrotoxicosis can give rise to an enlarged thymus, has been decided in favor of the second possibility, because enlarged thymus glands can be reduced under conservative therapy in patients with thyrotoxicosis (ROSE and LAM 1982).

Tumorous enlarged thymus glands have also been observed following thyroxine therapy for primary hypothyroidism (FRANKEN 1968). An 11-year-old girl reported by YULISH and OWEN (1980) seems to be the only reported patient in whom exogenously administered thyroxine led to huge thymic enlargement (in fact in this case thoracotomy was necessary).

HARRIS et al. (1980) described a 12-year-old boy with recurrent thyroiditis, a cervicomediastinal mass density and swelling. Control examinations over a period of 21 months did not show any change in the size of the "tumor". Biopsy revealed normal thymic tissue.

TESSERAUX (1953) described an association between thymic hyperplasia and Addison's disease and acromegaly. Anencephaly, castration, and periods of increased growth have also been reported in connection with thymic hyperplasia, whereas periods of decreased growth lead to thymic diminution (YULISH and OWENS 1980).

The special relationship between thymic pathology, including thymic functional disorders, and histiocytosis X has been studied by NEWTON et al. (1987) and CONSOLINI et al. (1987) (see Chaps. 3 and 9.4). True thymic involvement, with enlargement of the organ, has been described in histiocytosis by SILVERMAN (1985) in a 2-year-old boy, by FASANELLI et al. (1987) in two infants aged 3 and 5 months, and by SHUANGSHOTI and SEKSARN (1987) in an 11-month-old boy. GOLDSTEIN and MACKAY (1969) also mentioned an association with lupus erythematosus.

Finally, tumorous infiltration of the thymus in cases of leukemia and non-Hodgkin's lymphoma can enlarge the organ, as will be explained in Sect. 8.4.

7.4.5 Imaging Procedures and Findings

In *young children*, plain chest radiography will normally be sufficient for primary diagnosis, although it does not permit differentiation of hyperplasia and thymoma. Usually bilateral enlargement of the mediastinal shadow is visible in hyperplasia (more rarely there is unilateral enlargement), in some cases filling the entire mediastinum from the jugulum to the apex of the heart (Fig. 5.2; COCCHI 1959; OLIVA 1973). The region of the heart base is particularly involved (LACK 1981). The outline of the enlarged mediastinum is clearly

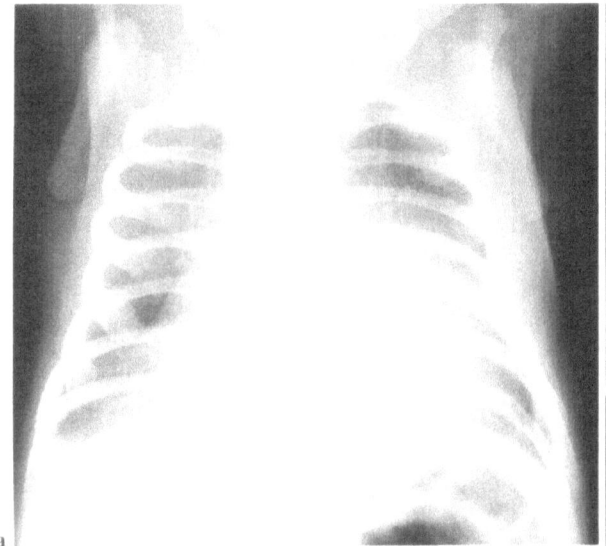

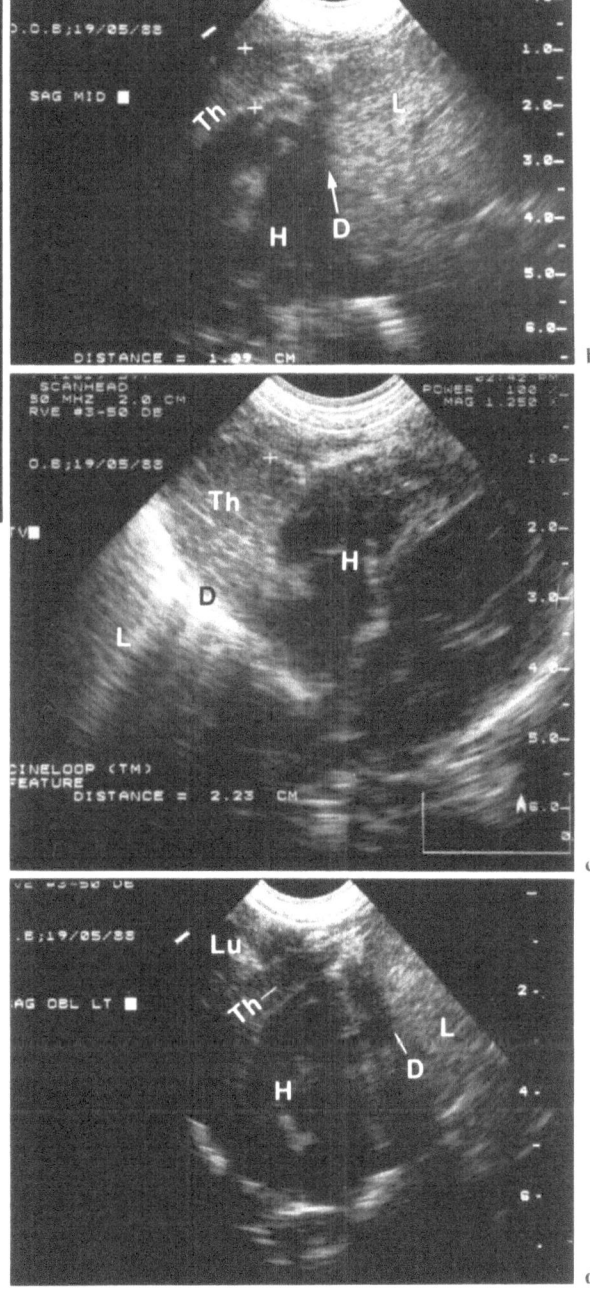

Fig. 7.16 a–d. Large thymus simulating cardiopathy. Routine examination of an infant (2 weeks old) preoperatively. a Plain chest radiograph of the thorax: giant mediastinal shadow overlapping the cardiac margins. b–d Ultrasonography. b Substernal longitudinal midline view: precardiac thymus extending to the diaphragm. c Substernal left oblique view: thymus adjacent to the heart, extending to the diaphragm. d Substernal transverse view: precardiac thymus. *Th*, thymus; *D*, diaphragm; *H*, heart; *L*, liver; *Lu*, lung. (Courtesy of Dr. K. Raschke, Universities of Cape Town, South Africa and Heidelberg, FRG)

defined and convex or straight. On conventional radiographs hyperplasia may appear as a tumor-like mass which, in contrast to normal thymic tissue, can lead to tracheal stenosis (EBEL 1980) (Fig. 7.14; table 7.3, cases 14 and 26). Shadowing of the retrosternal area is found on the lateral view. On *fluoroscopy* a large thymus should be visible, the size varying in accordance with respiration (PARKER et al. 1985).

In *adults* chest radiography in two planes is inefficient for the diagnosis of thymic hyperplasia if the organ is only slightly larger than normal. In our own series of patients (adolescents and adults), as in that of BARON et al. (1982), 50%–60% of those with myasthenia gravis did not show any pathologic process on chest radiographs, although thoracic surgery revealed thymic hyperplasia. *Conventional tomography* does not permit specific differential diagnosis against masses of other origin.

Enlarged thymic lobes with a smooth surface can be detected by *pneumomediastinography*. Definition of the gland is, however, more difficult cranially than caudally (SONE et al. 1980) (Fig. 5.24). Thymic hyperplasia situated immediately supracardially and extending caudally or paracardially may resemble cardiomegaly (see Sect. 7.4.7).

Ultrasonography should definitely be the imaging procedure of choice in children, ahead of invasive methods or procedures entailing exposure to radiation, because even an enlarged thymus displays typical density structures and echogenicity (KIM HAN et al. 1989; VON LENGERKE and SCHMIDT 1988; PARKER et al. 1985) (Fig. 7.16; see also Figs. 5.10, 5.11, 8.43, 8.44, and 8.46).

Computed tomography (CT) has been successfully used by many authors because it also visualizes the neighboring organs (trachea, lungs, great vessels, bronchi) and is of greater diagnostic value than plain radiography. In thymic hyperplasia CT reveals a retrosternally and/or paracardially situated mass or a generally sharp outline (Fig. 7.7 d, 7.12 c). The organ is larger than appropriate for the age (BARON et al. 1982). The solid, homogeneous, and dense tissue portions display attenuation values equivalent to those of normal thymic tissue (WALTER and HÜBENER 1980; BARON et al. 1982). Heterogeneous attenuation values are sometimes obtained due to the presence of areas of fatty degeneration.

Figure 7.14 shows the results of imaging procedures in a 6-month-old infant with stridor, in whom thoracotomy and extirpation of a giant thymus were required to secure the diagnosis and eliminate the stridor.

In *adults*, diagnosis can be very difficult because of the problem of differential diagnosis against tumors (see Chap. 8).

The value of CT is still a subject of controversy today. This while some publications concerning adults emphasize the importance of CT (e.g., SCHNYDER and CANDARDJIS 1987), others deny it (e.g., GLATHE et al. 1989). In children, however, CT has become of prime importance in the diagnosis of hyperplasia (KOBAYASHI et al. 1986).

Magnetic resonance imaging (MRI) allows reliable diagnosis (Fig. 7.8). In children with rebound thymic hyperplasia, the thymus may be increased in size as measured on MRI, relative to the normal range, but the appearance of the thymus on T1- and T2-weighted imaging sequences, and presumably their T1 and T2 values, are unchanged (SIEGEL et al. 1989).

In adults with myasthenia gravis, thymic hyperplasia may also be difficult to distinguish from normal thymus (BATRA et al. 1987). Hyperplastic thymus need not be enlarged. The MR characteristics of normal and hyperplastic thymus in adults do not appear to be significantly different.

In one study (BATRA et al. 1987) of patients with myasthenia gravis who had both CT and MRI, 7 of 16 patients had thymic hyperplasia proven surgically. In five of these seven, both CT and MRI showed normal thymic size and morphology; both thymic lobes were visible in three of these five, and thymic thickness measured from 3 to 9 mm on CT and from 3 to 19.5 mm on MRI. In one of the seven patients with hyperplasia, thicknesses of the right and left lobes were thought to be abnormally increased for the patient's age of 11 years (14 and 17.5 mm on CT, and 12 and 24 mm on MRI, respectively). In the remaining patient with hyperplasia, the thymus appeared normal on CT, but was poorly seen on MRI.

Ventilation and perfusion scintigraphy of the lungs can only determine their function and volume reduction (THOMAS and GUPTA 1988).

7.4.6 Regenerative Hyperplasia (Regrowth, Rebound Phenomenon, see also Sect. 7.4.2.3)

The term "regenerative hyperplasia" describes the regrowth of the thymus subsequent to its diminution or (radiologic) disappearance owing to exogenous stress factors.

Animal experiments have shown that the restitution or recovery of lymphopoietic or immunologic functions after stress situations is dependent on thymus-controlled mechanisms (LAW 1966) and is to be regarded as a prognostically positive sign.

– Regenerative hyperplasia occurs in children upon *recovery after diseases*. It is especially evident after: fever or starvation, tuberculosis (BERTOYE et al. 1956; SILVERMAN 1985), pneumonia (Fig. 7.17) (PARKER et al. 1985) and other consumptive diseases, burns (GELFAND et al. 1972; see also Table 7.3, case 13), surgery for cyanotic cardiac defects (the cyanosis, representing a chronic anoxic stress situation, keeps the thymus small) (SILVERMAN 1985; HOEFFEL et al. 1988), and transposition of the great vessels (RIZK et al. 1972). In general, regenerative hyperplasia can also occur after operations (LAMESCH 1983) and after birth (see Table 7.2, case 7, and Table 7.3, cases 12, 13, 15, 18, 25, and 26).

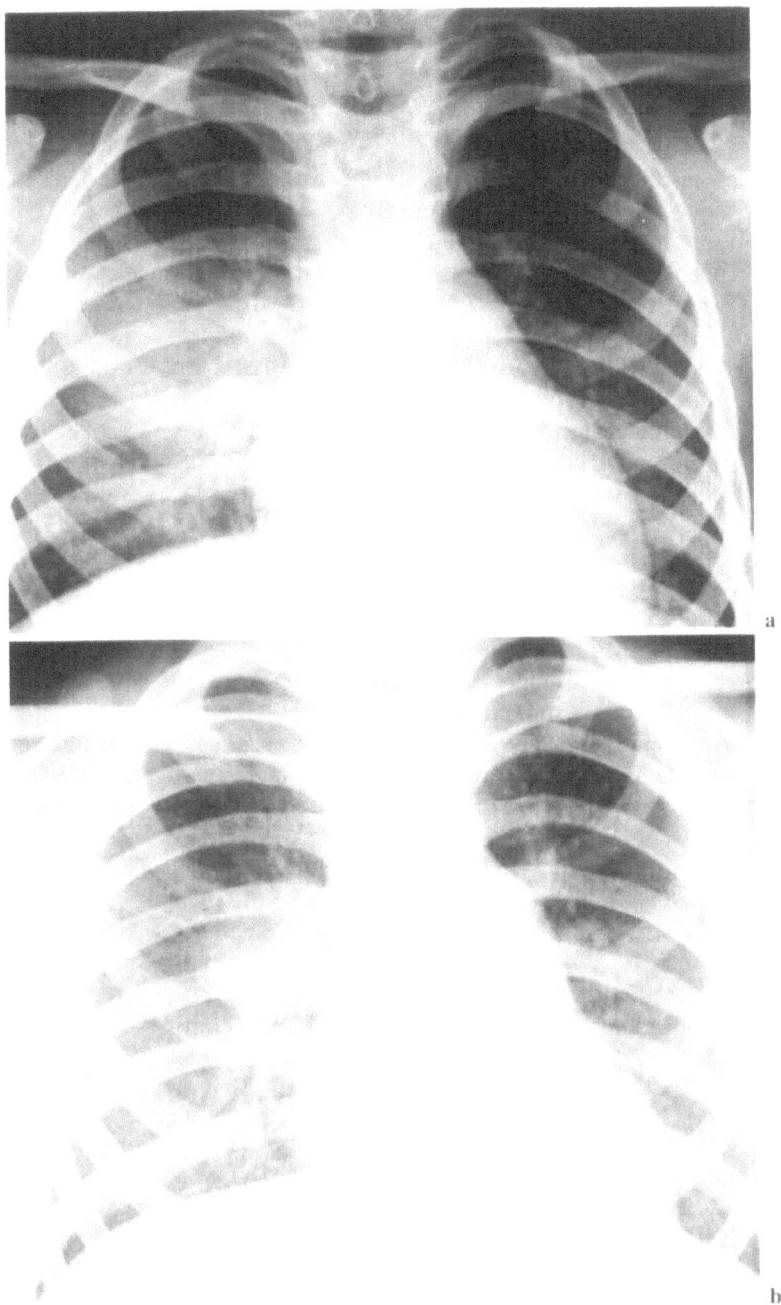

Fig. 7.17 a,b. Regenerative thymic hyperplasia after pneumonia in a 5-year-old boy. **a** Chest radiograph shows pneumonic infiltrations in the posterior parts of the right lower lobe. The pulmonary segment is straight, and suggestive of persistent thymus. **b** Control radiograph 2$^{1}/_{2}$ weeks later: healing pneumonia. Despite the lower positioning of the diaphragm, the shadow of the enlarged thymus is prominent above the left cardiac margin up to the aortic arch. Rebound phenomenon

– The second group in whom regenerative hyperplasia is seen comprises patients of all age groups who have received *chemotherapy for malignant tumors*. It has been reported, for example, in patients with nonseminomatous, metastasizing testicular cancers (HENDRICKX and DÖHRING 1989; ABILDGAARD et al. 1989) in adolescents and adults aged 16–52 years with metastatic testicular teratoma (KISSIN et al. 1987), and in children and adults with Hodgkin's disease (SHIN and HO 1983; GRISSOM et al. 1983; TARTAS et al. 1985; FORD et al. 1987). Corresponding observations have been reported in children with malignant tumors (Wilm's tumors, malignant lymphomas, etc.) or undergoing treatment for leukemia; in some such children the reduction in the size of the thymus occurred during and after radiation, i.e., before chemotherapy, while in those treated without radiation it occurred during chemotherapy (HILL and DODD 1970; HAL-LER et al. 1980; COHEN et al. 1980; BELL et al. 1984; CHOYKE et al. 1987; BODE and SCHEIDT 1988). During chemotherapy the thymus may be reduced to half its original size; regenerative hyperplasia in children occurs at the earliest 2–3 weeks after discontinuation of therapy, and in most cases 2–3 months thereafter. In adults regenerative hyperplasia can develop up to 1 year after therapy and regression usually takes 2 years.

While reduction in the size of the thymus occurred in the majority of patients (approximately 80%) undergoing chemotherapy, regenerative hyperplasia has been observed more often in children than in adults (25%).

In the published cases the regrowth of the thymus varied in extent in some cases it did not reach the original size, while in others it exceeded the original size to a considerable extent. During a second course of chemotherapy the thymic diminution and subsequent regrowth repeated itself, though in a smaller percentage. CHOYKE et al. (1987) differentiate thymic regrowth as any increase in volume relative to the previous scan, and thymic rebound as a greater than 50% increase in volume over baseline.

Analysis of 104 cases of regenerative thymic hyperplasia after treatment for malignancies, detailed in Table 7.4, yields the following results: The age structure shows 37 children and 62 adults; 5 further patients represent a mixed group. With regard to the reaction of the patients to corticoids, children displayed a shorter average interval until the appearance of the rebound phenomenon than did adults (6 months vs 9.3 months, respectively). When the time of appearance of the rebound phenomenon was analyzed in relation to therapy, the interval from *termination* of therapy until discovery of the rebound phenomenon was found to be 2–14 months in 38 of 39 patients (97%) in whom the relevant details were available; only in one patient was the interval longer. In one group of adult patients without individual case details, the interval was 6 months to 2 years (HENDRICKX and DÖHRING 1989).

In 87 patients data were available on the appearance of the rebound phenomenon in relation to the *commencement* of therapy. The interval until regenerative thymic enlargement was found to be 3–

14 months in 76 (87%); in five patients the interval was longer (15–31 months) and in six, shorter[1].

– Patients treated by *steroid therapy* for different reasons and for different lengths of time constitute a third group in whom regenerative hyperplasia occurs. From preceding comments regarding the steroid test (see Sect. 6.2) it follows that the thymus decreases in size within a few days; the regenerative thymic enlargement, which may be so pronounced as to entail excessive growth, occurs in children within just 2 or 3 weeks after discontinuation of the steroid therapy, while in adults it occurs a little later. Occasionally, nevertheless, the previously radiologically invisible thymus can be recognized only as a slight "mediastinal enlargement" after termination of long-term steroid therapy, i.e., without hyperplasia (HALLER et al. 1980; COHEN et al. 1980; BELL et al. 1984). This mediastinal enlargement can, however, occur a long time after the termination of therapy: intervals of 4 months to 5 years have been described.

Rebound hyperplasia after treatment of Cushing's syndrome also belongs to this third group, because endogenous or exogenous secretion of ACTH occurs in these patients. Pathogenetic mechanism are thought to include an exhaustion of steroids as a consequence of high blood plasma concentrations of glucocorticoids, the reduction of which might cause regenerative thymic hyperplasia. Adrenal adenomas and adrenal carcinomas are chiefly responsible, but an ACTH-producing pituitary gland adenoma may also be the cause.

This phenomenon was demonstrated by DOPPMAN et al. (1986) in a 15-year-old patient after transsphenoidal resection of an ACTH-producing pituitary gland adenoma and in another two patients with ectopic ACTH syndromes (a 27-year-old female and a 35-year-old male), in one instance following a successfully resected bronchogenic carcinoid and in the other following an idiopathic positive reaction to glucocorticoid antagonists. In these cases the thymic enlargement was observed 3–4 weeks after a decrease in steroid levels, and lasted for a few months. FINDLING and TYRELL (1986) reported a similar finding.

7.4.7 Differential Diagnosis

The importance of differential diagnosis of the large thymus increases with age to the same degree as the thymus usually decreases in size; in other

---

[1] The total number of cited patients exceeds the figure of 104 shown in Table 7.4 because some authors give data pertaining to both the beginning and the end of therapy.

words, a large thymus is so common in the first 2 years of life that, when clinical data are taken into account, invasive diagnostic methods "to exclude a tumor" are typically unnecessary. Only at school age do such methods become more important.

Differentiation between normal thymic tissue and thymic hyperplasia by CT is very complicated (BARON et al. 1982). Because of the fatty atrophy of the tissue, volume measurements by CT are not successful. Thus MOORE et al. (1983) found histologic proof of thymic hyperplasia in 15 of 53 patients in whom the thymus had been classified as normal by previous CT.

Differential diagnosis between an enlarged or hyperplastic thymus and a tumor can be very difficult (see also Sect. 8.2.2.4). This is especially so:

- In children past infancy, especially those with a persistent thymus at school age
- When the thymus has an atypical position
- When the thymus has an unusual shape
- In adults, because of the higher incidence of thymomas in comparison to children

These difficulties have long been taken as an indication for thymectomy, which is reliable in securing the diagnosis of a normal thymus or thymic hyperplasia (SCHRAMM et al. 1968; OH et al. 1971; GUBBAWAY and HOFMANN 1974; SCHNELL 1975; BARTH et al. 1976; EBEL 1980; PARKER et al. 1985). Important criteria are age, clinical symptomatology, and placement of the mass. It should be borne in mind that most of the masses in the anterior mediastinum in children represent thymic hyperplasia (POKORNY and SHERMAN 1974).

Numerous radiodiagnostic methods, as described in Chap. 4, have now been superseded by CT. However, even CT does not always provide confirmation of the diagnosis, as reported by BROWN et al. (1983) in two patients aged 14 and 21 years. Both cases showed soft tissue density and thymic hyperplasia histologically. Radiologically the first case was described as normal tissue, but the second as thymoma (see also Fig. 7.14).

In imaging diagnostics the following facts and signs are relevant to differential diagnosis between a tumor and normal or hyperplastic thymus:

1. The frequency of tumors increases with age; tumors are most seldom when the thymus is still large, especially in the first 2 years of life. The converse is true in the case of thymic hyperplasia.
2. Calcifications are always suggestive of a tumor (Fig. 9.3).

3. The normal of hyperplastic thymus consists of soft and flexible tissue and therefore causes neither displacement nor compression of adjacent organs; thus in general no clinical symptoms will be present (for exceptions, see Sect. 7.4.3.2). By contrast tumors do tend to give rise to clinical and radiologic symptoms such as stridor, compression, impression, displacement of the esophagus and trachea, and, rarely, hoarseness.
4. On radiographs and CT scans, the thymus is more translucent than a thymic tumor, i.e., the latter displays a higher density.
5. Accompanying pleural effusions, be they slight or massive, suggest leukemic infiltration or a non-Hodgkin's lymphoma (Fig. 8.41).
6. A positive steroid test generally excludes a tumor since the tumor will not decrease in size (exceptions: leukemia, non-Hodgkin's lymphoma). If the test results are negative, a steroid-resistant thymus might be the underlying cause.
7. Finally the following signs on CT scans should be mentioned (HEIBERG et al. 1982):
- A normal thymus shows molding to the mediastinum and the anterior chest wall, while a tumor does not.
- The lateral contours of the thymus are smooth whereas the margins of a tumor are mostly lobulated or irregular, and adjacent organs or structures are deformed or displaced.
- Symmetrical thymic enlargement is suggestive of hyperplasia rather than thymoma, which tends to be focal or asymmetric in character (SIEGEL et al. 1982).
- Qualitative assessment of the shape of the thymus has proven useful (FRANCIS et al. 1985).
- Measurement of the thymic lobes has been used by FRANCIS et al. (1985) in order to differentiate a normal thymus from hyperplastic thymus (Fig. 5.27).

Differential diagnosis between tumorous *thymic infiltration or thymic involvement in leukemia and hyperplasia* can be very difficult, and sometimes impossible, using radiologic methods. This is of clinical importance, since the thymus will initially be involved in 15% of cases of childhood leukemia (GILMARTIN 1963). This involvement can be so pronounced that the heart and great vessels are completely obscured by the high thymic density (Fig. 8.41 a).

Pleural or mediastinal effusions, which occur frequently in non-Hodgkin's lymphomas and in leukemia but never in hyperplasia, are of consider-

Table 7.4. Thymic rebound hyperplasia after treatment for malignancies. Summary of 104 published cases, compiled by E. WILLICH and W.J. HOFMANN

Case no.	No. of pts with rebound; age/sex[a]	Malignancy	Treatment of the malignancy	Time from treatment to, or duration of, thymic hyperplasia	Clinical and radiologic findings, methods of examination	Treatment of thymic hyperplasia	Reference
1	19 yr, f	Hodgkin's disease II s B	Chemotherapy incl. corticosteroids[b]	10 mo 8 mo 3 mo	Interstitial lung disease Herpes zoster Nonproductive cough Definite left hilar mass Chest radiography	Partial resection (6 × 4 cm)	GRISSOM et al. 1983
2	4.5 yr, m	Wilms' tumor	Nephrectomy Radiotherapy Vincristine	12 mo 11 mo 8 mo	Widening of the mediastinum Chest radiography	Thymectomy	HILL and DODD 1970
3	3 yr, m	Wilms' tumor	Nephrectomy Radiotherapy Vincristine	12 mo 9 mo	Lobulated mass in a widened mediastinum Chest radiography	Thymectomy	COHEN et al. 1980
4	32 mo, f	Lymphoblastic leukemia	Chemotherapy	Several months	Definite widening of the anterior mediastinum Chest radiography	Biopsy	COHEN et al. 1980
5	9 yr, m	Osteosarcoma of the distal femur	Amputation Chemotherapy	17 mo 1 mo	Anterior mediastinal mass Chest radiography	None[c]	COHEN et al. 1980
6	5 yr, f	Malignant teratoma	Resection Chemotherapy	5 mo	Widened anterior mediastinum Chest radiography	None[d]	COHEN et al. 1980
7	4 yr, m	Malignant lymphoma	Radiotherapy Chemotherapy	During	Mediastinal widening Chest radiography	None[e]	COHEN et al. 1980
8	4 yr, f	Poorly diff. lymphocytic lymphoma (convoluted type)	Chemotherapy	10 mo	Polyarthritis[f] Widening of the mediastinum Chest radiography	Corticosteroids[g]	COHEN et al. 1980
9	23 mo, f	Wilms' tumor	Nephrectomy Radiotherapy Chemotherapy	10 mo	Large left mediastinal mass Chest radiography	Corticosteroids[h]	COHEN et al. 1980
10	2.5 yr, m	Embryonal rhabdomyosarcoma of left testicle	Orchiectomy Chemotherapy	12 mo	Enlargement of the superior mediastinum CT	Resection of the right thymic lobe (28 g)	BELL et al. 1984
11	33 yr, f	Hodgkin's disease II B	Chemotherapy Radiotherapy	22 mo	Anterior mediastinal soft tissue mass seemed to be of thymic origin. Laboratory findings normal	Partial resection[i]	TARTAS et al. 1985
12	23 yr, m	Hodgkin's disease III$_2$A	Chemotherapy	During	Persistent anterior mediastinal mass CT, chest radiography	Thymectomy 10 × 6 × 2 cm	CARMOSINO et al. 1985
13	23 yr, f	Endodermal sinus tumor of left ovary	Hysterectomy with bilateral salpingo-oophorectomy, chemotherapy	10 mo	Widened mediastinum, anterior mediastinal mass CT, chest radiography	Thymectomy 75 g 10 × 9 × 2 cm	CARMOSINO et al. 1985

No.	Age, sex	Diagnosis	Treatment	Time	Findings	Procedure	Reference
14	16 yr, m	Mixed germ cell tumor with elevated tumor markers (α-FP, β-HCG)	Orchiectomy Chemotherapy	6 mo	Anterior mediastinal mass 3 cm in diameter; tumor markers negative CT	Thymectomy 58 g 120×80×20 cm	DÜE et al. 1988
15–44[j]	30/50 pts. 17–49 yr, m	Testicular cancer	Orchiectomy Chemotherapy (Einhorn scheme)	13 mo after beginning, 6 mo after end of chemotherapy; duration of thymic hyperplasia up to 2 years	Metastatic disease, diffuse enlargement of the anterior mediastinum with a soft tissue-like density CT	None	HENDRICKX and DÖHRING 1989
45–51[j]	7/21 pts. 17–50 yr, m	Nonseminomatous testicular cancer	Chemotherapy	3–12 mo after beginning of chemotherapy	Enlargement of the thymus. Serum tumor markers normalized during follow-up CT	None	ABILDGAARD et al. 1989
52	8 yr, m	Hodgkin's lymphoma III	Chemotherapy	18 mo after diagnosis	Persistent anterior mediastinal enlargement until 1 yr CT	Thoracotomy	FORD et al. 1987
53	3 yr	Wilms' tumor	Extirpation Chemotherapy Irradiation	9 mo	Mediastinal mass Chest radiography	Prednisone	FORD et al. 1987
54	4 yr	Burkitt's lymphoma	Chemotherapy Surgery	2 yr 7 mo into chemotherapy	Mediastinal mass Chest radiography	Prednisone	FORD et al. 1987
55	4 yr	Lymphoma of bones	Chemotherapy	10 mo into chemotherapy	Mediastinal mass. No evidence of disease after 7½ yr	Prednisone	FORD et al. 1987
56	23 mo	Wilms' tumor	Surgery Chemotherapy Irradiation	10 mo into chemotherapy	Mediastinal mass, persistent	Open biopsy	FORD et al. 1987
57	7 yr	B cell lymphoma	Chemotherapy	During last course of chemotherapy	No evidence of disease at 1 year	Prednisone	FORD et al. 1987
58	5 yr	Non-Hodgkin's lymphoma	Chemotherapy	2 mo after chemotherapy	Chest radiograph stable at 2½ yr	Prednisone	FORD et al. 1987
59	2½ yr	Acute lymphatic leukemia	Chemotherapy	3 mo after chemotherapy	Chest radiography No evidence of disease at 5 yr	Mediastinoscopy and biopsy	FORD et al. 1987
60	8 yr	Lymphoma	Chemotherapy	10 mo after chemotherapy	Chest radiography	Open biopsy	FORD et al. 1987
61	15 yr	Hodgkin's lymphoma	Chemotherapy	–	No evidence of disease at 7 mo	Open biopsy	FORD et al. 1987
62	7 yr	Hodgkin's lymphoma	Chemotherapy	1 yr after chemotherapy	Chest radiography No evidence of disease at 3 mo	Open biopsy	FORD et al. 1987
63	17 yr	Hodgkin's lymphoma	Chemotherapy	–	No evidence of disease at 3 mo	Open biopsy	FORD et al. 1987
64	15 yr	Hodgkin's lymphoma	Chemotherapy	1 yr after chemotherapy	–	Open biopsy	FORD et al. 1987
65	5 yr	Malignant teratoma, dysgerminoma	Operation Chemotherapy	5 mo into chemotherapy	Chest radiography Stable at 1 yr	None	FORD et al. 1987

Table 7.4. (continued)

Case no.	No. of pts with rebound; age/sex[a]	Malignancy	Treatment of the malignancy	Time from treatment to, or duration of, thymic hyperplasia	Clinical and radiologic findings, methods of examination	Treatment of thymic hyperplasia	Reference
66	9 yr	Osteosarcoma	Chemotherapy	1 yr after chemotherapy	Chest radiography No evidence of disease at 7 yr	None	Ford et al. 1987
67–80[i]	14/120 pts. 17–39 yr, m	Testicular teratoma	Orchiectomy Chemotherapy	3–14 mo after beginning of therapy	Metastatic disease CT	Resection in one case. Thymus weighing 160 g	Kissin et al. 1987
81	20 yr, f	Osteosarcoma	Chemotherapy	8.5 mo after end of therapy	Enlarged thymus CT	None	Bode and Scheidt 1988
82	16 yr	Osteosarcoma	Chemotherapy	9 mo after therapy	Enlarged thymus CT	None	Bode and Scheidt 1988
83	15 yr, m	Osteosarcoma	Chemotherapy	5–11 mo after therapy	Enlarged thymus CT	None	Bode and Scheidt 1988
84	14 yr, m	Osteosarcoma	Chemotherapy	11 mo after therapy	Enlarged thymus CT	None	Bode and Scheidt 1988
85	13 yr, f	Osteosarcoma	Chemotherapy	16 mo after therapy	Enlarged thymus CT	None	Bode and Scheidt 1988
86	13 yr, f	Osteosarcoma	Chemotherapy	7 mo after therapy	Enlarged thymus CT	None	Bode and Scheidt 1988
87	11 yr, f	Osteosarcoma	Chemotherapy	4 mo after end of therapy	Enlarged thymus CT	None	Bode and Scheidt 1988
88	7 yr, m	Osteosarcoma	Chemotherapy	9 mo after start and 1 mo after end of therapy	Enlarged thymus CT Relapse	None	Bode and Scheidt 1988
89	2 yr, f	Wilms' tumor	Surgery Irradiation Chemotherapy	3 mo after chemotherapy	Enlarged thymus CT	None	Bode and Scheidt 1988
90	21 yr, m	Testicular carcinoma	Orchiectomy Chemotherapy	9 mo after chemotherapy	Enlarged thymus CT	None	Bode and Scheidt 1988
91	25 yr, m	Testicular carcinoma	Orchiectomy Chemotherapy	30 mo after chemotherapy	Enlarged thymus CT	None	Bode and Scheidt 1988
92	14 yr, f	Ewing's sarcoma	Chemotherapy	6 mo after therapy	Enlarged thymus CT	None	Bode and Scheidt 1988
93	10 yr, m	Neuroblastoma	Surgery Chemotherapy	2 mo after chemotherapy	Enlarged thymus CT	None	Bode and Scheidt 1988
94	17 yr, m	Hemangiopericytoma	Chemotherapy	13.5 mo after the start and 2–14 mo after the end of chemotherapy	Enlarged thymus Two relapses CT	None	Bode and Scheidt 1988

95–99[j]	5/22 pts. 2–35 yr	Several malignancies (osteosarcoma, malignant fibrous histiocytoma, Hodgkin's disease)	Chemotherapy Partial extirpation	3–8 mo after the end of chemotherapy	Enlarged thymus CT	3 × biopsy	CHOYKE et al. 1987
100	18 yr, f	Hodgkin's disease	Chemotherapy	7 mo after the end of chemotherapy course	Fever, night perspiration, bilateral hilar lymphadenopathy and circular mass in the left apex. Bleomycin-induced pulmonary interstitial fibrosis	Mediastinotomy Partial resection of the thymus (100 g, normally 46 g) 3 × 4 × 8 cm	SHIN and HO 1983
101	26 yr, m	Metastatic germ cell tumor	Orchiectomy Chemotherapy	8 mo after the end of chemotherapy	Left testicular swelling. Mass in the anterior mediastinum. Multiple metastases in the lung and retroperitoneal space CT	Mediastinotomy Excision	TOBISU et al. 1987
102	27 yr, m	Malignant teratoma	Orchiectomy Chemotherapy	7 mo after the end of chemotherapy	Slight mediastinal widening CT: thickening in the anterior superior mediastinum	2 mo observation, then excision; 160 g	TAIT et al. 1986
103	4 yr, f	Wilms' tumor Lung metastases	Irradiation	1 yr	Puzzling mass extending from the right mediastinum to the right hilum Tomography: typical triangular shape of the thymic lobe	None	HARRIS et al. 1980
104	13 yr, m	Ewing's sarcoma of the right upper arm	Radiotherapy Five courses of chemotherapy	3 months after completing chemotherapy	Aching pain in the right lower humerus Chest radiography, CT	None	WOODHEAD 1984

a Sex unknown in some cases
b Corticosteroids were given as part of therapy for Hodgkin's disease and to treat drug-induced interstitial lung disease
c The mediastinal contour returned to normal after 1 year
d No significant change in the mediastinal silhouette
e Observation (no change)
f Therapy with corticosteroids
g Prednisone (60 mg/m^2); 24 h after the first dose a definite shrinking of the mediastinal mass was evident; the mediastinal shadow was entirely normal by 48 h
h Striking reduction of the mass after 7 days of oral prednisone therapy
i The mediastinal mass disappeared in 2 months
j Details not published

able radiologic importance (Fig.8.41c). Another possible differential diagnostic criterion consists in the different reactions to cytostatic treatment: leukemia and non-Hodgkin's lymphomas respond promptly to cytostatic treatment, so that complete regression of the lesion occurs within a few days, whereas thymic hyperplasia does not react. However, each of these conditions can improve under steroid treatment.

In this context, also, differences according to age should be noted: thymic hyperplasia decreases continually after the 1st year of life, whereas leukemia and non-Hodgkin's lymphomas tend to increase.

Finally other tumors of the anterior mediastinum must be mentioned, especially *mediastinal teratoma,* which accounts for 18% of all mediastinal tumors in children but only 11% in adults. Although benign in nature, it becomes more malignant with increasing age. In contrast to thymomas it grows more often on the left than on the right side, and occasionally occurs in association with extensive pleural effusions. It may present as a rapidly growing lesion in infancy but there are also asymptomatic cases that occur in young children or at school age. Since this tumor contains elements of all three germ layers, calcifications (bone, teeth) in the tumor shadow are radiologically pathognomonic (Fig.8.55).

In patients treated because of malignant disease, other differential diagnostic problems must be considered if, during or after chemotherapy, a solid mass appears in the anterior mediastinum. Such masses can represent:

– A relapse of the underlying mediastinal disease
– Mediastinal metastases because of a primary tumor located elsewhere or systemic lymphatic disease
– Reactive thymic hyperplasia after chemotherapy (rebound phenomenon)

These problems occur mostly in children, adolescents, and young adults with malignant lymphomas, leukemia, Wilms' tumors, testicular carcinomas, sarcomas, and malignant teratomas. Except in patients with lymphomas and leukemia, the steroid test can be useful, if symptoms or other clinical indications of a relapse are not present. FORD et al. (1987), for example, recommended use of the steroid test carefully controlled by chest radiography after 1 week (Table 7.4, cases 52–66). KOBAYASHI et al. (1986) used the test in three of four cases but reached the conclusion that it is only indicated if no acute respiratory symptoms are

present, since they only once observed a reduction in thymic size in an infant (Table 7.3, cases 22–25). If the solid mass does not decrease following steroid therapy or if there is thymic enlargement, the situation must be clarified by open biopsy.

Differential diagnosis against *cardiopathies* has already been discussed in Sect.7.3 (vis-à-vis stridor, see Sect.7.4.3.2). Figure 7.16 shows a 2-week-old infant with "cardiomegaly", in whom ultrasonography confirmed a hyperplastic thymus.

In infants and young children, *mediastinal lymphadenopathies* usually can be easily distinguished because they are situated in the middle mediastinum on chest radiography in the lateral projection (Fig.7.18). In toddlers and schoolchildren a persistent thymus can resemble a systemic lymphatic disease such as Hodgkin's disease in the sagittal projection because of the unilateral or bilateral mediastinal enlargement of the chimney shape (Figs.7.5, 7.7). A lateral radiograph or, even better, a CT scan can be useful in such cases (Fig.7.7d). Involvement of the thymus in systemic diseases and leukemias causes difficulties because infiltrated lymph nodes, together with the enlarged thymus and sometimes even a mediastinal effusion, from a conglomerate tumor which can be identified on CT scans but cannot always be attributed to a specific disease. Therefore further diagnostic procedures such as bone marrow biopsy, lymph node biopsy, and differential blood analysis must be used (Figs.8.41–8.45).

Mediastinal and interlobar pleuritis have already been discussed. Differentiation of the thymus from mediastinal pleurisy must be determined on the lateral radiologic plane. An enlargement of the midshadow due to effusion can be radiologically verified by spot-film radiographs in the head-down position. The pleural fluid will flow off cranially (Fig.8.41c). CT can be employed to clarify smaller or doubtful effusions in older children if the new information would have therapeutic consequences.

Although imaging procedures alone cannot always yield pathognomonic findings, the rare mediastinal pleurisy should nowadays not be mistaken for the thymus when clinical and anamnestic data (Fig.7.19) and the patient's age are taken into account (WILLICH 1975).

Interlobar pleurisy (pleurisy of the small lobe fissure) used to be another frequent misdiagnosis as far as the thymus is concerned, this because it was taken as proof of "anterior superior mediastinal pleurisy." A relatively dense interlobar line is indeed sometimes found in connection with the

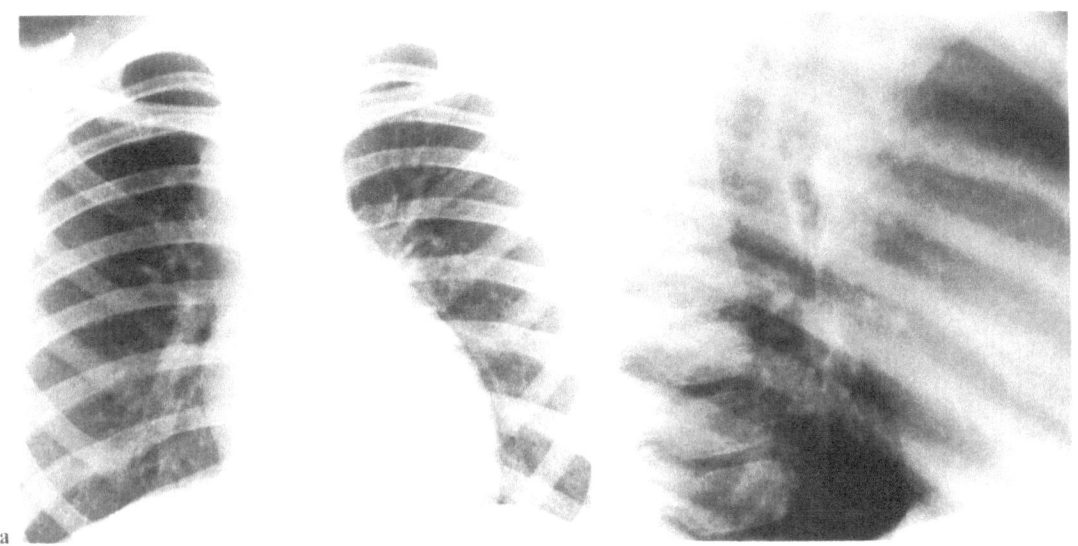

Fig. 7.18 a, b. Lymphadenopathy of the paratracheal lymph node due to tuberculosis in a 7-year-old boy. **a** Chest radiograph: chimney-like configuration of the superior mediastinum (similar to findings in Figs. 7.5, 7.7, 8.42, and 8.45).

b Lateral view: the "mediastinal enlargement" is projected to the middle mediastinum in the form of shadowing. Tuberculin test positive

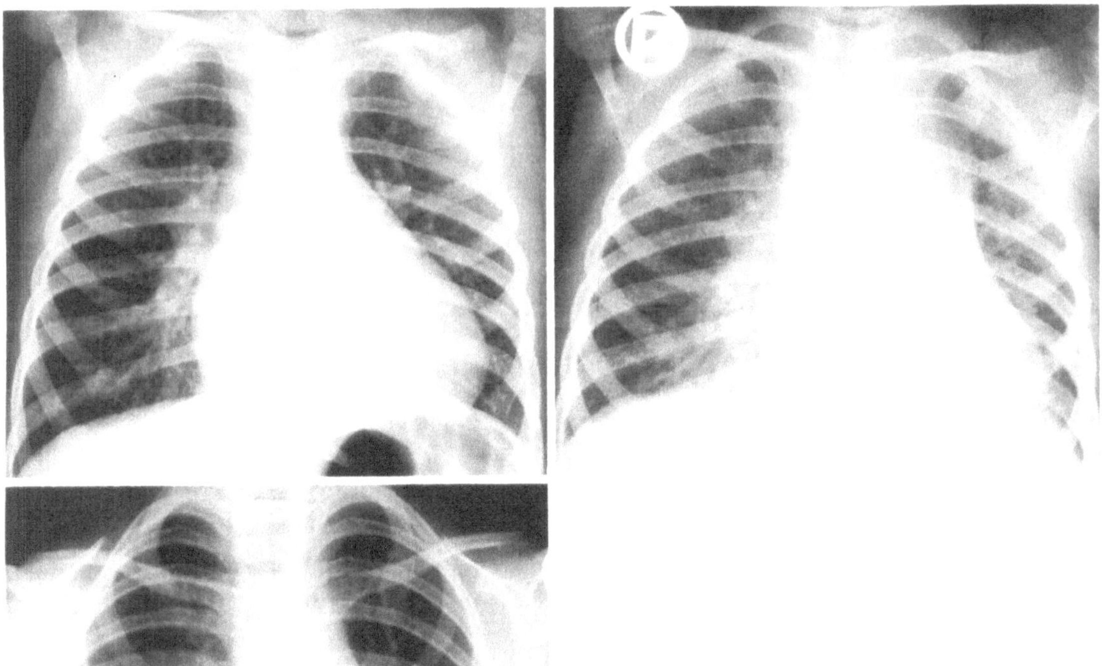

Fig. 7.19 a–c. Mediastinal effusion in a 4-year-old girl with a defect of the atrial septum and incomplete atrioventricular canal. **a** Preoperative anteroposterior chest radiograph: left-sided dilatation of the heart. **b** Postoperative control radiograph after patch closure: enlargement of the mediastinum due to left-sided (sanguinous?) effusion. (The lateral view yielded no diagnostic information.) **c** 16 days after operation resorption of the effusion has taken place and the appearance has normalized (posteroanterior projection)

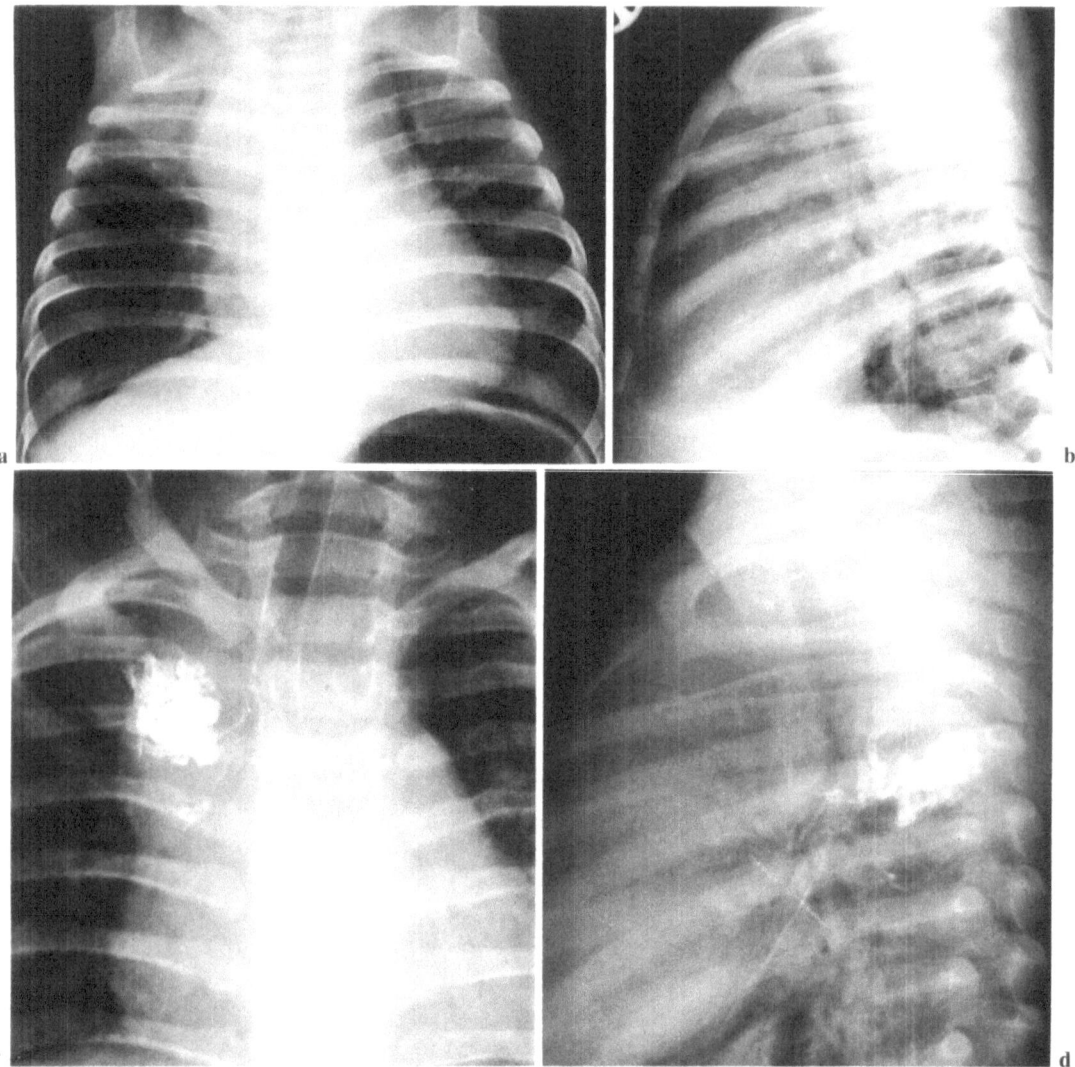

Fig. 7.20 a–d. Large thymus and upper lobe compression atelectasis in a 10-month-old infant with chronic recurrent infections of the upper airways. **a** Chest radiograph shows a dense enlargement of the right superior mediastinum; laterally discreet homogeneous shadowing of the right upper lung lobe is present. The interlobar space is displaced cranially. There is slight cardiomegaly due to a defect of the ventricular septum. **b** Lateral view: inhomogeneous shadow in the thymic space. **c,d** Bronchography due to continuous infections over several months: severe stenosis of the apical and posterior segmental bronchi. Total occlusion of the anterior upper lobe bronchus

thymus, but in 1958 ZSEBÖK was able to prove that this is due to growth of a thymic tip into the interlobar fissure.

Upper lobe atelectases can also simulate thymic hyperplasia. In infants atelectases are in any case relatively common because of the soft and elastic bronchial walls, the narrow bronchial lumina, and the tendency toward a strong reaction of the bronchial lymph nodes, the enlargement of which can cause to compression of the bronchial and segmental lumina and yield appearances resembling the thymus (see Table 7.2, case 7, and 7.3, cases 16 and 27).

As a consequence P.C. SCHMID (1956) defended the hypothesis of upper lobe atelectasis in pediatric and radiologic journals until ESSER and HILGERT (1956) pointed out that the most important criterion for diagnosis of upper lobe atelectasis is the position of the small lobe fissure, and that a horizontal course is incompatible with upper lobe atelectasis.

There are four differential diagnostic possibilities in respect of the thymus and upper lobe atelectasis when an increase in density is observed in the upper lung area:

1. *Pure atelectasis.* This can usually be distinguished from the thymus by its density, homogeneity, sharp contours, and typical shape and position. In addition there may be vicarious emphysema of the adjacent middle and lower lobes.

2. *Coincidental combination of thymus and atelectasis.* When the diagnosis is not clear-cut, the steroid test can be used or one can await the further course (involution of the atelectasis with persistence of the thymus will clarify the diagnosis). Clinical data, e.g., upper respiratory tract infection, are often of diagnostic value.

3. *A large thymus compressing the upper lobe bronchus* or an upper lobe segmental bronchus, thus causing compression atelectasis. GUBBAWAY and HOFMANN (1974) reported two such cases. Steroid therapy had failed in one case. Both had undergone bronchotherapy and thoracotomy; one showed hyperplastic and the other normal thymic tissue. A similar case is shown in Fig. 7.20. For further information see Sect. 7.4.3.2.

4. *Thymus simulating atelectasis.* An atypical shape and unusual density are prerequisites for this diagnosis. LANNING and HEIKKINEN described one such a case in 1980 in a 7-month-old boy in whom bronchoscopy did not show atelectasis. Thoracotomy was nevertheless performed, and normal thymic tissue found.

Awareness of possible thymic enlargement at all ages, with radiologic appearances from "mediastinal enlargement" to "mediastinal tumor," is very important in avoiding misinterpretations and especially diagnostic thoracotomy.

7.4.8 Therapy

Radiotherapy of the enlarged thymus was first advocated in 1907 by an American author, FRIEDLÄNDER (cited by BIRK 1918). It was used from 1911 in France (D'OELSNITZ), from 1913 in Germany (DUTOIT, EGGERS), and from 1914 in Italy (LUZZATTI, cited by BIRK 1918; COZZOLINO). The late effects forced such therapy to be abandoned (see Sect. 6.2).

Steroid test. Another form of therapy was developed from the already mentioned steroid test

(Sect. 6.2); this therapy is, however, still the subject of controversy. The effect is only temporary and therefore regrowth must be expected after discontinuation of the therapy. A longlasting therapeutic effect thus cannot be achieved in the rare cases with clinical symptoms of a giant thymus (Fig. 5.2). *Probative steroid therapy* was used successfully in two of four cases by DANILEWICZ-WYTRYCHOWSKA (1981) and BLASIMANN et al. (1977), and also by HARRIS et al. (1980: one of five cases), COHEN et al. (1983: two of seven cases), and KOBAYASHI et al. (1986: one of three cases). This treatment was used without success, i.e., without any reduction in the size of the thymus, by LAMESCH (1983) and HALLER et al. (1980). Because of the possible lymphatic or leukemic involvement of the thymus, most authors have not used steroids. HALLER et al. (1969) treated conservatively eight children (four newborns and four aged from 3 months to 3 years) out of a series of 80 children with mediastinal tumors. Conservative treatment, i.e., a wait and see attitude, was also employed in one of seven children aged 2 weeks to 28 months by POKORNY and SHERMAN (1974), and in three of five children aged between 4 and 11 years by HARRIS et al. (1980).

Of interest in this context is ATTAR et al.'s report of an infant who suffered from respiratory symptoms caused by thymic hyperplasia which had been proven by biopsy. A right-sided upper lobe atelectasis existed at the same time. During 8 months' treatment with prednisolone a respiratory distress syndrome again developed, together with a "relapse" of giant thymus which at operation turned out to be a malignant mesenchymoma arising from the thymus (see Table 7.3, case 27).

Oncologists warn of possible confusion of the thymus with malignant lymphomas and leukemia since these generally react to steroids in the same manner. Nevertheless, some thymus glands do not react at all to steroids; they are, so to speak, steroid resistant. Therefore in the differential diagnosis of thymoma the absence of a reduction in the size of mass is not a reliable indicator of a tumor. Only a positive reaction, i.e., a diminution of the thymus, is of diagnostic import (see Sect. 6.2).

Especially if there are not clinical symptoms which call for special treatment, patients with thymic hyperplasia should in the first instance be treated *conservatively*. The younger the patient, the greater the weight that must be given to the possibility of harmless hyperplasia, and the weaker the necessity to exclude a tumor! Doubtful cases must be closely controlled if therapeutic consequences are expected. Computed tomography sometimes can be of assistance, as in four cases reported by KOBAYASHI et al. (1986) and in five reported by COHEN (1980); magnetic resonance imaging may also be of value (Figs. 5.17, 7.8).

Thoracotomy with extirpation of the thymus is justified when there is a clear causal connection with the clinical symptoms or in cases with strong suspicion of malignancy. However, rapid intraoperative biopsy must be performed to exclude a systemic disease requiring radio- or chemotherapy.

Thoracotomy and open biopsy, and in some cases extirpation of the thymus, have in the past been performed on the basis of the excessive size of the thymus when there was accompanying compression or displacement of a lung lobe without clinical symptoms (HALLER et al. 1969; EBEL 1980; BLASIMANN et al. 1977; Fig. 7.20). Other published cases suspicious for tumor revealed only huge thymus glands which were extirpated (O'SHEA et al. 1978: thymus weight 420 g; LEE et al. 1979: 22-month-old child, thymus weight 550 g; KATZ et al. 1977: infant with a thymus weight of 224 g; BARTH et al. 1976: 8-month-old infant; LACK 1981: two cases; see Tables 7.2, 7.3).

JUDD reported the case of a 12-year-old boy with asthmatic-like symptoms, dysphagia and an extended anterior mediastinal shadow on the chest radiograph. Resection yielded a large thymus weighing 245 g (average for this age 34 ± 10 g), with normal thymic parenchyma and a myoid component (see Table 7.2, case 12).

THOMAS and GUPTA (1988) described a 7-week-old infant with massive compression of the left lung lobe caused by a giant thymus, with corresponding respiratory symptoms and displacement of the heart. Extirpation revealed a thymus of normal structure, weighing 72 g (Table 7.3, case 26).

Further cases of hyperplasia that led to thoracotomy have been described by RASORE-QUARTINO et al. (1979), LAMESCH (1983), NEZELOF and NORMAND (1986), and ARLISS et al. (1988) (see Table 7.2). Naturally, pathologists also recommend thoracotomy (see Sect. 7.4.2).

The therapeutic approach in 104 cases of regenerative thymic hyperplasia following treatment for malignancies is shown in Table 7.4. Seventysix cases were treated conservatively, i. e., without any treatment of the thymus. In nine cases thymectomy was performed, in eight diagnostic biopsy, and in four partial resection. In seven cases steroids were used.

In summary, on the basis of past experience it must be concluded that even a giant thymus (especially when presenting in the first years of life)

does not justify therapeutic measures if it does not cause severe clinical symptoms or if it is merely an incidental finding without underlying general disease.

7.4.9 Follow-up

KUZMENKO (1986) reported the subsequent case histories of 143 children with thymomegaly in infancy and early childhood. The follow-up examinations took place from a few months to 16 years later; 10 % had died in the meantime. It was found that more than one-third had suffered from chronic recurrent upper respiratory tract infections, and 17 % from infectious-allergic or allergic diseases (e. g., bronchial asthma). In four children tumors of various type had appeared. The high incidence of autoimmune, infectious-allergic, and tumorous diseases is thought not to be accidental but rather the result of impairment of cellular immunity. However, precise characterization of the repeatedly postulated cellular immunodeficiency in thymic hyperplasia is still lacking. Moreover, in this study (at least in the general overview) the findings of chronic recurrent infections or infectious-allergic diseases do not appreciably exceed the normal average.

Figure 5.2 shows follow-up radiographic examinations of a newborn until the age of 12 years.

References

Abildgaard A, Lien HH, Fosså SD, Høie J, Langholm R (1989) Enlargement of the thymus following chemotherapy for non-seminomatous testicular cancer. Acta Radiol 30: 259

Alpert LI, Papatestas A, Kark A, Osserman RS, Osserman K (1971) A histologic reappraisal of the thymus in myasthenia gravis. A correlative study of thymic pathology and response to thymectomy. Arch Pathol 91: 55

Alt W, Hochman HJ (1982) Thyrotoxicosis and myasthenia gravis. Clin Pediatr 21: 749

Amann L (1962) Der Thymus beim Säugling und Kleinkind aus heutiger Sicht. Pädiatr Prax 1: 385

Arliss J, Scholes J, Dickson PR, Messina JJ (1988) Massive thymic hyperplasia in an adolescent. Ann Thorac Surg 45: 220

Attar Z, Muraji T, Matsumoto Y et al. (1988) Malignant mesenchymoma of the mediastinum initially presenting as benign thymic hyperplasia. Pediatr Surg Int 4: 56

Balcom RH, Hakanson DO, Werner A, Gordon LP (1985) Massive thymic hyperplasia in an infant with Beckwith-Wiedemann syndrome. Arch Pathol Lab Med 109: 153

Barcia PJ, Nelson TG (1979) Hyperplasia of the thymus and thymic neoplasms in children. Milit Med 144: 799

Baron RL, Lee JKT, Sagel SS, Peterson RR (1982) Computed tomography of the normal thymus. Radiology 142: 121

Barth K, Schnauffer L, Kaufmann HJ (1976) Giant idiopathic thymomegaly. Pediatr Radiol 4: 117

Bar-Ziv J, Barki Y, Itzchak Y, Mares AJ (1984) Posterior mediastinal accessory thymus. Pediatr Radiol 14: 165

Batra P, Herrmann C, Mulder D (1987) Mediastinal imaging in myasthenia gravis: correlation of chest radiography, CT, MR and surgical findings. AJR 148: 515

Bell BA, Esseltine DW, Azouz EM (1984) Rebound thymic hyperplasia in a child with cancer. Med Pediatr Oncol 12: 144

Bertoye A, Beraud C, Depierre A, Duc H, Beraud A (1956) Hypertrophie thymique et primo-infection du nourrisson. Pédiatrie 11: 545

Bierich JR, Schmidt-Grimminger V (1966) Untersuchungen über die Bedeutung des großen Thymus im Säuglings- und Kleinkindalter. Pädiatr Grenzgeb 5: 179

Birk W (1918) Beiträge zur Klinik und Behandlung der Thymushyperplasie bei Kindern. Monatschr Kinderheilkd 14: 363

Bistritzer T, Tamir A, Oland J, Varsano D, Manor A, Gall A, Aladjem M (1985) Severe dyspnea and dysphagia resulting from an aberrant cervical thymus. Eur J Pediatr 144: 86

Blasimann B, Kuffer F, Bettex M (1977) Chirurgische Betrachtungen über die Thymushyperplasie. Z Kinderchir 21: 214

Bode U, Scheidt W (1988) Change of thymic size during and following cytotoxic therapy in young patients. Pediatr Radiol 18: 20

Bofill M, Janossy G, Willcox N, Chilosi M, Trejdosiewicz LK, Bagott M, Newsom-Davic J (1985) Microenvironments in the normal and myasthenia gravis thymus. Am J Pathol 199: 462

Bower RJ, Kiesewetter WB (1977) Mediastinal masses in infants and children. Arch Surg 112: 1003

Brown LR, Muhm JR, Sheedy II PF, Unni KK, Bernatz PE, Hermann RC (1983) The value of computed tomography in myasthenia gravis. AJR 140: 31

Bruce JW, Graves S (1922) Respiratory obstruction resulting in death. Case report with necropsy findings. Am J Dis Child 23: 438

Caffey J (1950) Pediatric X ray diagnosis, 2nd edn. Year Book Publishers, Chicago, pp 322 and 327

Caffey J, Silbey R (1960) Regrowth and overgrowth of the thymus after atrophy induced by the oral administration of adrenocorticosteroids to human infants. Pediatrics 26: 762

Capper A, Schless RA (1934) Thymic gland and thymic symptoms: investigation of 1074 newborn babies. J Pediatr 4: 573

Carmosino L, DiBenedetto A, Feffer S (1985) Thymic hyperplasia following successful chemotherapy. A report of two cases and review of the literature. Cancer 56: 1526

Castleman B (1966) The pathology of the thymus gland in myasthenia gravis. Ann NY Acad Sci 135: 496

Castleman B, Norris EH (1949) The pathology of the thymus in myasthenia gravis. Medicine (Baltimore) 28: 27

Choyke PL, Zeman RK, Gootenberg JE, Greenberg JN, Hoffer F, Frank JA (1987) Thymic atrophy and regrowth in response to chemotherapy: CT evaluation. AJR 149: 269

Ciba Foundation Symposium, No. 84 (1981) Microenvironments in haemopoietic and lymphoid differentiation. Pitman, London

Cocchi U (1959) Röntgendiagnostik und Strahlentherapie des Thymus. Strahlentherapie [Sonderb] 109: 426

Cohen M, Hill CA, Cangir A, Sullivan MP (1980) Thymic rebound after treatment of childhood tumors. AJR 135: 151

Cohen MD, Weber TR, Sequeira FW, Vane DW, King H (1983) The diagnostic dilemma of the posterior mediastinal thymus: CT manifestations. Radiology 146: 691

Consolini R, Cini P, Cei B, Bottone E (1987) Thymic dysfunction in histiocytosis-X. Am J Pediatr Hematol Oncol 9: 146

Cozzolino O (1914) Il trattamento radioterapeutico della iperplasia timica nell'infanzia. Pediatria 22: 292

Dalakas MC, Engel WK, McClure JE, Goldstein AL, Askanas V (1981) Immunocytochemical localization of thymosin-α_1 in thymic epithelial cells of normal and myasthenia gravis patients and in thymic cultures. J Neurol Sci 50: 239

Danilewicz-Wytrychowska T (1981) Zur Röntgendiagnostik und Differentialdiagnose der Thymuserkrankungen im Kindesalter. Radiologe 21: 542

Dieckmann K-P, Düe W, Bauknecht K-J, Hamm B (1988) Reaktive benigne Thymushyperplasie nach zytostatischer Chemotherapie. Dtsch Med Wschr 113: 598–601

d'Oelsnitz PL, Pachetta L (1911) Les charactères de l'image radioscopique dans l'hypertrophie du thymus. Bull Soc Pédiatr 462

Doppmann JL, Oldfield EH, Chrousos GP, Nieman L, Udelsmar R, Cutler GB, Loriaux DL (1986) Rebound thymic hyperplasia after treatment of Cushing's syndrome. AJR 147: 1145

Düe W, Dieckmann K-P, Stein H (1988) Thymic hyperplasia following chemotherapy of a testicular germ cell tumor. Cancer 63: 446

Dutoit A (1913) Die Radiotherapie der Thymushyperplasie. Dtsch Med Wochenschr 39: 515

Ebel KD (1980) Zur Röntgendiagnostik des Thymus im Kindesalter. Radiologe 20: 379

Eggers F (1913) Experimentelle Beiträge zur Einwirkung der Röntgenstrahlen auf den Thymus. Z Röntgenkd 15

Esser C, Hilgert F (1956) Zur Frage: Thymus, Atelektase oder mediastinaler Pleuraerguß? ROFO 84: 3

Fasanelli S, Barbuti D, Grazioni M (1987) Thymic involvement in acute disseminated histiocytosis. X-rays 12: 39

Filler RM, Simpson JS, Ein SH (1979) Mediastinal masses in infants and children. Pediatr Clin North Am 26: 677

Findling JW, Tyrell JP (1986) Occult ectopic secretion of corticotropin. Arch Intern Med 146: 929

Fischl R (1923) Physiologie und Pathologie der Thymusdrüse im Kindesalter. In: Pfaundler M von, Schlossmann A (eds) Handbuch der Kinderheilkunde, 3rd edn, vol 1. FCW Vogel, Leipzig, p 919

Ford EG, Lockhart SK, Sullivan MP, Andrassy RY (1987) Mediastinal mass Hodgkin's disease: recurrent tumor or thymic hyperplasia? J Pediatr Surg 22: 1155

Francis JR, Glazer GM, Bookstein FL, Gross BH (1985) The thymus: reexamination of age-related changes in size and shape. AJR 145: 249

Franken EA Jr (1968) Radiologic evidence of thymyic enlargement in Graves' disease. Radiology 91: 20

Friedjung JK (1910) Der Thymus. In: Pfaundler M, Schlossmann A (eds) Handbuch der Kinderheilkunde, 2nd edn, vol 3. FCW Vogel, Leipzig, p 448

Gelfand DW, Goldman AS, Law EJ, MacMillan BG, Larson D, Abston S, Schreiber JT (1972) Thymic hyperplasia in children recovering from thermal burns. J Trauma 12: 813

Gilmartin D (1963) Leukemic involvement of the thymus in children. Br J Radiol 36: 211

Glanzmann E (1949) Einführung in die Kinderheilkunde, 3rd edn. Springer, Wien

Glathe S, Neufang KFR, Haupt FW (1989) Was leistet die radiologische Thymusdiagnostik bei der Myasthenia gravis? Röntgenblätter 42: 455

Goldstein G, Mackay IR (1969) The human thymus. Heinemann Medical, London, pp 13, 134, 242, 290

Graham CB, Berdon WE, Patriquin HB, Kuhn JP (1990) Thymic hyperplasia. film panel cases Soc. of Pediatr. Radiol: Pediatr Radiol 20: 371

Grissom JR, Duran JR, Whitley RJ, Flint A (1983) Thymic hyperplasia in a case of Hodgkin's disease. South Med J 76: 1189

Grody WW, Jobst S, Keesey J, Herrmann C, Maeim F (1986) Pathologic evaluation of thymic hyperplasia in myasthenia gravis and Lambert-Eaton syndrome. Arch Pathol Lab Med 110: 843

Gubbawy H, Hofmann A (1974) Der Thymus im Säuglings- und Kindesalter. Prax Pneumol 28: 615

Haller JA Jr, Mazur DO, Morgan WW Jr (1969) Diagnosis and management of mediastinal masses in children. J Thorax Cardiovasc Surg 58: 385

Haller JO, Schneider M, Kassner EG, Friedman AP, Waldroup LD (1980) Sonographic evaluation of the chest in infants and children. AJR 134: 1019

Harris VJ, Ramilo J, White H (1980) The thymic mass as a mediastinal dilemma. Clin Radiol 31: 263

Heiberg E, Wolverson MK, Sundaram M, Nouri S (1982) Normal thymus: CT characteristics in subjects under age 20. AJR 138: 491

Hendrickx P, Döhring W (1989) Thymic atrophy and rebound enlargement following chemotherapy for testicular cancer. Acta Radiol 30: 263

Hill CA, Dodd GD (1970) Thymic hyperplasia simulating mediastinal metastasis. Tex Med 66: 78

Hochsinger C (1903) Stridor thymicus infantum. Wien Med Wochenschr 2106: 2162

Hoeffel JC, Pernot C, Worms AM, Bretagne MC, Bernard C (1988) L'hypertrophie thymique post-opératoire dans les cardiopathies congénitales graves. Ann Pédiatr (Paris) 35: 440

Hofmann WJ, Möller P, Momburg F, Moldenhauer G, Otto HF (1984) Struktur des normalen Thymus, der lymphofollikulären Thymushyperplasie und der Thymome, dargestellt mit Lectinen, S-100-Proteinen und Keratin-Antiseren und monoklonalen (epithelitropen) Antikörpern. Verh Dtsch Ges Pathol 68: 504

Hofmann WJ, Möller P, Manke H-G, Otto HF (1985) Thymoma – a clinicopathologic study of 98 cases with special reference to three unusual cases. Pathol Res Pract 179: 337

Hofmann WJ, Möller P, Otto HF (1987) Thymic hyperplasia. II. Lymphofollicular hyperplasia in the thymus. An immunohistologic study. Klin Wochenschr 65: 53

Hofmann WJ, Momburg F, Möller P, Otto HF (1988a) Intra- and extrahepatic B cells in physiological study on normal thymus and lymphofollicular hyperplasia of the thymus. Virchows Arch [A] 412: 431

Hofmann WJ, Momburg F, Möller P (1988b) Thymic medullary cells expressing B-lymphocyte antigens. Hum Pathol 19: 1280

Hofmann WJ, Möller P, Otto HF (1990) Thymushyperplasia. In: Givel JC, Merlini M, Clarke DB, Dusmet M (eds) Surgery of the thymus, Springer, Berlin Heidelberg New York Tokyo, p 59

Hope JW, Borns PF, Koop CE (1963) Radiological diagnosis of mediastinal masses in infants and children. Radiol Clin North Am 1: 17

Janossy G, Thomas JA, Bollum FJ et al. (1980) The human thymic microenvironment: an immuno-histologic study. J Immunol 125: 202

Janossy G, Bofill M, Trejdosiewicz LK, Willcox HNA, Chilosi M (1986) Cellular differentiation of lymphoid subpopulations and their microenvironments. In: Müller-Hermelink H-K (ed) Current topics in pathology 75. The human thymus. Histophysiology and pathology. Springer, Berlin Heidelberg New York, p 89

Judd RL (1987) Massive thymic hyperplasia with myoid cell differentiation. Hum Pathol 18: 1180

Katz SM, Chatten J, Bishop HC, Rosenblum H (1977) Massive thymic enlargement. Am J Clin Pathol 68: 786

Keuth U (1974) Thymushyperplasie. Pädiatr Prax 14: 447

Kim M, Martrou P, Nedele G, Saint-Macary M, Tchertoff C (1972) Les détresses respiratoires d'origine thymique chez le nouveau-nè et le nourrisson. A propos deux observations. Arch Fr Pédiatr 29: 556

Kim Han B, Babcock DS, Oestreich AF (1989) Normal thymus in infancy: sonographic characteristics. Radiology 170: 471

Kirchner T, Schalke B, Melms A, von Kügelgen T, Müller-Hermelink HK (1986) Immunohistological patterns of non-neoplastic changes in the thymus in myasthenia gravis. Virchows Arch [B] 62: 237

Kirks DR, Korobkin M (1980) Chest computed tomography in infants and children. An analysis of 50 patients. Pediatr Radiol 10: 75

Kissin CM, Husband JE, Nicholas D, Eversman W (1987) Benign thymic enlargement in adults after chemotherapy: CT demonstration. Radiology 163: 67

Kobayashi T, Hirabayashi Y, Kobayashi Y (1986) Diagnostic value of plain chest roentgenogram and CT scan findings in four cases of massive thymic hyperplasia. Pediatr Radiol 16: 452

Kook Sang Oh, Weber AL, Borden S (1971) Normal mediastinal mass in late childhood. Radiology 101: 625

Kornstein MJ, Brooks JJ, Anderson AO, Levinson AI, Lisak RP, Zweiman B (1984) The immunohistology of the thymus in myasthenia gravis. Am J Pathol 117: 184

Kuzmenko LG (1986) The subsequent case-history of thymomegalic pediatric patients. Pediatrija (Mosk) 12: 31

Lack EE (1981) Thymic hyperplasia with massive enlargement. J Thorac Cardiovasc Surg 81: 741

Lamesch AJ (1983) Massive thymic hyperplasia in infants. Z Kinderchir 38: 16

Lamesch AJ, Capesius C, Theisen-Aspesberro MC (1974) Cervical thymic cysts in infants and children. Z Kinderchir 14: 213

Lanning R, Heikkinen E (1980) Thymus simulating left upper lobe atelectasis. Pediatr Radiol 9: 177

Law LW (1966) Studies of thymic function with emphasis on the role of the thymus in oncogenesis. Cancer Res 26: 551

Lee Y, Moallem S, Clauss RH (1979) Massive hyperplastic thymus in a 22-month-old infant. Ann Thorac Surg 27: 356

Leinisch HD (1963) Untersuchungen zur topographischen Anatomie des Thymus in Beziehung zum plötzlichen Säuglingstod. Thesis, Erlangen

Levine GD, Rosai J (1978) Thymic hyperplasia and neoplasia: a review of current concepts. Hum Pathol 9: 495

Mitchell-Nelson, ed by Nelson EW (1945) Textbook of pediatrics, 4th edn. WB Saunders, Philadelphia, p 925

Moore AV, Korobkin M, Powers B et al. (1982) Thymoma detection by mediastinal CT: patients with myasthenia gravis. AJR 138: 217

Moore AV, Korobkin M, Olanow W, Heaston DK, Ram PC, Dunnick NR, Silverman PM (1983) Age-related changes in the thymus gland: CT-pathologic correlation. AJR 141: 241

Müller-Hermelink H-K (ed) (1986) The human thymus. Histophysiology and pathology. Springer, Berlin Heidelberg New York (Current topics in pathology, vol 75)

Newton WA, Hamondi AB, Shannon BT (1987) Role of the thymus in histiocytosis-X. Hematol Oncol Clin North Am 1: 63

Nezelof C, Normand C (1986) Tumor-like massive thymic hyperplasia in childhood: a possible defect of T-cell maturation, histological and cytoenzymatic studies of three cases. Thymus 8: 117

Nicholson RL (1978) Thymic hyperplasia in thyrotoxicosis. J Can Assoc Radiol 29: 264

Oliva L (1973) Erkrankungen des Mediastinums. In: Schinz HR, Baensch WE, Frommhold W, Glauner R, Uehlinger E, Wellauer J (eds) Lehrbuch der Röntgendiagnostik, vol IV/2, 6th edn. Pleura, Mediastinum und Lunge. Thieme, Stuttgart

O'Shea PA, Pansatiankul B, Farnes P (1978) Giant thymic hyperplasia in infancy: immunologic, histologic, and ultrastructural observations. Lab Invest 38: 391

Otto HF (1984) Pathologie des Thymus. In: Doerr W, Seifert G, Uehlinger E (eds) Spezielle pathologische Anatomie, vol 17, Springer, Berlin Heidelberg New York

Paltauf A (1910) Erkrankungen des Thymus, Status lymphaticus und plötzliche Todesfälle. In: Pfaundler M von, Schlossmann A (eds) Handbuch der Kinderheilkunde, 2nd edn, vol 3. FCW Vogel, Leipzig, p 448

Pardo-Mindan FJ, Crisci CD, Serrano M, Arcas R (1980) Immunological aspects of sarcoidosis with true thymic hyperplasia. Allergol Immunopathol (Madr) 8: 91

Parker LA, Gaisie G, Scatliff JH (1985) Computed tomography and ultrasonographic findings in massive thymic hyperplasia. Clin Pediatr 24: 90

Pfaundler M von (1948) Pathologie des Blutes und der Blutungsbereitschaft. In: Feer E, Kleinschmidt H (eds) 4. Lehrbuch der Kinderheilkunde, 16th edn. Fischer, Jena, p 167

Pokorny WJ, Sherman JO (1974) Mediastinal masses in infants and children. J Thorac Cardiovasc Surg 68: 869

Potter EL, Craig JM (1975) Pathology of the fetus and infant, 3rd edn. Year Book Medical, Chicago, p 321

Rasore-Quartino A, Rebizzo F, Romagnoli G (1979) Iperplasia gigante del timo nell'infanzia. Pathologica 71: 711

Rizk G, Cueto L, Amplatz K (1972) Rebound enlargement of the thymus after successful corrective surgery for transposition of the great vessels. AJR 116: 528

Rosai J, Devine GD (1976) Tumors of the thymus. In: Atlas of tumor pathology, 2nd series, fasc 13. Washington DC. Armed Forces Institute of Pathology p 26–33; 133–137

Rose JS, Lam C (1982) Thymic enlargement in association with hyperthyroidism. Pediatr Radiol 12: 37

Saegesser F, Zoupanos G (1970) Thymomas, tumors of the thymic site, and the paraneoplastic immunological syndromes associated with them. In: Saegesser F, Pattavee J

(eds) Surgical oncology. Hans Huber, Bern (Current problems in surgery, vol 14, p 447)

Sato T, Tamaoki N (1989) Myoid cell in the human thymus and thymoma revealed by three different immunohistochemical markers for striated muscle. Acta Pathol Jpn 39: 509

Scadding GK, Vincent A, Newsom-Davis J, Henry K (1981) Acetylcholine receptor antibody synthesis by thymic lymphocytes: correlation with thymic histology. Neurology 31: 935

Scheiff JM, Cordier AC, Haumont S (1977) Epithelial cell proliferation in thymic hyperplasia induced by triiodothyronine. Clin Exp Immunol 27: 516

Schmid PC (1956) Thymushyperplasie oder Oberlappenatelektase? ROFO 84: 20

Schnell VY (1975) Probleme der Thymusdiagnostik bei atypischer Lage und seltenen Begleitumständen. Thesis, Cologne

Schnyder P, Candardjis G (1987) Computed tomography of thymic abnormalities. Eur J Radiol 7: 107

Schramm H, Danz M, Bartel M (1968) Klinik und Morphologie thymogener Mediastinaltumoren. Med Bild 11: 83

Sealy WC, Weaver WL, Young WG (1965) Severe airway obstruction in infancy due to thymus gland. Ann Thorac Surg 1: 389

Shackelford GD, McAlister WH (1974) The aberrantly positioned thymus. A cause of mediastinal or neck masses in children. AJR 120: 291

Shin MS, Ho KJ (1983) Diffuse thymic hyperplasia following chemotherapy for nodular sclerosing Hodgkin's disease. Cancer 51: 30

Shuangshoti S, Seksarn P (1987) Histiocytosis X: overlapping form between Letterer-Siwe disease and Hand-Schüller-Christian disease with advanced thymic involvement and obstructive jaundice. J Med Assoc Thai 70: 344

Siegel MJ, Sagel SS, Reed K (1982) The value of computed tomography in the diagnosis and management of pediatric mediastinal abnormalities. Radiology 142: 149

Siegel MJ, Glazer HS, Wiener JI, Molina PL (1989) Normal and abnormal thymus in childhood: MR imaging. Radiology 172: 367

Silverman NA, Sabiston DC Jr (1980) Mediastinal masses. Surg Clin North Am 60: 757

Silverman FN (1985) Caffey's Pediatric X-ray diagnosis: an integrated imaging approach, 8th edn. Year Book Med Publ, Chicago

Slowikowski J, Kubrakiewicz Z, Zielinski S (1968) Giant hypertrophy of the thymus in three siblings. Pol Med J 7: 634

Sone S, Higashihara T, Morimoto S et al. (1980) Normal anatomy of the thymus and anterior mediastinum by pneumomediastinography. AJR 134: 81

Strobl K (1985) Congenitaler und erworbener kindlicher Stridor und seine radiologische Abklärung. Thesis, Cologne

Szakáll S (1973) Zur Bedeutung der Thymushyperplasie im Säuglings- und Kleinkindesalter. Pädiatr Grenzgeb 12: 337

Tait D, Goldstraw P, Husband J (1986) Thymic rebound in an adult following chemotherapy for testicular cancer. Eur J Surg Oncol 12: 385

Tartas NE, Korin J, Dengra CS, Barazutti LM, Blasetti A, Avalos JCS (1985) Diffuse thymic enlargement in Hodgkin's disease. JAMA 19: 406

Tesseraux H (1953) Physiologie und Pathologie des Thymus unter besonderer Berücksichtigung der pathologischen Morphologie. Barth, Leipzig

Thal W (1972) Kinderbronchologie. Barth, Leipzig, p 187

Thomas E, Kochenrath J (1922) Zur Klinik des Säuglings-Stridors. Z Hals-Nasen-Ohrenheilkd 1: 34

Thomas JA, Willcox HNA, Newsom-Davis J (1982) Immunohistological studies of the thymus in myasthenia gravis: correlation with clinical state and thymocyte culture responses. J Neuroimmunol 3: 319

Thomas NB, Gupta SC (1988) Unilobar enlargement of normal thymus gland causing mass effect. Br J Radiol 61: 244

Thurmond AS, Brasch RC (1978) Radiologic evaluation of the thymus in juvenile myasthenia gravis. Pediatr Radiol 7: 136

Tischer W (1967) Diagnostische und therapeutische Möglichkeiten bei Thymushyperplasie im Säuglingsalter. Kinderärztl Prax 35: 333

Tobisu K, Kakizoe T, Takai K, Matsumoto K, Tsuchiya R (1987) Thymic enlargement following treatment for a metastatic germ cell tumor. A case report. J Urol 137: 520

Tridente G (1985) Immunopathology of the human thymus. Semin Hematol 22: 56

van Herle AJ, Chopra IJ (1971) Thymic hyperplasia in Graves' disease. J Clin Endocrinol Metab 32: 140

von Lengerke HJ, Schmidt H (1988) Mediastinal-Sonographie im Kindesalter. Ergebnisse bei 310 Untersuchungen. Radiologe 28: 460

Waldbott GL (1934) So-called "thymic death": pathologic process in 34 cases. Am J Dis Child 47: 41

Walter E, Hübener K-H (1980) Computertomographische Charakteristika raumfordernder Prozesse im vorderen Mediastinum und ihre Differentialdiagnose. ROFO 133: 391

Whittaker LD, Lynn HB (1973) Mediastinal tumors and cysts in the pediatric patient. Surg Clin North Am 53: 893

Willich E (1975) Mediastinalpleuritis. Pädiatr Prax 15: 45

Woodhead PJ (1984) Thymic enlargement following chemotherapy. Br J Radiol 57: 932

Wychulis AR, Payne WS, Clagett OT, Woolner LB (1971) Surgical treatment of mediastinal tumors. J Thorac Cardiovasc Surg 62: 379

Yulish BS, Owens RP (1980) Thymic enlargement in a child during therapy for primary hypothyroidism. AJR 135: 157

Zsebök Z (1958) Röntgenanatomie der Neugeborenen- und Säuglingslunge. Thieme, Stuttgart, p 118

8 Tumors of the Thymus

E. Walter, E. Willich, W. J. Hofmann, H. F. Otto, W. R. Webb, and G. de Geer

8.1 Introduction

E. Walter

As would be expected from studies of developmental anatomy, the thymus consists of heterogeneous material, which naturally can give rise to various benign and malignant tumors.

A large number of lists of tumors of the thymus have been published. Otto (1984) described 20 different pathoanatomic classifications. While Tesseraux (1953) differentiated between benign and malignant tumors of the thymus, today the tumors are differentiated according to their cell structure, hormone production, and function. This method of differentiation is favored by the fact that it is seldom possible to differentiate between benign and malignant forms of thymoma unless there is invasive growth in the surrounding tissue or metastases are found.

During the past two decades, substantial progress has been made in understanding the biology of the thymus and, therefore, the pathology and clinical behavior of thymic tumors (Levine and Rosai 1978; Janossy et al. 1980; Ciba Foundation Symposium, No. 84, 1984). Such tumors include those arising from thymic epithelial cells (thymomas), neuroendocrine cells (carcinoid tumors of the thymus), lymphoid cells (malignant non-Hodgkin's lymphomas and Hodgkin's disease), and adipose tissue (thymolipomas). All other tumors (myoid and histiocytic) and tumor-like lesions (cysts, hyperplasia) are extremely rare (Rosai and Levine 1976; Otto 1984).

The different tumors of the thymus discussed here reflect the surveys of Otto and Hüsselmann (1978) and Otto (1984), supplemented by recent reports of the more seldom tumors:

1. Epithelial tumors (encapsulated and invasive thymomas, squamous cell carcinoma etc.)
2. Carcinoids
3. Malignant lymphoma and leukemia
4. Mesenchymal tumors (thymolipoma)
5. Germ cell tumors
6. Rare tumors (hemangioma, choristoma etc.)
7. Metastases

References

CIBA Foundation Symposium No. 84 (1981) Microenvironments in haemopoietic and lymphoid differentiation. Pitman, London

Janossy G, Thomas JA, Bollum FJ et al. (1980) The human thymic microenvironment: an immunohistologic study. J Immunol 125: 202

Levine GD, Rosai J (1978) Thymic hyperplasia and neoplasia: a review of current concepts. Hum Pathol 9: 495

Otto HF (1984) Pathologie des Thymus. In: Doerr W, Seifert G, Uehlinger G (eds) Spezielle pathologische Anatomie, vol 17. Springer, Heidelberg, Berlin, New York

Otto HF, Hüsselmann (1978) Klinisch-pathologische Studie zur Klassifikation und Prognose von Thymustumoren. Z Krebsforsch 91: 81

Rosai J, Levine GD (1976) Tumors of the thymus. In: Atlas of tumor pathology, sec. series, fasc. 13. AFIP, Washington, DC

Tesseraux H (1953) Physiologie und Pathologie des Thymus unter besonderer Berücksichtigung der pathologischen Morphologie. Barth, Leipzig

8.2 Epithelial Tumors of the Thymus

8.2.1 Pathologic Features

W. J. HOFMANN and H. F. OTTO

8.2.1.1 Macroscopic Appearance

8.2.1.1.1 Location

Most thymomas are located in the anterior mediastinum. About 4% of thymomas are located in the lateral cervical region (ROSAI and LEVINE 1976; SALYER and EGGLESTON 1976; GRAY and GUTOWSKY 1979; WICK et al. 1990), which might be a consequence of fetal maldevelopment that led to an undescended thymus (RIDENHOUR et al. 1970). There are, however, some rare locations like the posterior mediastinum (ROSAI and LEVINE 1976), the thyroid gland (ASA et al. 1988), within the pleura, or spread out like a mesothelioma (Fig. 8.1) (ROSAI and LEVINE 1976; HARTMANN and HANKE 1984; HOFMANN et al. 1985b; KUNG et al. 1985; FUKAYAMA et al. 1989).

8.2.1.1.2 Size and Cut Surface

The diameter of thymomas varies considerably within the range of 1 mm in a fortuitously detected lesion (ROSAI and LEVINE 1976) and 20–30 cm (BERNATZ et al. 1961; SALYER and EGGLESTON 1976; LEGOLVAN and ABELL 1977; GRAY and GUTOWSKY 1979). ROSAI and LEVINE (1976) reported a median diameter of 5–10 cm; in our own series of 98 thymomas (HOFMANN et al. 1985b) we found a range from 2 to 20 cm. A diameter of 20 cm seems to be the upper limit since the findings of most authors do not exceed this value (BATATA et al. 1974; SALYER and EGGLESTON 1976; LEGOLVAN and ABELL 1977; GRAY and GUTOWSKY 1979; LEIPNER et al. 1982). This could be due to the fact that tumors of that size are detected by the local symptoms they cause.

The average tumor weight is 120–150 g. GRAY and GUTOWSKY (1979), for example, reported a median weight of 130 g (range, 30–250 g). BERGH and co-workers (1978) found that stage III tumors were heaviest 85–1700 g compared to 20–440g for stage I tumors.

Most of the thymomas are lobulated by fibrous bands resulting in a nodular surface and in a lobulated cut surface, one of the most characteristic but nevertheless nonspecific gross features of thymomas (Fig. 8.2). The consistency of the tumors varies from soft to very firm. Within the tumors, small areas of necrosis can be found, but these are less common than cysts. Smaller cysts might be filled with a clear fluid, larger ones with a thick, brown, blood-like fluid (Fig. 8.3). Foci of hemorrhage of varying extent occur in about 30% of the tumors (ROSAI and LEVINE 1976; SALYER and EGGLESTON 1976; LEGOVAN and ABELL 1977; GRAY and GUTOWSKY 1979).

8.2.1.1.3 Encapsulation

One of the most important prognostic parameters of the tumor in situ is whether it is encapsulated or not, as will be discussed below. About 60%–70% of the thymomas are encapsulated; the rest grow into the surrounding fat tissue or organs like pleura and lungs, pericardium, or great vessels (FRIEDMAN 1967; BATATA et al. 1974; SALYER and EGGLESTON 1976; LEGOLVAN and ABELL 1977; BERGH et al. 1978; GRAY and GUTOWSKY 1979; HOFMANN et al. 1985b; VERLEY and HOLLMANN 1985).

ROSAI and LEVINE (1976) observed that the surgeon is usually in a better position than the pathologist to assess the invasive nature of a thymoma from the findings at thoracotomy, but it is sometimes difficult to differentiate macroscopically between fibrous adhesions and invasion by the tumor. In these cases an intraoperative cryostat section or a filament marking of the suspected site would be desirable to enable the pathologist to examine the histology of this site.

8.2.1.2 Histologic Appearance

8.2.1.2.1 The Epithelial Component

The epithelial cells of thymoma can occur as round to oval, large cells with vesicular nuclei and small, inconspicuous or prominent nucleoli. In our series of 98 thymomas, 55.1% were primarily composed of these epitheloid cells (Fig. 8.4). The other feature of epithelial cells is their markedly elongated spindle-shaped and elongated nuclei: 17.4% in our series were primarily composed of that spindle cell type (Fig. 8.5). If a thymoma is a combination of the cell types mentioned above, it is classified as a mixed thymoma. In our series 20.4% were of that type (HOFMANN et al. 1985b).

Most thymomas are of these three types. There are, however, some other rare differentiations of thymoma epithelial cells reported in the literature:

Fig. 8.1. Malignant thymoma; invasive growth like that of a mesothelioma. The tumor, which is composed of solid nodules of various size separated by fibrous septa, surrounds the lobe of a lung. 28-year-old man without myasthenia gravis. (compare Hofmann et al. 1985 b)

Fig. 8.2. Thymoma totally surrounded by a fibrous capsule and lobulated by fibrous bands. Regressive changes with a focus of hemorrhage and small cysts (left and right lower side). Female, 60 years, myasthenia gravis, thymomectomy specimen 80 g

Fig. 8.3. Malignant thymoma with large cystic degeneration. Male, 54 years, myasthenia gravis, thymectomy specimen

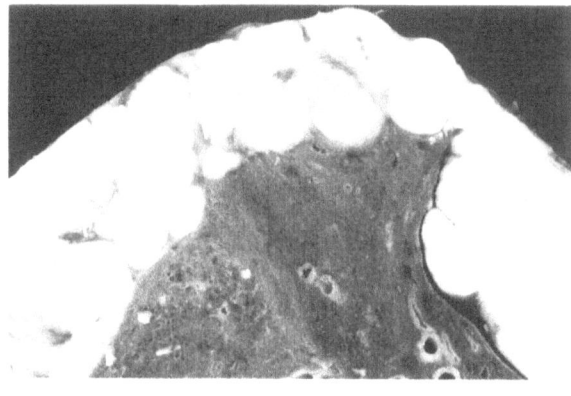

8.1

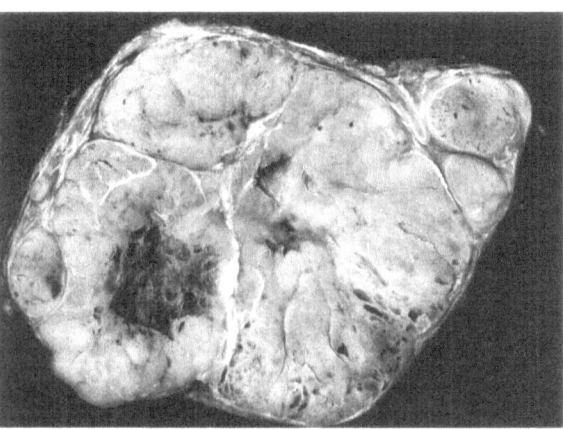

8.2

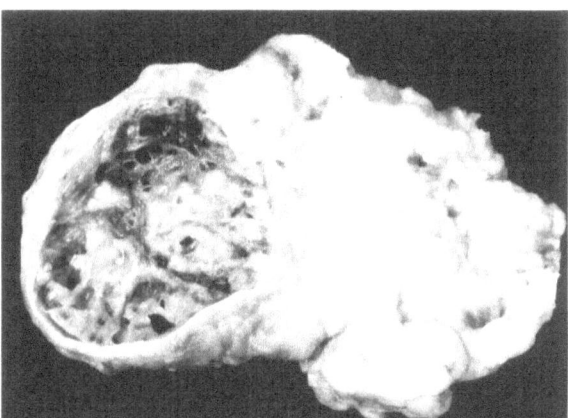

8.3

Table 8.1. Classification of thymomas according to Rosai and Levine (1976) and to Levine and Rosai (1978)

1. Benign encapsulated thymomas ("circumscribed thymomas")
   Well encapsulated, without invasion and distant metastases
   With no or minimal cytologic atypia
     a) Large/epitheloid cell type
     b) Spindle cell type   With or without associated lymphocytic component
     c) Mixed cell type

2. Malignant thymomas (category I by Levine and Rosai 1978)
   Locally invasive or with distant metastases
   With no or minimal cytologic atypia
     a) Large/epitheloid cell type
     b) Spindle cell type   With or without associated lymphocytic component
     c) Mixed cell type

3. Thymic carcinomas (category II by Levine and Rosai 1978)
   With cytologic atypia
   Encapsulated or invasive or metastatic[a]
     a) Undifferentiated
     b) Lymphoepithelioma-like
     c) Squamous
     d) Basaloid   With or without associated lymphocytic component
     e) Clear cell
     f) Sarcomatoid
     g) Mucoepidermoid

[a] Compare: Thomson and Thackray 1957; Shimosato et al. 1977; Levine and Rosai 1978; Snover et al. 1982; Wick et al. 1982; Hofmann et al. 1985 b

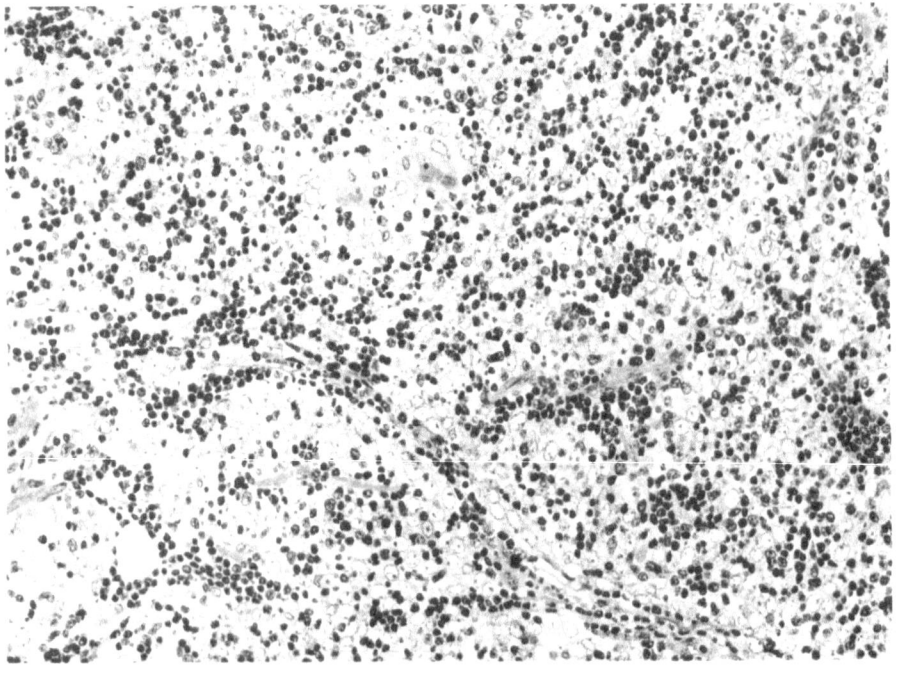

Fig. 8.4. Large epithelioid cell type thymoma (thymoma of cortical type). Epithelial cells with large, vesicular nuclei and inconspicuous cytoplasmic outlines. Predominant lymphocytic association almost covering the epithelial tumor cells. H & E, ×270

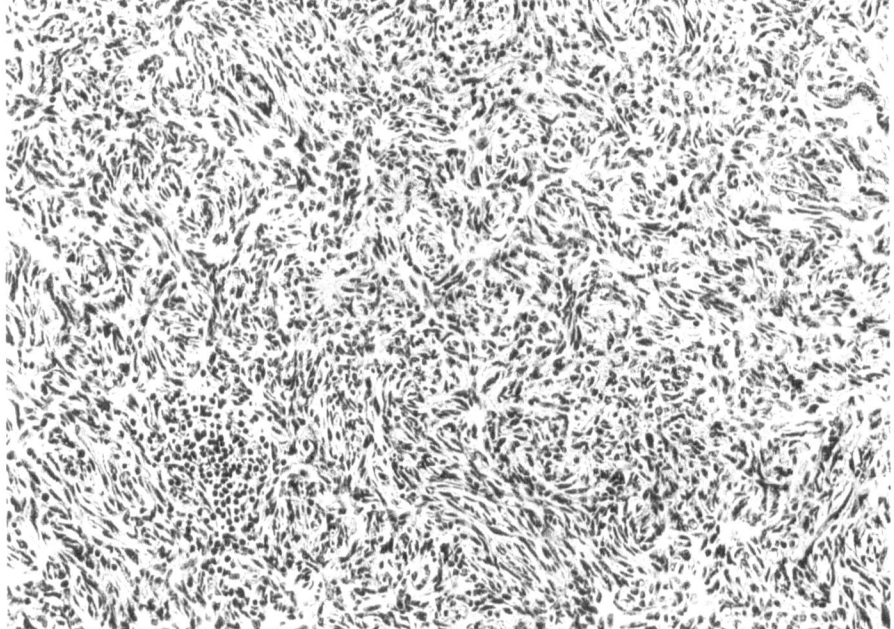

Fig. 8.5. Spindle cell type thymoma. Elongated cells with elongated nuclei are arranged in whorls resembling fibrous histiocytoma. H & E, ×135

small cell (LEGG and BRADY 1965), reticular-shaped, squamoid (Fig. 8.6), and true squamous differentiation (LEVINE and ROSAI 1978).

Cytologic malignant features are missing or extremely rare in the formerly mentioned types of thymoma, whereas the types listed in Table 8.1 are characterized by well-documented cytologic malignant features and are therefore called thymic carcinoma (LEVINE and ROSAI 1978). Numbers, in relation to the thymomas with minimal cytologic atypia or none, are small. They can occur in the morphologic variants outlined in the table: undifferentiated, lymphoepithelioma-like, squamous, basaloid (Fig. 8.7), clear cell, sarcomatoid, and

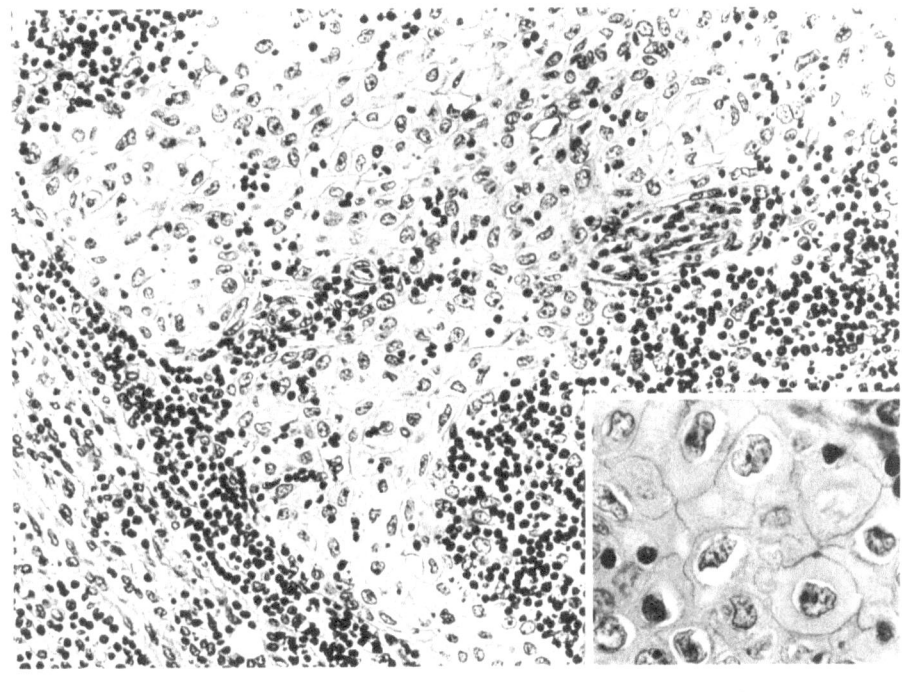

Fig. 8.6. Thymoma with an epidermoid appearance. Note the distinct cytoplasmic out-lines of tumor cells. Moderate lymphocytic association. Papanicolaou stain, × 200. *Inset,* × 400

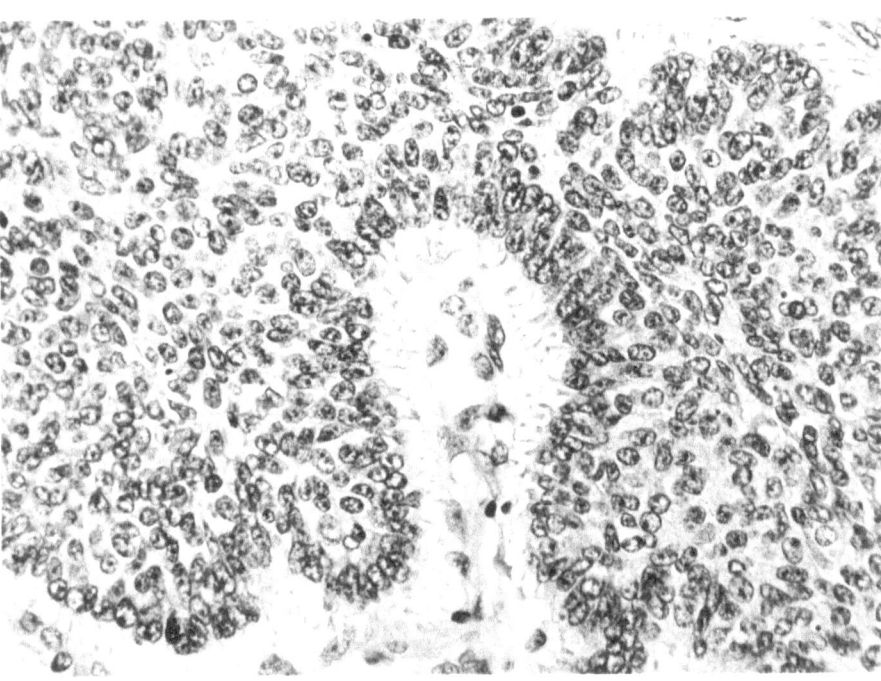

Fig. 8.7. Basaloid carcinoma of the thymus. Palisading of the cells at the periphery of tumor lobules is a characteristic feature of this type. H & E, × 340

mucoepidermoid thymus carcinoma (THOMSON and THACKRAY 1957; SHIMOSATO et al. 1977; LEVINE and ROSAI 1978; SNOVER et al. 1982; WICK et al. 1982; CHEN 1984; HOFMANN et al. 1985b; MORINAGA et al. 1987; KUO et al. 1990; TRUONG et al. 1990; y CAJAL and SUSTER 1991).

8.2.1.2.2 Lymphocytic Association

Thymomas can be associated with a variable number of lymphocytes (Figs. 8.4, 8.8). Most authors describe the association in a semiquantitative manner (ROSAI and LEVINE 1976; GRAY and GUTOWSKY 1979; MASAOKA et al. 1981; MONDEN et al. 1985). If

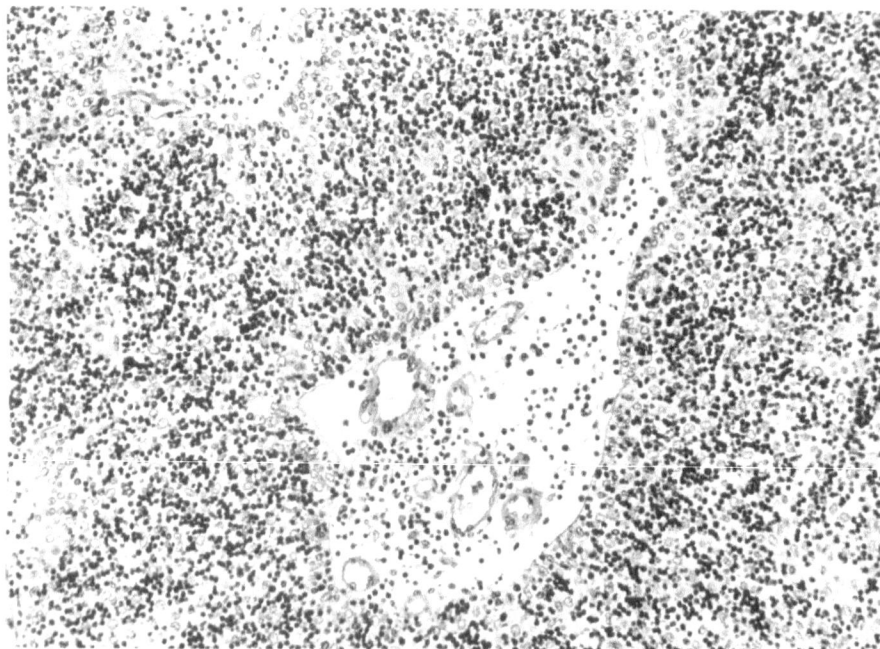

Fig. 8.8. Epitheloid cell type thymoma with a perivascular space that contains mature lymphocytes. Papanicolaou stain, ×240

the lymphocytic association is so great that it becomes difficult to recognize the epithelial component, it is classified as predominant. If there is an equal distribution of epithelial cells and lymphocytes, the lymphocytic association is called moderate. If few lymphocytes are associated with the epithelial cells, the association is scant. In a thymoma without lymphocytes the association is absent.

Some authors referred to the lymphocytic association and classified thymomas as epithelial, lymphoepithelial, and lymphocytic according to the number of lymphocytes and as spindle shaped according to the epithelial component (LATTES and JONAS 1957; LATTES 1962; SALYER and EGGLESTON 1976; LEGOLVAN and ABELL 1977). Since this classification mingles epithelial cell characteristics and lymphocytic association and since it assumes there is no lymphocytic association in the case of spindle cell thymoma (which is not true), we prefer the classification based on that of ROSAI and LEVINE (1976).

8.2.1.2.3 Structural Differentiation

Beside the characteristics of the epithelial component and the different lymphocytic association, there are a number of structural differentiations of thymomas. These can be helpful in the differential diagnosis of anterior mediastinal tumors if they are

imitations of structures occurring in normal thymic tissue. But they can also be a challenge if they resemble structures of anterior mediastinal tumors other than thymomas.

Tumor cells can be arranged like HASSALL's corpuscles and imitate them in the way they occur in the normal thymus (Fig. 8.9). Perivascular spaces (Figs. 8.8, 8.10) are areas around blood vessels filled with lymphocytes, macrophages, foamy cells, plasma cells, and mast cells and are sometimes hyalinized. Lymphocyte-rich thymomas may display areas with no or minimal lymphocytic association, mimicking the appearance of normal thymic medulla (medullary differentiation).

Epithelial cells of thymoma can be arranged along blood vessels like a hemangiopericytoma. The cells of the spindle cell thymoma can grow in whorls or in a storiform pattern resembling fibrous histiocytoma. Rosette formation and gland-like formation of epithelial tumor cells might occur and must then be distinguished from metastatic adenocarcinoma spreading into the anterior mediastinum. Finally, microcystic degeneration can occur.

8.2.1.3 Classification

There are many different classifications of thymomas (for review see OTTO 1984), a consequence of the small number of tumors, on the one hand, and

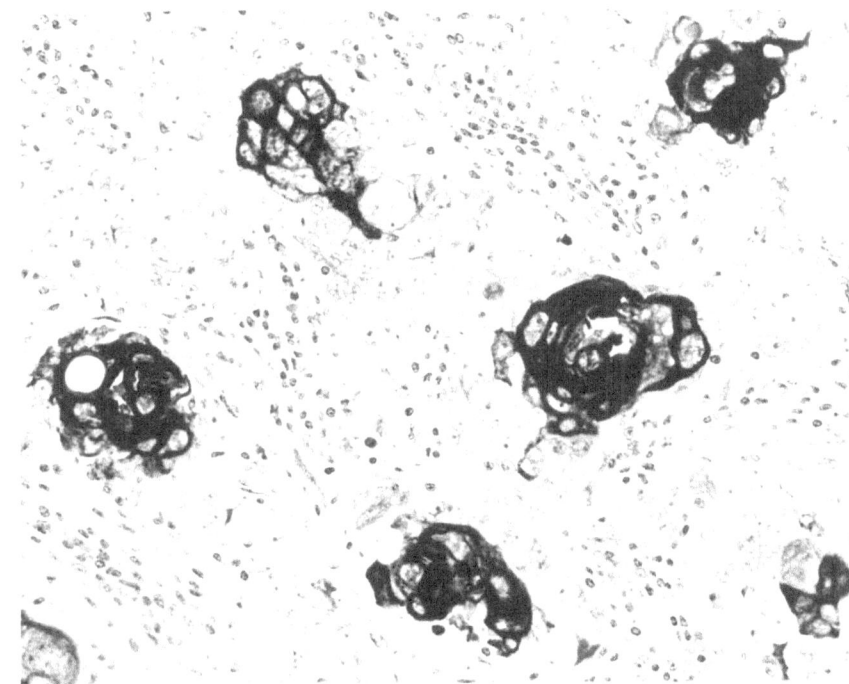

Fig. 8.9. Structural differentiation of thymoma. Thymoma epithelial cells are arranged like Hassall's corpuscles. Keratin, × 300

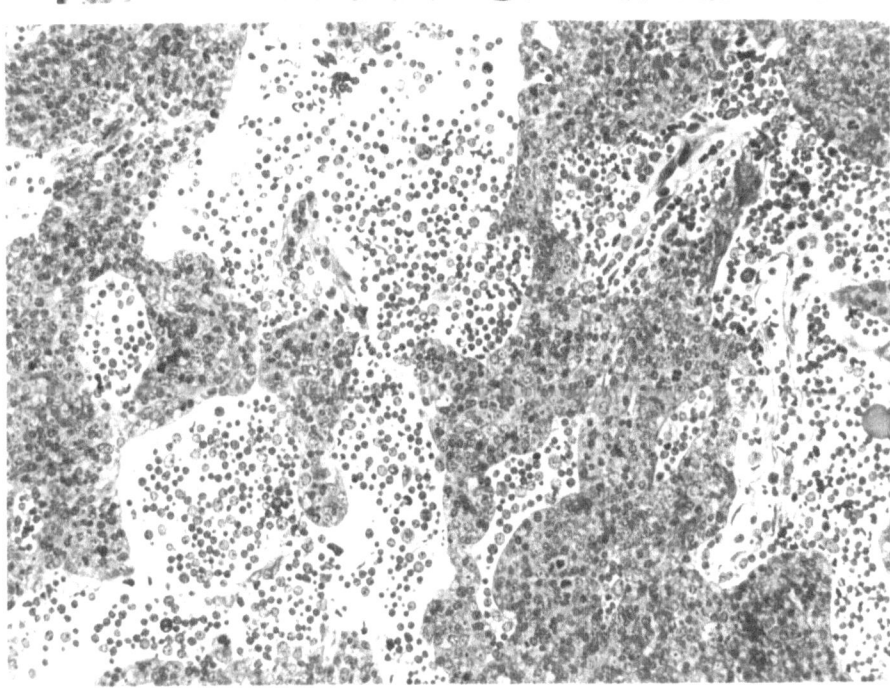

Fig. 8.10. Epitheloid cell thymoma with perivascular spaces that contain mature lymphocytes. Semithin section, toluidine blue, × 320

of longstanding neglect of the special histology of the normal thymus on the other. The difficulty with every classification lies in the enormous variability of the histologic appearance of thymomas, which can be observed even in a single tumor (FRIEDMAN 1967; ROSAI and LEVINE 1976; SALYER and EGGLESTON 1976). We believe that at least ten different sites of a tumor have to be examined to get a survey of the histologic appearance. Therefore one must be aware of the fact that a descriptive diagnosis of a thymoma cannot cover all aspects and is restricted to its predominant part. This is true for every feature of the tumor. To be practical clinically, a classification should be easily re-

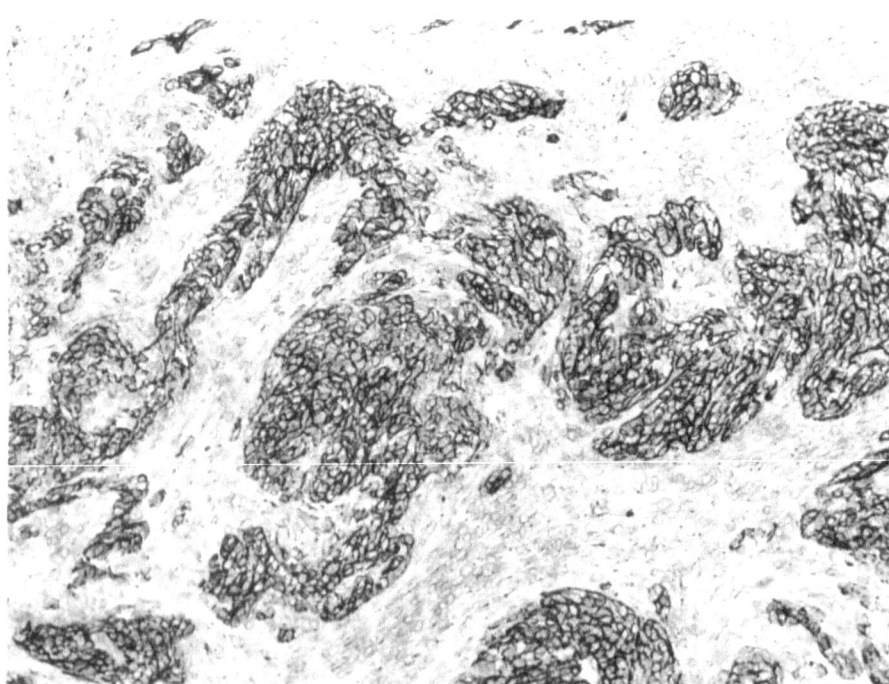

Fig. 8.11. Epitheloid cell type thymoma. Intense staining of tumor cells by antikeratin antibody. Fibrous bands are not stained. Cryostat section, keratin labeling, × 160

producible. In addition it should correspond with certain clinical and functional characteristics of the tumor. So far, the descriptive classification of LEVINE and ROSAI (1978) is the most accepted in the literature. It clearly distinguished between epithelial differentiation, lymphocyte association, and structural differentiation.

As mentioned earlier, only tumors of thymic epithelial cell origin are classified as thymomas. According to the shape of these epithelial cells, the thymomas are classified as large or epitheloid cell type and spindle cell type. If both cell types can be found in equal distribution, they are classified as mixed type thymomas. The degree of lymphocytic association does not serve as a classification parameter but only provides additional information within the descriptive diagnosis.

In the overwhelming number of thymomas, cytologic atypias of tumor cells (i.e., high numbers of mitoses, atypical mitosis, pleomorphic nuclei) are absent or extremely scarce. Nevertheless, thymomas of this group are classified into a "benign" subgroup, the benign encapsulated thymoma, if they are surrounded by a totally intact capsule, and into a "malignant" subgroup, the malignant thymoma [category I of malignant thymomas according to LEVINE and ROSAI (1978)], if tumors show local invasion or actually have lymphatic or hematogenous spread. The reason for this differentia-

tion into two groups lies in the different clinical outcome of patients with invasive thymomas.

Furthermore, as mentioned, a small number of thymomas exhibit clear-cut malignant cytologic features and are therefore called thymic carcinomas [category II of malignant thymomas according to LEVINE and ROSAI (1978)]. Different morphologic variants of these tumors are described in the literature as follows: undifferentiated, lymphoepithelioma-like, squamous, basaloid, clear cell, sarcomatoid, and mucoepidermoid carcinoma of the thymus (for numbers and references see Table 8.1). If a tumor of the above-mentioned histologic pattern is found in the anterior mediastinum, a primary tumor (for example, of the nasopharynx, lung, skin, thyroid gland, kidney, salivary gland, or lung) must be excluded before diagnosing thymic carcinoma, which histologically resembles tumors of these regions.

8.2.1.4 Immunohistology

Although in most cases of thymoma this diagnosis can be made by conventional light microscopic methods, there are cases, especially if the tumor is undifferentiated, when it is difficult to decide whether or not a tumor is a thymoma. In this situation immunohistologic methods can serve as a di-

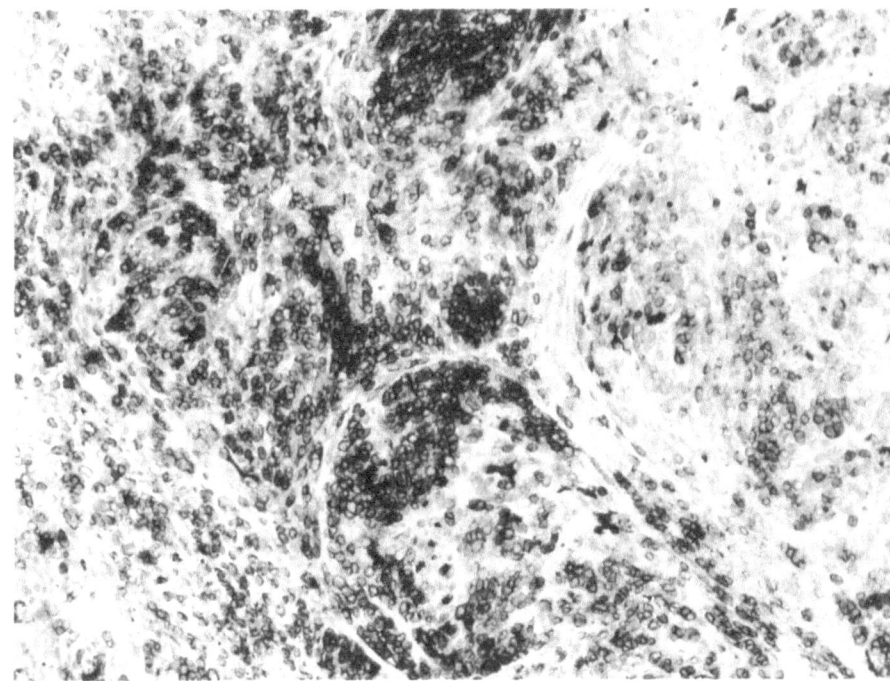

Fig. 8.12. Lymphocytic compartment of a thymoma stained by anti-T6 antibody: majority of lymphocytes express CD1 antigen. Dentritic CD1-positive cells are interspersed. Cryostat section, T6 labeling, × 160

agnostic tool because the epithelial cells of thymomas can be detected by antikeratin antibodies (Fig. 8.11) (BATTIFORA et al. 1980; LÖNING et al. 1981; HIROKAWA et al. 1988; NABARRA et al. 1989; KUO et al. 1990).

Beside the descriptive classification of thymomas by conventional light microscopy, there have always been attempts to classify thymomas histogenetically. LEVINE and ROSAI (1978), for example, held that the thymoma epithelial cells differentiate toward either the normal cortical or the normal medullary cells. Thymoma cells with indistinct cytoplasmic outlines that appear only as vesicular nuclei – with sometimes conspicuous nucleoli – resemble those of normal thymus cortex. In most cases thymomas are composed of these cells. OTTO (1984) distinguished between "cortical" and "medullary" types of epithelioid thymoma cells: cells of the cortical type have indistinct cytoplasmic outlines and seem to be noncohesive; cells of the medullary type have conspicuous cytoplasmic outlines and seem to be cohesive.

MARINO and MÜLLER-HERMELINK (1985) have published a more recent classification of thymomas with cortical, medullary, or mixed types by conventional light microscopic and immunohistologic (MÜLLER-HERMELINK et al. 1985 and 1986; KIRCHNER and MÜLLER-HERMELINK 1989) methods. Immunohistologic methods have intensified the efforts to set up such a classification. In order to classify thymomas as cortical, medullary, or mixed, interest was focused on the immunohistologic properties of normal thymic epithelial cells (KORNSTEIN et al. 1988).

Despite the differential expression of epithelial antigens on normal thymic medullary and cortical epithelial cells (see Chap. 2), the classification of thymomas into the medullary or the cortical type by means of the expression of those antigens is only possible in a minority of cases. Different studies (TAKACS et al. 1987; WILLCOX et al. 1987; HOFMANN et al. 1989) have revealed a coexpression of normal medullary and cortical epithelial antigens on thymoma epithelial cells, thus making it impossible to classify all the tumors on that basis.

This coexpression of both medullary and cortical epithelial antigens on the tumor cells indicates a disturbance of the normal immunophenotype of thymic epithelial cells and thus in gene regulation in such tumors. This phenomenon of antigen disturbance in certain thymomas may indicate their higher degree of dedifferentiation in comparison to those tumors where the antigen expression is not disturbed (HOFMANN et al. 1989). However, whether this phenomenon is of any practical and clinical importance remains to be elucidated in further experimental work.

In addition, immunologic methods have been

applied in determining the lymphocytic component of thymomas. Earlier research, based on the sheep erythrocyte rosette-forming test, revealed that the majority of the thymoma-associated lymphocytes are T lymphocytes (Levine and Polliak 1975; Shirai et al. 1976; Cossman et al. 1978; Fukayama et al. 1989). These results could be confirmed by surface membrane antigen determination by means of monoclonal antibodies. Furthermore, it could be demonstrated that most of the associated T lymphocytes belong to the group of immature thymocytes of normal thymic cortex (Fig. 8.12) (Chilosi et al. 1984; Mokhtar et al. 1984; Hofmann et al. 1985a, 1989; Kornstein et al. 1985). Only some of the lymphocytes, mainly located in areas with few lymphocytes, belong to the group of mature T lymphocytes (Chilosi 1984; Mokhtar et al. 1984; Hofmann et al. 1985a, 1989).

It has been suggested that parts of thymoma lymphocytes might be normal bone marrow precursors that have migrated to the thymus (Lauriola et al. 1981), an assumption that is supported by detecting prothymocytes in a thymoma (Piantelli et al. 1983). Thus, malignant cells that are derived from normal thymic epithelial cells still possess the ability to attract prothymocyte-like cells and to form a distinct thymus-like microenvironment which to a certain degree allows the differentiation of the attracted lymphocytes.

8.2.1.5 Clinicopathologic Correlations

There have been many attempts at the time of diagnosis to correlate a clinical or pathologic feature of the thymoma with the clinical outcome of the disease.

8.2.1.5.1 Histology and Prognosis

There are only slight indications of the correlation between any histologic feature of the current classifications and the prognosis of thymoma (Castleman 1955; Lattes 1962; Wilkins et al. 1966; Batata et al. 1974; Rosai and Levine 1976; Salyer and Eggleston 1976; LeGolvan and Abell 1977; Levine and Rosai 1978; Gray and Gutowsky 1979; Masaoka et al. 1981; Pescarmona et al. 1990). Thymomas classified as thymic carcinoma because of evident cytologic atypia are more likely to be invasive and to metastasize (LeGolvan and Abell 1977; Levine and Rosai 1978;

Gray and Gutowsky 1979). Thymomas associated with a small number of lymphocytes have a less favorable prognosis and seem to be more aggressive than those associated with a high number of lymphocytes (LeGolvan and Abell 1977; Gray and Gutowsky 1979; Masaoka et al. 1981; Monden et al. 1985). Spindle cell thymomas tend to grow slowly (Levine and Rosai 1978). Patients with spindle cell thymoma seem to have a better survival rate than patients with other thymomas (Verley and Hollmann 1985). But in citing Lattes (1962) the attempts to predict the outcome of a thymoma on purely histologic grounds are useless guesswork; another, more important factor is necessary.

8.2.1.5.2 Gross Pathology and Prognosis

One of the most important factors in the prognosis of a thymoma is encapsulation (Bernatz et al. 1961; Lattes 1962; Legg and Brady 1965; Wilkins et al. 1966; Batata et al. 1974; Rosai and Levine 1976; Salyer and Eggleston 1976; LeGolvan and Abell 1977; Gray and Gutowsky 1979), a fact that has led to the development of different staging schemes. The first was designed by Bergh and co-workers (1978) (Table 8.2) and was later modified by Masaoka and co-workers (1981), who intro-

Table 8.2. Staging of thymoma according to Bergh and co-workers (1978)

Stage	Description
I	Intact capsule or growth within the capsule
II	Pericapsular growth into mediastinal fat tissue
III	Invasive growth into the surrounding organs, intrathoracic metastases, or both

Table 8.3. Staging of thymoma according to Masaoka and co-workers (1981)

Stage	Description
I	Macroscopically completely encapsulated and microscopically no capsular invasion
II	Macroscopic invasion into surrounding fatty tissue or mediastinal pleura or microscopic invasion into capsule
III	Macroscopic invasion into neighboring organs (i.e., pericardium, great vessels, or lung)
IV a	Pleural or pericardial dissemination
IV b	Lymphatic or hematogenous metastases

Table 8.4. Staging of thymoma according to VERLEY and HOLLMANN (1985)

Stage	Description
I	Encapsulated, noninvasive tumor; total excision
I a	Without adhesions to the environment
I b	With fibrous adhesions to mediastinal structures
II	Localized invasiveness (e. g., perivascular growth into the mediastinal fat tissue or adjacent pleura or pericardium)
II a	Complete excision
II b	Incomplete excision with local remnants of tumor
III	Largely invading tumor
III a	Invasive growth into the surrounding organs and/or intrathoracic tumorous grafts (pleura pericardium)
III b	Lymphatic or hematogenous metastases

duced the microscopic examination of the tumor capsule (Table 8.3). More recently, VERLEY and HOLLMANN (1985) proposed a staging classification that, in addition to the macroscopic findings, includes the extent of surgical treatment (Table 8.4).

An evaluation of the three classifications reveals an incremental decline in survival rates as the clinical stage advances. Statistical analysis based on the classification of MASAOKA and associates, however, indicates significant differences only between the 5-year survival rates of stages I and III, and of stages I and IV, respectively. As to the classification of VERLEY and HOLLMANN (1985), the statistical analysis reveals a significant difference only between noninvasive stage I tumors and invasive stage II or III tumors. Thus, invasiveness is an important prognostic factor, but the degree of invasion at the time of operation does not seem to influence the survival rate.

8.2.1.5.3 Associated Myasthenia Gravis and Prognosis

About 30% of thymomas are associated with myasthenia gravis (OTTO 1984). Some investigation series have indicated that myasthenia gravis-associated thymomas have a more unfavorable prognosis than thymomas without associated myasthenia gravis (WILKINS et al. 1966; BATATA et al. 1974; SALYER and EGGLESTON 1976; LEGOLVAN and ABELL 1977; GRAY and GUTOWSKY 1979; TANDAN et al. 1990) but this seems to be owing to the existence of two potentially lethal diseases rather than to a more aggressive behavior of thymoma as-

sociated with myasthenia gravis (LEGOLVAN and ABELL 1977).

On examining the causes of death it can be stated that death owing to tumor occurs less often in patients with myasthenic thymomas than in those with nonmyasthenic thymomas (SALYER and EGGLESTON 1976; MASAOKA et al. 1981). Therefore thymomas in myasthenic patients not only are less lethal than in nonmyasthenic patients (BERNATZ et al. 1961), they even appear slightly less aggressive (VERLEY and HOLLMANN 1985). A recent report indicates a more favorable 5-year survival rate in myasthenic patients (94%) than in nonmyasthenic patients (68%) with thymomas (WILKINS and CASTLEMAN 1979). Improved long-term medical treatment of myasthenic patients together with discovery of thymoma at an earlier stage when associated with myasthenia gravis could explain this fact.

References

Asa SL, Dardick I, van Nostrand AWP, Bailey DJ (1988) Primary thyroid thymoma: A distinct clinicopathologic entity. Hum Pathol 19: 1463–1467

Batata MA, Martini N, Huvos AG, Aguilar RI, Beattie EJ (1974) Thymomas: clinico-pathologic features, therapy, and prognosis. Cancer 34: 389–396

Battifora H, Sun T-T, Bahu RM, Rao S (1980) The use of antikeratin serum as a diagnostic tool – thymoma versus lymphoma. Hum Pathol 11: 635–641

Bergh NP, Gatzinsky P, Larsson S, Lundin P, Ridell B (1978) Tumors of the thymus and thymic region. I. Clinicopathological studies on thymomas. Ann Thorac Surg 25: 91–98

Bernatz PE, Harrison EG, Clagett OT (1961) Thymoma – a clinicopathological study. J Thorac Cardiovasc Surg 42: 424–444

Castleman B (1955) Tumors of the thymus gland. In: Atlas of tumor pathology, second series, fascicle 19. Washington DC: Armed Forces Institute of Pathology

Chen KTK (1984) Squamous carcinoma of the thymus. J Surg Oncol 25: 61–63

Chilosi M (1984) Immunohistochemical analysis of thymoma – evidence for medullary origin of epithelial cells. Am J Surg Pathol 8: 309–318

Ciba foundation symposium, No. 84 (1981) Microenvironments in haemapoietic and lymphoid differentiation. Pitman, London

Cossman J, Deegan MJ, Schnitzler B (1978) Thymoma: an immunologic and electron microscopic study. Cancer 41: 2183–2191

Friedman NB (1967) Tumors of the thymus. J Thorac Cardiovasc Surg 53: 163–182

Fukayama M, Maeda Y, Funata N, Koike M, Saito K, Sakai T, Ikeda T (1989) Pulmonary and pleural thymoma. Diagnostic application of lymphocyte marker to the thymoma of unusual site. Am J Clin Pathol 89: 617–621

Gray GF, Gutowsky WT (1979) Thymoma – a clinicopathologic study of 54 cases. Am J Surg Pathol 3: 235–249

Hartmann C-A, Hanke S (1984) Ungewöhnliche Pleurabe-
teiligung eines metastasierenden Thymoms. Pathologe 5:
169–172
Hartmann C-A, Roth Chr, Minck C, Niedobitek G (1990)
Thymic carcinoma. Report of five cases and review of the
literature. J Cancer Res Clin Oncol 116: 69–82
Hirokawa K, Utsuyama M, Moriizumi E, Hashimoto T,
Masaoka A, Goldstein AL (1988) Immunohistochemical
studies in human thymomas. Localization of thymosin
and various cell markers. Virchows Arch [B] 55: 371–380
Hofmann WJ, Möller P, Otto HF (1985 a) Immunohistolo-
gische Charakterisierung von Thymomen mit Hilfe mo-
noklonaler Antikörper, polyklonalem Anti-Keratinse-
rum und Lektinen. Verh Dtsch Ges Pathol 69: 641
Hofmann WJ, Möller P, Manke H-G, Otto HF (1985 b)
Thymoma – a clinicopathologic study of 98 cases with
special reference to three unusual cases. Pathol Res Pract
179: 337–353
Hofmann WJ, Pallesen G, Möller P, Kunze W-P, Kayser K,
Otto HF (1989) Expression of cortical and medullary
thymic epithelial antigens in thymomas. An immunohistochemical study of 14 cases including a characterization
of the lymphocytic compartment. Histopathology 14:
447–463
Janossy G, Thomas JA, Bollum FJ et al. (1980) The human
thymic microenvironment: an immunohistologic study.
J Immunol 125: 202–212
Kirchner Th, Müller-Hermelink KH (1989) New ap-
proaches to the diagnosis of thymic epithelial tumors.
Progr Surg Pathol 10: 167–189
Kornstein MJ, Hoxie JA, Levinson AJ, Brooks JJ (1985)
Immunohistology of human thymomas. Arch Pathol Lab
Med 109: 460–463
Kornstein MJ, Curran WJ Jr, Turrisi AT III, Brooks JJ
(1988) Cortical versus medullary thymomas: a useful
morphologic distinction? Hum Pathol 19: 1335–1339
Kung I, Loke SL, So SY, Lam WK, Mok CK, Khin MA
(1985) Intrapulmonary thymoma: report of two cases.
Thorax 40: 471–474
Kuo TT, Chang J-P, Lin F-J, Wu W-C, Chang C-H (1990)
Thymic carcinomas: histopathological varieties and im-
munohistochemical study. Am J Surg Pathol 14: 24–34
Lattes R (1962) Thymomas and other tumors of the thymus:
An analysis of 107 cases. Cancer 15: 1224–1260
Lattes R, Jonas S (1957) The pathological and clinical fea-
tures in eighty cases of thymoma. Bull NY Acad Med 33:
145
Lauriola L, Maggiano N, Marino M, Carbone A, Piantelli
M, Musiani P (1981) Human thymoma: immunologic
characteristics of the lymphocytic components. Cancer
48: 1992–1995
Legg MA, Brady WJ (1965) Pathology and clinical behavior
of thymomas. A survey of 51 cases. Cancer 18: 1131–1144
LeGolvan DP, Abell MR (1977) Thymomas. Cancer 39:
2142–2157
Leipner N, Cremer H, Engel C (1982) Thymome: klinisch-
pathologische Aspekte. Onkologie 5: 196–205
Levine GD, Polliak A (1975) The T-cell nature of the lymphocytes in two human epithelial thymomas: a comparative immunologic, scanning and transmission electron microscopic study. Clin Immunol Immunopathol 4:
199–208
Levine GD, Rosai J (1978) Thymic hyperplasia and neoplasia: a review of current concepts. Hum Pathol 9: 495–515
Löning T, Caselitz J, Otto HF (1981) The epithelial frame-

work of the thymus in normal and pathological condi-
tions. Virchows Arch [A] 392: 7–20
Marino M, Müller-Hermelink H-K (1985) Thymoma and
thymic carcinoma – relation of thymoma epithelial cells
to the cortical and medullary differentiation of thymus.
Virch Arch [A] 407: 119–149
Masaoka A, Monden Y, Nakahara K, Tanioka T (1981)
Follow-up study of thymomas with special reference to
their clinical stages. Cancer 48: 2485–2492
Mokhtar N, Hsu SM, Lad RP, Haynes BF, Jaffe ES (1984)
Thymoma: lymphoid and epithelial components mirror
the phenotype of normal thymus. Hum Pathol 15: 378–
384
Monden Y, Nakahara K, Ioka S et al. (1985) Recurrence of
thymoma: clinicopathological features, therapy, and
prognosis. Ann Thorac Surg 39: 165–169
Morinaga S, Sato Y, Shimosato Y, Sinkai T, Tsuchiya R
(1987) Multiple thymic squamous cell carcinomas associated with mixed type thymoma. Am J Surg Pathol 11:
982–988
Müller-Hermelink KH, Marino M, Palestro G (1986) Pathology of thymic epithelial tumors. In: Müller-Hermelink KH (ed) The human thymus. Histophysiology and
pathology. Curr Top Pathol 75: 207–268
Müller-Hermelink HK, Marino M, Palestro G, Schumacher U, Kirchner Th (1985) Immunohistological evi-
dences of cortical and medullary differentiation in thymoma. Virchows Arch A 408: 143–161
Nabarra B, Manganella G, Savino W (1989) Differential diagnosis between undifferentiated tumor and thymoma by
electron microscopy and immunohistochemical labelling.
Pathol Res Pract 185: 257–263
Otto HF (1984) Pathologie des Thymus. In: Doerr W, Seifert G, Uehlinger E (eds) Spezielle pathologische Anatomie, vol 17. Springer, Berlin Heidelberg New York
Pescarmona E, Rendina EA, Venuta F, Ricci C, Ruco LP,
Baroni CD (1990) The prognostic implication of thymo-
ma histologic subtyping. A study of 80 consecutive cases.
Am J Clin Pathol 93: 190–195
Piantelli M, Ranelletti FO, Musiani P, Lauriola L, Maggia-
no N (1983) A human thymoma with promyelocyte-like
infiltration. Clin Immunol Immunopathol 28: 350–360
Ridenhour CE, Henzel JH, DeWeese MS, Kerr SE (1970)
Thymoma arising from undescended cervical thymus.
Surgery 67: 614–619
Rosai J, Levine GD (1976) Tumors of the thymus. In: Atlas
of tumor pathology, second series, fascicle 13. Armed
Forces Institute of Pathology, Washington, DC
Salyer WR, Eggleston JC (1976) Thymoma – a clinical and
pathological study of 65 cases. Cancer 37: 229–249
Shimosato Y, Kameya T, Nagai K, Suemasu K (1977) Squa-
mous cell carcinoma of the thymus. An analysis of eight
cases. Am J Surg Pathol 1: 109–121
Shirai T, Miyata M, Nakase A, Itoh T (1976) Lymphocyte
subpopulation in neoplastic and non-neoplastic thymus
and in blood of patients with myasthenia gravis. Clin Exp
Immunol 26: 118–123
Snover DC, Levine GD, Rosai J (1982) Thymic carcinoma:
five distinct histological variants. Am J Surg Pathol 6:
451–470
Takacs L, Savino W, Monostori E, Ando J, Bach J-F, Dardenne M (1987) Cortical thymocyte differentiation in
thymomas; an immunohistologic analysis of the pathologic microenvironment. J Immunol 138: 687–698
Tandan R, Raylor R, DiConstanzo DP, Sharma K, Fries T,

Roberts J (1990) Metastasizing thymoma and myasthenia gravis. Favorable response to glucocorticoids after failed chemotherapy and radiation therapy. Cancer 65: 1286–1290

Thomson AD, Thackray AC (1957) The histology of tumours of the thymus. Br J Cancer 11: 348–364

Truong LD, Mody DR, Cagle PT, Jackson-York GL, Schwartz MR, Wheeler TM (1990) Thymic carcinoma. A clinicopathologic study of 13 cases. Am J Surg Pathol 14: 151–166

Verley JM, Hollmann KH (1985) Thymoma – a comparative study of clinical stages, histologic features and survival in 200 cases. Cancer 55: 1074–1086

Wick MR, Simpson RW, Niehans GA, Scheithauer BW (1990) Anterior mediastinal tumors: A clinicopathologic study of 100 cases, with emphasis on immunohistochemical analysis. Progr Surg Pathol 11: 79–119

Wick MR, Weiland LH, Scheithauer BW, Bernatz PE (1982) Primary thymic carcinomas. Am J Surg Pathol 6: 613–630

Wilkins EW, Castleman B (1979) Thymoma: a continuing survey at the Massachusetts General Hospital. Ann Thorac Surg 28: 252–255

Wilkins EW, Edmunds LH, Castleman B (1966) Cases of thymoma at the Massachusetts General Hospital. J Thorac Cardiovasc Surg 52: 322–330

Willcox N, Schluep M, Rittr MA, Schuurman HJ, Newsom-Davis J, Christensson B (1987) Myasthenic and nonmyasthenic thymoma. An expansion of a minor cortical epithelial cell subset? Am J Pathol 127: 447–460

y Cajal SR, Suster S (1991) Primary thymic epithelial neoplasms in children. Am J Surg Pathol 15: 466–474

8.2.2 Encapsulated and Invasive Thymomas

E. WALTER

8.2.2.1 Occurrence and Clinical Symptoms

8.2.2.1.1 Occurrence

Although tumors of the thymus are relatively rare, they account for approximately 5%–16% of all tumors of the mediastinum (LENNERT and HEPP 1968; KRAUS et al. 1970; DÜX 1977; OTTO and HÜSSELMANN 1978). Between 20% and 30% of tumors of the anterior mediastinum are primary tumors of the thymus (SALAYER and EGGLESTON 1976; LEVASSEUR et al. 1976).

Age Distribution. Thymomas are found at all ages. They are rare in children, but can be found directly following birth (OPPERMANN and BRANDEIS 1975). Whereas HASSE and WALDSCHMIDT (1967) found thymomas in 18% of 4074 patients of all age groups with a tumor of the mediastinum, only 12%

of 1191 tumors of the mediastinum in children were found to originate from the thymus (HASSE 1968). OPPERMANN and WILLICH (1978) reported in their statistical collation that thymoma could be found in 10%–18% of children with tumors of the mediastinum. Collation of six reports with large case numbers (HECKER et al. 1967; HALLER et al. 1969; WILLICH 1970; POKORNY and SHERMAN 1974; KING et al. 1982; SCHWEISGUTH and CHAPUIS 1962) shows that in 627 children with mediastinal lesions, 31 thymomas (4.9%) were found. The frequency varied in the different reports between 0.8% and 10%.

Thymomas are found mainly in adults. In the cases studied by ELLIS et al. (1988) only 3% of the patients with thymoma were younger than 20 years. Most authors have found that the majority of thymomas occur between the ages of 50 and 60 (BERNATZ et al. 1961; HASNER and WESTENGÅRD 1963; ROSAI and LEVINE 1976; SALYER and EGGLESTON 1976; LEGOLVAN and ABELL 1977; BERGH et al. 1978; OTTO 1984; ELLIS et al. 1988); only in rare cases have tumors been found in patients over 60 (KEMP HARPER and GUYER 1965). ELLIS et al. (1988) found in their studies that 5% of thymomas occur in patients between the ages of 21 and 30, 20% in patients aged between 33 and 45, and 35% in patients above 46 years of age. LEWIS et al. (1987) calculated an average age of 52 based on an analysis of 283 thymomas.

Sexual Predilection. Thymomas are found equally in men and women (ROSENTHAL et al. 1974; BATATA et al. 1974; LEWIS et al. 1987; COHEN et al. 1988). LEGOLVAN and ABELL (1977) found the epithelial type to be twice as prevalent in men than in women, whereas the lymphoepithelial type was twice as prevalent in women.

Localization. At least 81%–88% of thymomas are located in the middle and anterior superior mediastinum (GREMMEL and VIETEN 1961; KEMP HARPER and GUYER 1965); DEWES et al. (1986) even found between 85% and 95% to be located there.

Ectopic positions are possible (COCCHI 1959). According to ROSAI and LEVINE (1976), 4% of thymomas are found in the neck, extending as far as the submandibular gland cranially. GÖRICH et al. (1988) described a thymoma in the angle of the left jaw. JUARBE et al. (1989) found that 12 ectopic cases have been reported, with an even spread between men and women; only two of these thymomas were invasive. Accompanying parathymic symptoms have not been reported.

BLADES (1946), COOPER and NARODICK (1972), and FUKAYAMA et al. (1988) have described thymoma in the posterior mediastinum. Of the thymomas seen by BATATA et al. (1974), 7% were in the caudial third of the mediastinum, most of them situated paracardially. GOOD (1947) and BARBIERI and LENTINIS (1948) described thymomas on the ventral side of the right ventricle. KAPLAN et al. (1988) found a thymoma in the angle of the left diaphragm.

Thymomas within the trachea (WADON 1934) or lung are rare (MCBURNEY et al. 1951; THORBURN et al. 1952; CRANE and CARRIGAN 1953; HORANYI and KORENYI 1955; KALISH 1963; YEOH et al. 1966; PAPLINSKI and SZYSZKO 1967; GULYA and KHAIDARLY 1968; KUNG et al. 1985; GREEN et al. 1987). To the author's knowledge only 12 thymomas have been reported within the lung. Five occurred in women and seven in men; their ages ranged from 14 to 74 years (Table 8.5). Four of the 12 tumors were found near the hilum, three on the left and one on the right side. The remaining thymomas within the lung showed no special position. The size and histologic structure can be seen in Table 8.5.

Tumor Status. Thymomas are potentially malignant: between 10% and 37% are described as malignant (SEYBOLD et al. 1950; CASTLEMAN and NORRIS 1959; GOLDMAN et al. 1975; BROWN et al. 1980; FON et al. 1982; BARAT et al. 1988). Only BATATA et al. (1974), HALLER et al. (1969), and WILLNOW and TISCHER (1973) report a higher proportion of malignant tumors in their studies, i.e., from 50% to a maximum of 67% (BATATA et al. 1974). Invasive calcified thymomas of the epithelial type are especially malignant (GÖRICH et al. 1988). Thymomas are not usually invasive in children, i.e., they are benign, as described by WERNITZ (1976) and CHATTEN and KATZ (1976). Occasional malignant forms have, however, been reported. BOWIE et al. (1979) described a lymphoepithelial malignant thymoma infiltrating the pericardium and the great vessels in a 9-year-old boy. WILLNOW and TISCHER (1973), and WILLICH (1988) have also reported such tumors in children.

The probability of malignant degeneration of a thymoma increases with age (MILLER 1985). Growth outside the organ of origin is usually to be expected only from the third decade onward.

8.2.2.1.2 Clinical Symptoms (Local Findings)

The clinical symptoms are dependent on the size, type, and localization of the thymoma and its duration of existence.

Orthotopic Position of the Thymoma. The tumor usually has a slow growth rate (BRINK and DELUCA 1987). Thus in 30%–40% of patients clinical symptoms are absent, the thymoma being discovered accidentally following routine chest radiography (LENNERT and HEPP 1968; THIES and THIES 1972; ROSENTHAL et al. 1974; BATATA et al. 1974; SALYER and EGGLESTON 1976; LEIPNER et al. 1982; ROSENBERG 1985; HOFMANN et al. 1985; COHEN et al. 1988, etc.); some authors even describe a lack of symptoms in up to 60% of cases (LEWIS et al. 1987).

Of patients with myasthenia, 70% show no local symptoms due to the thymoma (BERNATZ et al. 1961); however the symptomatology of myasthenia usually causes the thymoma to be diagnosed after 3–6 months. In the absence of paraneoplastic symptoms or where local tumor-related symptoms are the reason for the use of tumor-identifying diagnostic methods, the tumor is not discovered until after a pathoanatomic existence of 5 years (BARAT et al. 1988). The diameter of the thymoma, 5–10 cm, is thus usually considerably larger in patients without myasthenia than in those with clinical symptoms of myasthenia gravis (LEWIS et al. 1987).

In children, the tumor manifests itself as a so-called mediastinal syndrome in about half the cases (HECKER et al. 1967), i.e., with inspiratory and expiratory dyspnea, hoarseness, Horner's syndrome, elevation of the diaphragm, and dysphagia (OPPERMANN et al. 1977).

The symptoms in adults vary considerably according to the size of the tumor and its infiltration of neighboring organs. As well as general unspecific symptoms indicating a tumor, vague complaints due to the local tumor growth indicate a tumor in the mediastinum. A compilation of results from BATATA et al. (1974), SALYER and EGGLESTON (1976), LEIPNER et al. (1982), ROSENBERG (1985), DEWES et al. (1986), and SPÄTH et al. (1987) shows that symptoms such as retrosternal pressure, chest pain, cough, dyspnea, and a blockage of the superior vena cava are found, their individual frequency varying between 9% and 29% (LEIPNER et al. 1982). Symptoms such as hoarseness, dysphagia, tachycardia, fever, pulmonary infections, shoulder pain, loss of weight, loss of energy, and increased salivation are more seldom;

Table 8.5. Details of the 12 pulmonary thymomas reported in the literature

Author	Age/sex of patient	Symptoms at presentation	Localization	Shape/size	CT findings	Histology
THORBURN et al. 1952	37 yr; f	Accidental finding on routine chest radiograph	Left hilus	Oval, clearly defined, smooth walled, homogeneous 2 × 2.5 × 4.5 cm	–	Op: thymoma; also suggested it could be called "thymic choristoma"
CRANE and CARRIGAN 1953	19 jr; f	General fatigue	Root of left lung	Homogeneous tumor, 4 × 5 cm	–	Op: thymoma
MCBURNEY et al. 1951	65 yr; f	Myasthenia gravis of 3 months' duration	Right middle lobe	On radiograph: round, homogeneously dense	–	Op: thymoma
KALISH 1963	72 yr; m	Identified on routine chest radiograph	Right upper lobe	Smooth, homogeneously dense tumor; Ø 2.5 cm; no calcification (2 yr previously: thorax normal)	–	Autopsy: benign thymoma, no encapsulation
YEOH et al. 1966	71 yr; f	Lesion revealed by chest radiograph for adenocarcinoma of colon 2 yr previously	Right lower lobe	Coin sized, round, sharply defined; Ø2.5 cm	–	Op: thymoma
YEOH et al. 1966	50 yr; m	Accidental finding	Right upper lobe	Well defined, homogeneous, Ø3 cm	–	Op: thymoma
PAPLINSKI and SZYSZKO 1967	39 yr; m	Thoracic pain	Left, parahilar	Poorly defined oval tumor, 8 × 12 cm	–	Op: epithelial thymoma
GULYA and KHAIDARLY 1968	14 yr; f	Myasthenia gravis; suspected pulmonary tuberculosis clinically	Left upper and lower lobes	Ø3–3.5 cm		Op: thymoma with fibrous capsule
KUNG et al. 1985	46 yr; m	Hemoptysis, dyspnea, compression of left main bronchus	Left lung (several foci); effusion on left	Largest mass 12 × 10 cm; calcified		Epithelial thymoma
KUNG et al. 1985	60 yr; m	Cough, muscle weakness, myasthenia gravis	Right hilum	Round, well-defined; on radiograph Ø4 cm	–	Lymphocyte-predominant thymoma
GREEN et al. 1987	50 yr; m	Nephrotic syndrome; tumor revealed by chest radiograph	Left upper lobe	Well-defined tumor	Homogeneous density, sharply demarcated; Ø1.5 cm	Op: thymoma
FUKAYAMA et al. 1988	74 yr; m	Syncopal attack; tumor revealed by chest radiograph	Right upper lobe	Smooth, clearly demarcated tumor	Sharply demarcated tumor; Ø2 cm; homogeneous density	Lymphocyte-predominant thymoma

pericarditis and cardiac tamponade are reported in isolated cases (CANEDO et al. 1977; NISHIMURA et al. 1982; VENEGAS and SUN 1988). COCCHI (1959) and ASAMURA et al. (1988) have described paresis of the phrenic nerve associated with a thymoma. Cough, hoarseness, and increased JVP indicate infiltration of nerves and blood vessels by the tumor (OR et al. 1987). Where there is chest pain an invasive thymoma can be found in 68% of patients (BERNATZ et al. 1961).

An invasive thymoma can, in rare cases, break into the trachea or bronchial system. Using a bronchoscope ASAMURA et al. (1988) and SPAHR and FRABLE (1981) were able to identify thymomas as polypous tumors in the bronchial system, and obtained histologic confirmation by means of a biopsy. In all cases the main clinical symptom was sanguineous sputum.

Rarely, the clinical picture of pulmonary stenosis can be seen in cases of thymoma, owing to compression of the pulmonary trunk by the tumor (SOORAE and STEVENSON 1980; GOUGH et al. 1967; LITTLER et al. 1970). The pulmonary stenosis can occur either with (SHAVER et al. 1965) or without (NISHIMURA et al. 1982) cardiac murmur. Supraclavicular and cervical lymph node metastases are the first clinical symptom only in exceptional cases (BARAT et al. 1988). Infiltrative, i.e., malignant thymomas can spread in four different ways, whereby the tumor usually remains within the boundaries of the mediastinum:

1. Per continuitatem in the neighboring organs
2. Per continuitatem into the abdomen
3. Metastases in the regional and extrathoracic lymph nodes
4. Hematogenous distant metastases. An extrathoracic formation of metastases is rare.

Local infiltration per continuitatem in the neighboring organs is seen in (percentages according to: BATATA et al. 1974 / HARA et al. 1980 / BARAT et al. 1988) the esophagus, the trachea (2.8% / 5% / −), the lung (31% / − / −), the pleura (67% / 70% / 75%), the pericardium (47% / − / −), the heart (2.8% / − / −), the superior vena cava (− / 40% / −), the pulmonary artery (− / 5% / −), the aorta (− / 30% / −), the thoracic wall (− / 15% / −), the mediastinal fatty tissue (14% / − / −), mediastinal lymph nodes (11% / − / −), and the phrenic nerve (WICK et al. 1981 and others). Where there is caudal dystopia, the thymoma can infiltrate the diaphragm (BATATA et al. 1974; SALYER and EGGLESTON 1976), while with cervical dystopia it can infiltrate the thyroid gland (SALYER and EGGLES-

TON 1976). In 84% of cases one must reckon with infiltration of two neighboring structures at diagnosis, and in 54% of cases there is invasion of three such structures. Spreading per continuitatem below the diaphragm − observed in up to 31% of cases − can be seen in three ways (SCATARIGE et al. 1985):

1. Retroperitoneally via the intracrural space (Bochdalek's space): formation of pararenal and para-aortic metastases
2. Extraperitoneally via Morgagni's foramen with involvement of the abdominal cavity (KATZ 1953) as well as lymph node metastases in the celiac region (JOSE et al. 1980)
3. Directly through the diaphragm muscle: involvement the liver, typically with metastases of the margin

Formation of Metastases. The thymoma forms lymphogenous or hematogenous metastases in only about 6% of patients (KEMP HARPER and GUYER 1965). The results published vary between 1.5% and 15.5% (NICKELS and FRANSSILA 1976; ROSAI and LEVINE 1976; BERNATZ et al. 1961). Only ARRIAGADA et al. (1984) and GÖRICH et al. (1988) report the formation of metastases in a higher percentage of patients, 33%−38%, whereby GÖRICH et al. (1988) describe extrathoracic hematogenous metastases in 21%. According to a literature review by JOSE et al. (1980), metastases are more frequent in men than women.

No relationship exists between the histology of the tumor and the frequency of distant metastases (GRAVANIS 1968). Various organs can be involved:

Liver: BATATA et al. 1974; extensive literature sources in HIETALA et al. 1978; JOSE et al. 1980; LEWIS et al. 1987; THOMAS and MANIVEZ 1987; GÖRICH et al. 1988

Bone: BATATA et al. 1974; GÖLDEL et al. 1987; BARAT et al. 1988; JOSE et al. 1988; LEWIS et al. 1987; GÖRICH et al. 1988; STEVENS and BIGGS 1989

Kidneys: WILKINS et al. 1966; HIETALA et al. 1978

Brain and meninges: HASNER and WESTENGÅRD 1963; RACHMANINOFF and FENTRESS 1964; BATATA et al. 1974; SANDERS et al. 1976; JOSE et al. 1980; WICK et al. 1981; MEIGS and DE SCHWEINITZ 1984; DEWES et al. 1987; LEWIS et al. 1987; GÖRICH et al. 1988

Pleura: BROWN et al. 1980; GÖRICH et al. 1988, 1989

Spleen: WILKINS et al. 1966

Lymph nodes: mediastinal (GÖRICH et al. 1988) as well as extrathoracic: supraclavicular (in 25% of patients according to BATATA 1974; LEWIS et al.

1987; Görich et al. 1988), axillary, cervical (11% according to Batata et al. 1974; Barat et al. 1988)

Lungs: Lennert and Hepp 1968; Göldel et al. 1987; Wick et al. 1981; Or et al. 1987; Görich et al. 1988

Adrenal gland: Görich et al. 1988

Clinical Symptoms with an Ectopic Position of the Thymus. Where there has been insufficient descent of the thymus the thymoma is found in the neck. This can yield the clinical picture of a tumor with corresponding deformation of the neck. Salyer and Eggleston (1976) report a thymoma which was observed as a tumor at the side of the thyroid gland. Ridenhour et al. (1970) described a patient with a cervical tumor in whom the barium swallow was inconspicuous.

A rarity is the thymoma within the lung (see Table 8.5). Seven of the 12 thymomas reported were discovered following a routine chest radiograph; the rest caused uncharacteristic symptoms which led to the chest radiograph. Myasthenia was the reason for radiography in three cases (McBurney et al. 1951; Gulya and Khaidarly 1968; Kung et al. 1985).

8.2.2.2 Association of Thymoma with Other Syndromes and Diseases

Thymomas occur together with many systemic syndromes (Otto and Hüsselmann 1978; Otto 1984; Rosenberg 1985). Circa 70% of the patients are suffering from an immunologic phenomenon, approximately 10% from a malignant growth, 5% from an endocrinologic disease, and 15% from severe recurrent infections and diseases with no apparent connection to a thymoma. These are listed in Table 8.6.

Of the patients with parathymic syndromes, 25% suffer from more than one of the diseases cited in Table 8.6 (Souadjian et al. 1974). No correlation could be found between the histopathology of the thymus and the coexistence of accompanying systemic syndromes (Rosai and Levine 1976; Salyer and Eggleston 1976).

8.2.2.2.1 Autoimmune and Immune Disorders

Myasthenia gravis pseudoparalytica is by far the commonest concomitant affection: 40%–50% of all patients with parathymic syndromes suffer from myasthenia.

Table 8.6. Syndromes and disorders that can occur in combination with thymomas (after Rosenberg 1985)

Autoimmune and immune disorders	*Endocrine disorders*
Myasthenia gravis	Hyperthyroidism
Cytopenias	Addison's disease
Hypogammaglobulinemia	Panhypopituitarism
Polymyositis	
Systemic lupus erythematosus	*Malignoma*
Rheumatoid arthritis	*Severe infections and other illnesses*
Thyroiditis	Myocarditis
Sjögren's syndrome	Megaesophagus
Chronic ulcerative colitis	Chronic macrocutaneous candidiasis
Pernicious anemia	Others
Raynaud's disease	
Regional enteritis	
Rheumatic endocarditis	
Sarcoid	
Dermatomyositis	
Scleroderma	
Takayasu's disease	

According to which literature is studied, between 10% and 46% of thymomas are combined with this disease (Bernatz et al. 1961; Souadjian et al. 1974; Gray and Gutowsky 1979; Heilmann 1975; Salyer and Eggleston 1976; Brown et al. 1980; Lewis et al. 1987); only occasionally are higher values given (Wilkins et al. 1966: 58.7%), and usually values of between 10% and 15% are reported (Rosenthal et al. 1974; Heilmann 1975; Castleman 1966; Rosai and Levine 1976; Wechsler and Olanow 1980; Moore et al. 1982). Men and women are similarly affected [Lewis et al. (1987) reported that of 283 thymomas, 53% occurred in men and 47% in women]. Myasthenia gravis is found with thymomas of every histology (Salyer and Eggleston 1976). In 10% of cases it only appears after removal of the thymus (Martinez et al. 1987) – due to the special experience of the authors 7 weeks after thymectomy serum antibodies are found in almost all cases in which there is a combination of myasthenia and thymoma (Fischer et al. 1965). In 4% it is combined with a further thymogenic disease (Lewis et al. 1987). Apart from a thymoma in association with myasthenia gravis, Bailey et al. (1988), for example, found a pure red cell aplasia at the same time. Cruz et al. (1987) reported combination with lupus erythematosus and/or pemphigus.

The hematologic diseases that occur in combination with thymoma are also subsumed under the category of autoimmune or immunologic disorders. Thus the latter can be associated with different forms of hemopoietic insufficiency, especially with erythroblastic hypoplasia, agranulocytosis, pancytopenia, and hemolytic anemia (literature from Moskowitz et al. 1980; Lyonnais 1988). Therefore when aplastic anemia occurs in adults or children showing mediastinal spread, thymoma or thymic cysts should be thought of.

Pure red cell aplasia is found in 5% of patients with a thymoma (Barnes and O'Gorman 1962; Schmid et al. 1965; Hirst and Robertson 1967; Silverman and Sabiston 1977; Agarwal and Mehta 1980; Masaoka et al. 1989). Looking at it the other way round, when there is a pure red cell aplasia in 30%–50% of cases a thymoma can be found (Erslev 1983). Such a combination has even been described in a 5-year-old child (Talerman and Amigo 1968). The histology usually shows a lymphocytic or lymphoepithelial thymoma (Salyer and Eggleston 1976). The cause of the aplastic anemia is a pathologic increase in the erythropoietin level (Grips et al. 1976).

A third of the patients with pure red cell aplasia show a slight reduction in the lymphocytes and thrombocytes. An improvement in the disease following thymectomy can be expected in 20%–30% of cases (Zeok et al. 1979; Clark et al. 1984).

It is unclear why the combination of thymic tumors and isolated aplastic anemia is so seldom in children compared with adults, although the completely analogous congenital Diamond-Blackfan anemia is observed in the phase of greatest incidence of thymic hyperplasia, i.e., in the 1st year of life.

Along with pure red cell aplasia a pure white cell aplasia has been reported with metastasizing thymoma (Ackland et al. 1988).

Pancytopenia (Rogers et al. 1968; Lyonnaise 1988), Thrombocytopenia (Rogers et al. 1968), and pernicious anemia (Gibson and Muller 1987) are also found in association with thymoma (Rogers et al. 1968). In these cases also, an improvement can be expected following thymectomy (Braitman et al. 1971; Kaung et al. 1968).

A- or hypogammaglobulinemia is observed in 5%–10% of the patients (Bernatz et al. 1961; Barnes and O'Gorman 1962; Stillman and Baer 1972; Rosenthal et al. 1974; Souadjian et al. 1974).

Other associations between thymomas and other autoimmune and immune disorders have been reported. These are usually case reports with or without a summary of the literature:

Thymoma and dermatomyositis: Rundle and Spark 1963

Thymoma and polymyositis: Bonduelle et al. 1955; Klein et al. 1964; for further literature see Gibson and Muller 1987. Five percent of patients are supposed to suffer from this combination (Souadjian et al. 1974)

Thymoma and granulomatous myocarditis plus myositis: Mendelow and Jenkins 1934; Langston et al. 1959

Thymoma and lupus erythematosus disseminatus: Good cited in Larsson 1963; Larsson 1963; Thorlacius et al. 1989. According to Souadjian et al. (1974) this combination occurs in 2% of patients with thymoma

Thymoma and scleroderma: Ben-Shahar et al. 1987

Thymoma and autoimmune thyroiditis: Thorlacius et al. 1989 (five cases)

Thymoma and rheumatoid arthritis: Thorlacius et al. 1989 (two cases)

8.2.2.2.2 Endocrine Disorders

Kemp Harper and Guyer (1965) found thyrotoxicosis in four patients with thymoma, while Gibson and Muller (1987) reported two such cases.

8.2.2.2.3 Dermatologic Diseases

The connection between thymoma and dermatologic disorders was first studied by Gibson and Muller (1987). Of 172 patients, 34 suffered from dermatologic diseases, more than would have been expected statistically. In 19 cases clinical symptoms were already evident on discovering the thymoma: most cases (41.2%) were fungal infections of the skin (tinea capitis, onychomycosis, tinea pedis, saccharomycosis of the mouth), but shingles was also found (14.7%), and in rare cases there was pemphigus (Stillman and Baer 1972, Rothberg et al. 1989), lichen planus, basal cell carcinoma, malignant melanoma, aphthous ulcers, seborrheal keratosis, or immune disorders such as polymyositis. Sjögren's syndrome (Insler and Shelin 1987), and polyarthritis.

8.2.2.2.4 Malignancies

A combination of thymoma and other primary malignant growths is to be expected in up to 17% of patients (Souadjian et al. 1974; Lewis et al. 1987), whereby a combination of thymoma and neurogenic tumors is most often reported. ODA et al. (1987) found a combination of thymoma with myasthenia gravis, schwannoma, and gammopathy, SOUADJIAN et al. (1974) a combination with neurofibromatosis.

Gynecologic malignancies have also been reported in association with a thymoma (KEEN and LIBSHITZ 1987); thus carcinomas of the ovaries, the vulva, the endometrium, and the cervix have been found. Association with basal cell carcinoma has been described by KEEN and LIBSHITZ (1987) and MULLER and GIBSON (1987).

8.2.2.2.5 Limbic Encephalitis

A malignant thymoma can also be seen in combination with limbic encephalitis produced by a paraneoplastic syndrome (MCARDLE and MILLINEN 1988; INGENITO et al. 1990).

8.2.2.3 Diagnosis with Imaging Procedures

8.2.2.3.1 Conventional Radiology

The plain chest radiograph in two planes does not generally show pathologic findings. Due to their small size between 12% and 30% of thymomas cannot be seen on the sagittal view (BERNATZ et al. 1961; ELLIS and GREGG 1964; KEMP HARPER and GUYER 1965; BROWN et al. 1980). A soft lateral view is of more use (LENNERT and HEPP 1968; DÜX 1977; DEWES et al. 1986): 87.5% of thymomas should be recognized in this projection (BROWN et al. 1980). According to DEWES et al. (1986), 7.7% of thymomas can only be seen in the lateral view. Due to an even smaller size approximately 6% of the thymomas are missed on conventional chest radiography in two planes (BROWN et al. 1980).

Oblique views are especially useful. ELLIS et al. (1988) were able to identify 3 of 15 thymomas only on an oblique radiograph.

If the thymoma causes changes in the contour of the mediastinal border it can usually be seen on conventional chest radiographs as a round or oval, or in rare cases a lobular, deformation of the mediastinal shadow of constant density (Fig. 8.13). The homogeneous tumor usually shows a well-defined margin against the lung tissue, with a uni-rather than bilateral widening of the mediastinal shadow (see Fig. 8.14 for an example of the latter) (COCCHI 1959; KEMP HARPER and GUYER 1965; LEWIS et al. 1987); occasionally the border of the

tumor shadow is indistinct. Conclusions cannot be drawn as to whether the tumor is invasive or non-invasive on the basis of conventional films, since the extent of the tumor within the mediastinum cannot be revealed. Digital radiography likewise does not distinguish the tumor margin within the mediastinum and thus cannot demonstrate infiltrative growth (Fig. 8.15).

The thymoma usually shows an indistinct edge on the lateral radiograph; it lies retrosternally, usually ventral to the ascending thoracic aorta and the base of the heart. The tumor can displace the heart and great vessels and the trachea in a dorsal direction.

Calcifications are found in 20%–30% of cases and may occur both in the tumor periphery and in its center. The calcifications are usually patchy or amorphous and are not larger than 2×1 cm. They indicate tissue necrosis (KEYNES 1949; SEYBOLD et al. 1950; HEILMANN 1975; BROWN et al. 1980) but give no indication of the status of the thymoma (BATATA et al. 1974), even though GÖRICH et al. (1988) use them as a criterion of malignancy. Cystic thymomas sometimes show complete or partial ring-shaped calcifications (BERNATZ et al. 1961; KEMP HARPER and GUYER 1965). In such cases the differential diagnosis can involve a vascular process, a thymic cyst, a hydatid, or a dermoid.

A thymoma in the posterior mediastinum can be seen especially well on the lateral radiograph. Ventral displacement of the esophagus in its distal third is possible, whereby difficulty in swallowing need not necessarily occur. Stenosis of the bronchial system with widening of the carina (showing no clinical symptoms) has been reported (COOPER and NARODICK 1972).

Fluoroscopy should show a respiratory-dependent change in the size of the thymoma (ROSENTHAL et al. 1974) although no displacement of the tumor on coughing or swallowing can be seen (DÜX 1977).

Conventional tomography is disappointing (Fig. 8.13c). Demarcation of the thymoma against the heart or other mediastinal structures is, as with chest radiographs, not possible. No tumor has been found that could not be seen on the chest radiograph in two planes (KEMP HARPER and GUYER 1965). My own observations (WALTER 1988) show that conventional tomography provides no information over and above that obtained with conventional chest radiography in two planes. This is in agreement with the observations of KEESEY et al. (1980), BROWN et al. (1980), and DEWES et al. (1986). Only LIVESAY et al. (1979) have believed on

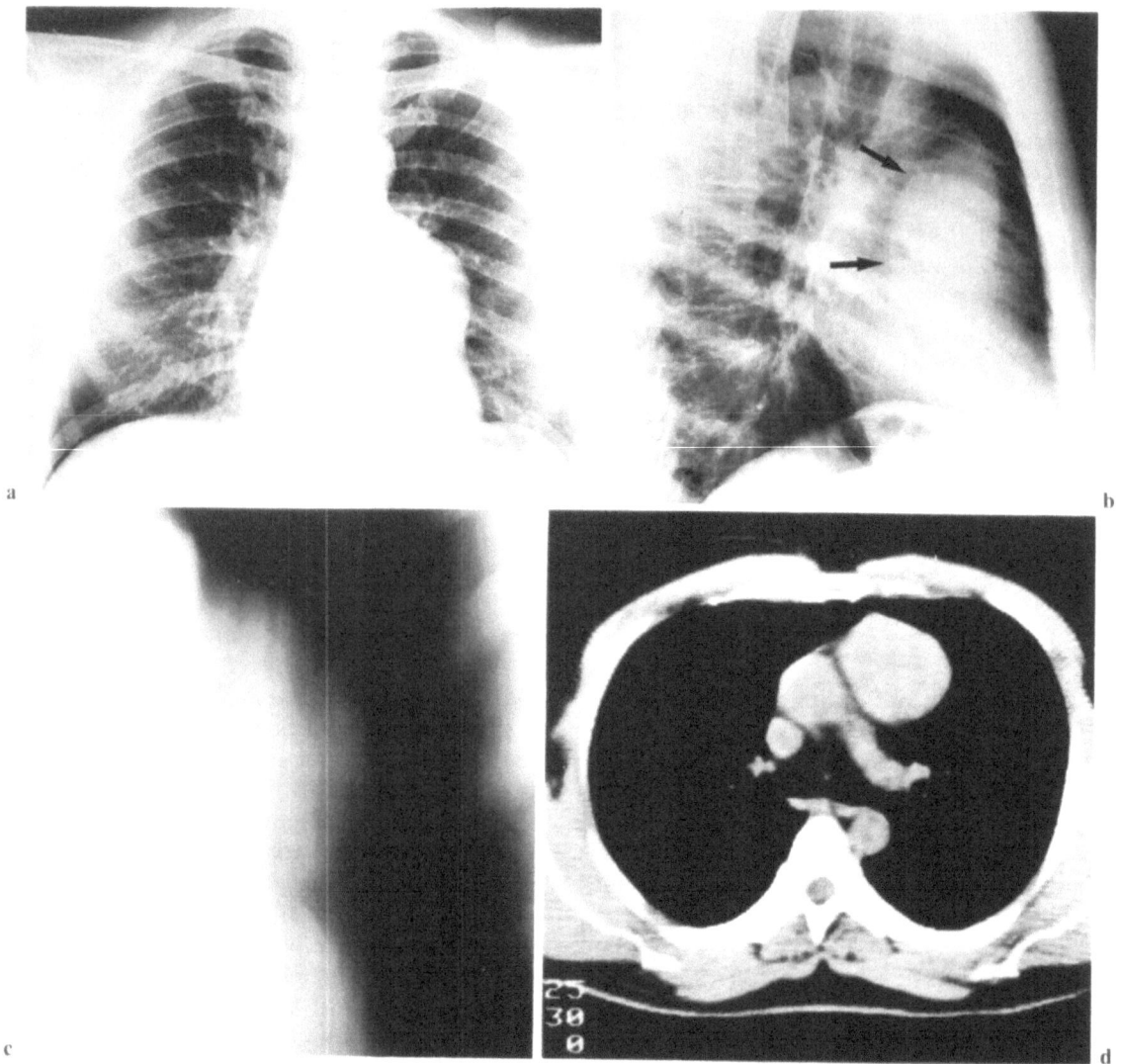

the basis of their analysis, that thymomas can be seen better on a lateral tomogram than on a plain radiograph. Stenosis and displacement of the bronchial system can be illustrated by conventional tomography; computed tomography, however, shows this in the same way.

Intrapulmonary thymomas have been described by GREEN et al. (1987) and other as a sharp-edged lesion of homogeneous density. Only in one of the 11 cases was calcification to be seen. No author has described pathognomonic results.

Fig. 8.13 a–d. Operatively confirmed noninvasive lympho-epithelial thymoma in a 42-year-old man. **a** The postero-anterior chest radiograph shows a tumor in the middle mediastinum. Distinction from the heart was possible neither on the plain radiograph nor on conventional tomography. The lateral radiograph (**b**) reveals a large retrosternal, para-aortic mass *(arrows)*, which in part shows a poorly demarcated margin (nevertheless, as already stated, the tumor proved to be noninvasive). **c** Conventional tomography: No additional diagnostic information is provided; no calcification is visible, and the tumor cannot be distinguished from the mediastinum. **d** CT scan. Differential diagnosis against a solitary lymphoma is not possible without additional clinical or CT characteristics

8.2.2.3.2 Ultrasonography

NISHIMURA et al. (1982) and WERNECKE et al. (1986) have reported on ultrasonographic experience in individual cases of thymoma. While NISHIMURA et al. (1982) examined the thymoma via the third intercostal space, WERNECKE et al. (1986) preferred the suprajugular approach. According to NISHIMURA et al. (1982) the thymoma could easily be differentiated from neighboring organs and ultrasonography enabled differential diagnosis between a cystic and a solid tumor. The thymoma was itself hyperechoic. WERNECKE et al. (1986), however, described a thymoma of 4 cm diameter as hypoechoic. Compression of the pulmonary trunk and adhesion to neighboring structures could be recognized ultrasonographically. This observation was confirmed by subsequent surgery (NISHIMURA et al. 1982).

The experiences of WERNECKE et al. (1986) show that ultrasonography cannot equal the results obtained with computed tomography as the region immediately retrosternal is difficult to judge using the suprajugular approach.

Ultrasonographic results are also available for a metastasis in the kidney of a spindle cell thymoma. It consisted of a solid, homogeneous hyperechoic structure (HIETALA et al. 1978).

8.2.2.3.3 Computed Tomography

In contrast to the conventional methods discussed above, computed tomography (CT) permits differentiation of the mediastinal structures owing to its higher density resolution and freedom from overlapping structures. Tumors of the thymus can

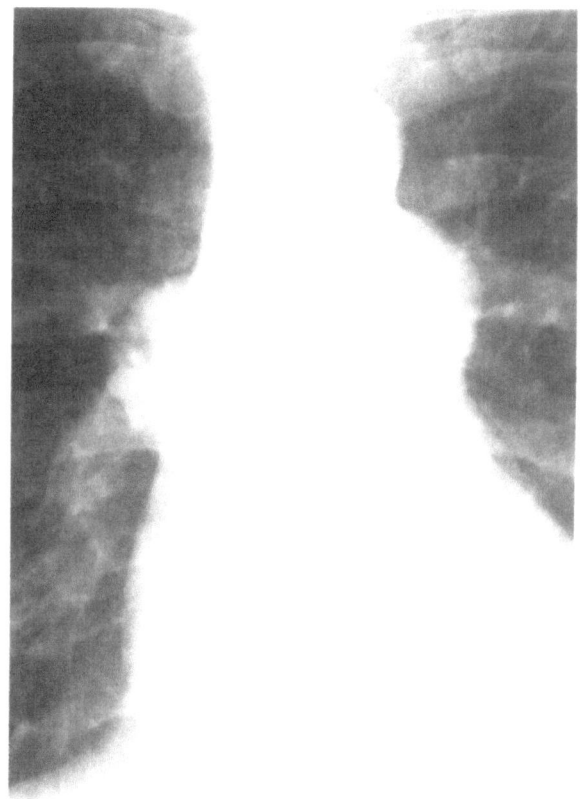

Fig. 8.14. Thymoma causing bilateral widening of the mediastinum (courtesy of Prof. Dr. DÜX, Mönchengladbach)

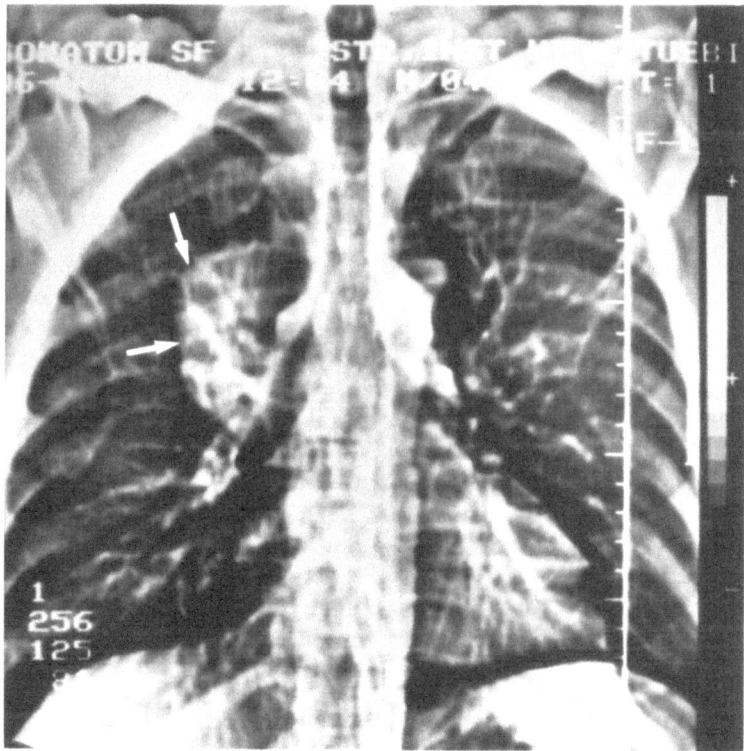

Fig. 8.15. Digital radiograph in a 38-year-old man with histologically invasive lymphoepithelial thymoma *(arrows)*. This digital technique does not permit the margin of the tumor to be distinguished; the invasive growth of the tumor is not recognizable

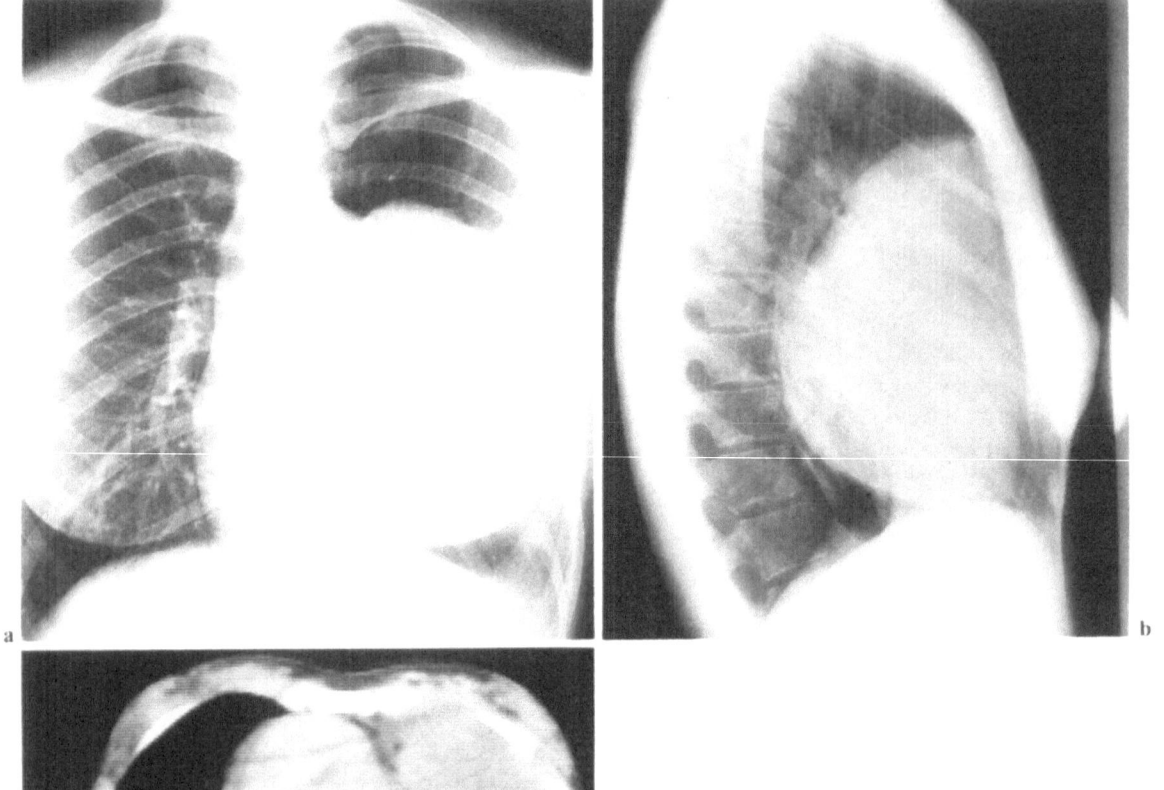

Fig.8.16a–c. Extensive invasive lymphoepithelial thymoma in a 26-year-old woman. **a,b** Chest radiography in two planes, showing the extremely large tumor. **c** Corresponding CT scan, illustrating infiltration of the chest wall and a central necrotic area *(arrow)*

be described as to their size, shape, homogeneity, tissue density, and relationship to the neighboring mediastinal organs. The serial section technique, possibly enhanced with a bolus of contrast medium, allows differentiation of a thymoma against vascular displacements such as aneurysms or ectatic or aberrant vessels (PUGATCH and FALING 1981).

Thymomas showing noninvasive growth, in the past thought to be benign, can be seen on a CT scan (Fig.8.13d) as spherical or possibly lobular (FON et al. 1982) tumors well defined against neighboring organs. Their size and extent can be exactly defined, and displacement of neighboring structures proved. Attenuation values of noninvasive thymomas vary between + 35 and + 60 HU, i.e., the values are similar to those of the chest wall

(WALTER 1982; BARON et al. 1982). The tumors are usually of a homogeneous density: the standard deviation of up to ± 5 HU in such cases is astonishingly small (WALTER 1982).

The lobular structure seen in pathologic sections of thymomas, with their connective tissue septa, is not visualized by CT. This is also true of the fibrous capsule. The attenuation values of epithelial, lymphoepithelial, and spindle cell thymomas show no significant difference (WALTER and HUEBENER 1980; WALTER 1982). Even a contrast medium bolus does not help to differentiate between these different histologic forms.

Sharp-edged cystic areas, described by OTTO and HÜSSELMANN (1978) as cystic softening, are typical in thymomas. The authors found them in 79% of the cases they saw, although only 5.5% could be

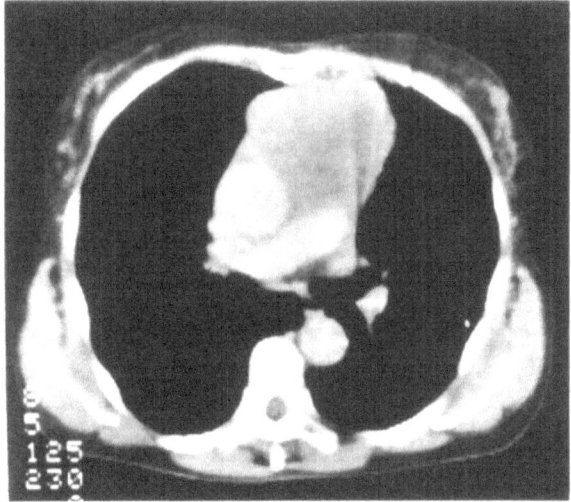

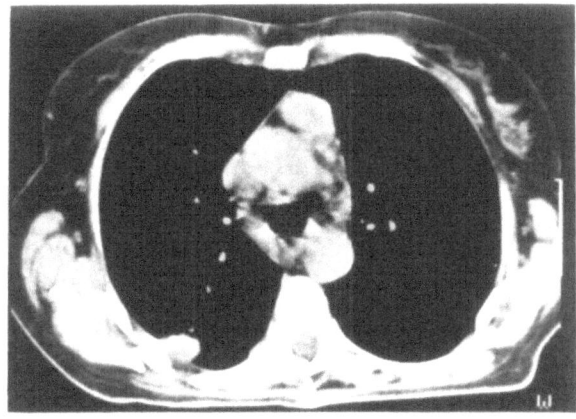

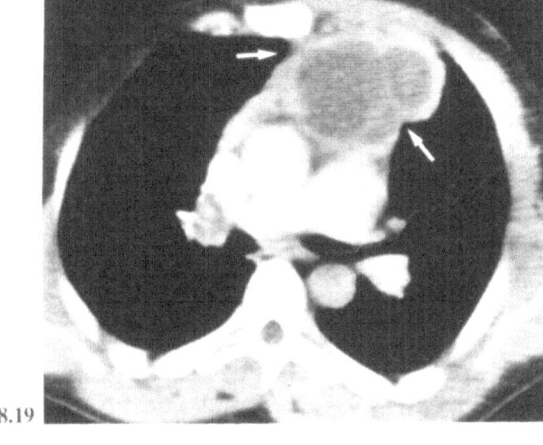

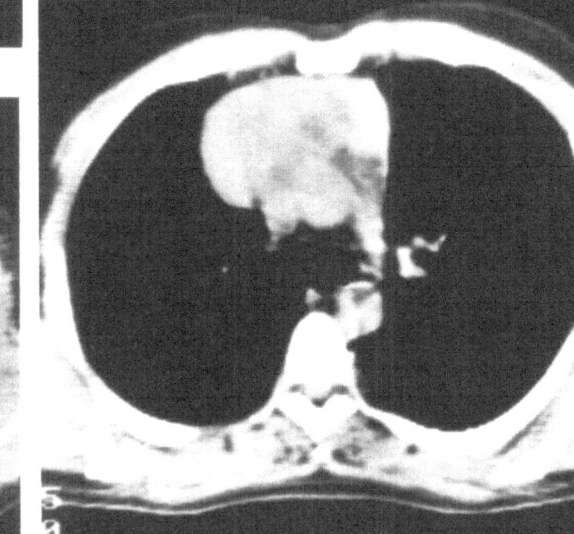

described as "large cystic" areas (OTTO 1984). BER-NATZ et al. (1961) also indicated in their pathoanatomic study that large cysts are much rarer than small cystic degeneration. Thus BATATA et al. (1974) found large cystic softening in about 15% of their cases. FON et al. (1982) found cysts in 9% of their CT-studied cases (and in only 11 patients with noninvasive thymoma). The regions of cystic softening show attenuation values of between +5 and +15 HU; this corresponds to values yielded by serous fluid (WALTER 1982). Invasive, i.e., malignant thymomas (Figs. 8.16, 8.17) are usually easy to differentiate from noninvasive forms. The infiltrative growth results in an ill-defined border against neighboring structures. The CT demonstration of local or distant metastases proves the malignancy of the lesion. Pleural metastases (Fig. 8.18) are commonest with malignant thymoma; they have been reported in up to 75% of cases (BARAT et al. 1980).

Fig. 8.17. CT of an invasive epithelial thymoma in a 68-year-old woman. The great vessels become distinguishable only after administration of a water-soluble contrast medium; this indicates that the vessels are infiltrated by the tumor

Fig. 8.18. Metastasizing thymoma: pleural metastases. CT scan in a 54-year-old woman with the clinical symptomatology of myasthenia gravis pseudoparalytica

Fig. 8.19. CT scan of an epithelial thymic carcinoma in a 40-year-old man with large cystic degeneration *(arrows)*

Fig. 8.20. Histologically invasive thymoma in a 38-year-old man. There is vascular invasion and extensive areas of necrosis

The attenuation values of the epithelial, lymphoepithelial, and spindle cell forms of the invasive thymoma all lie in the region of 35–60 HU. As with noninvasive thymoma, the different histologic forms cannot be differentiated.

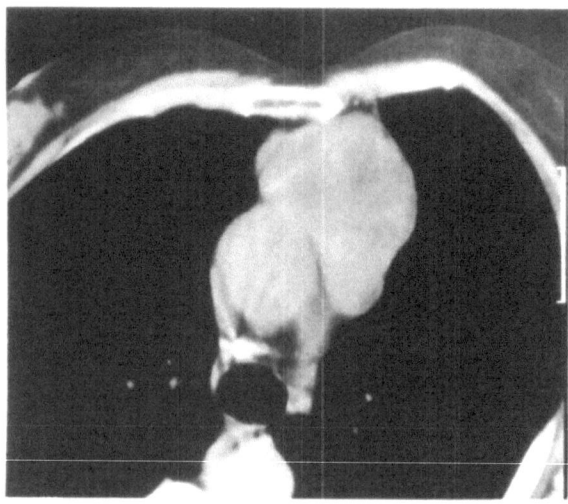

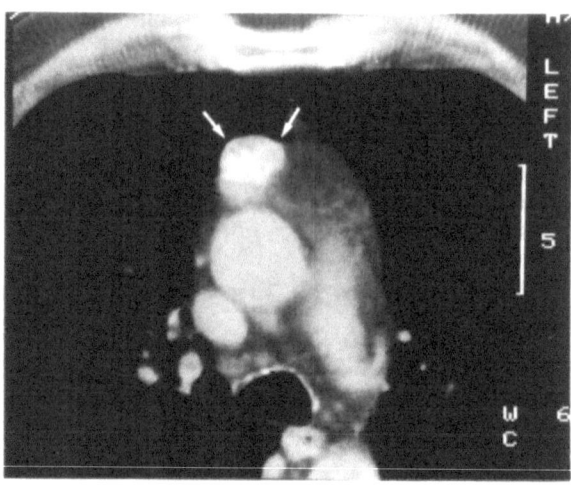

Fig. 8.21. CT scan of a 72-year-old woman without clinical signs of myasthenia gravis pseudoparalytica. Well-encapsulated lymphoepithelial thymoma with hypodense, i.e., necrotic areas

Fig. 8.22. CT scan of an epithelial thymoma *(arrows)* with typical calcifications in a 63-year-old man. At the dorsal circumference there is already invasive growth into the mediastinal fat

Malignant thymomas, like noninvasive thymoma, can show central cystic degeneration (Fig. 8.19). The CT appearance is similar to that of noninvasive thymoma. According to BATATA et al. (1974), 30% of invasive thymomas contain larger cysts, i.e., approximately twice as many as with benign thymoma. The margins are clearly defined and the resorption values are, as with noninvasive forms, the same as those of serous fluid, namely 5–15 HU.

Malignant, i.e., invasive thymomas can show necrotic liquefaction (Figs. 8.20, 8.21): pathoanatomic studies show that this can be expected in 17% of cases (SALYER and EGGLESTON 1976). On CT scans such lesions generally show a diffuse border; the attenuation values vary between +15 and +25 HU (WALTER 1982).

Following injection of a bolus of contrast medium (100 ml) an increase in the attenuation value to about 60–70 HU can be expected in the solid parts of the structure (DEWES et al. 1986). The cystic degenerations also show a somewhat delayed contrast medium enhancement due to diffusion into the cyst.

Calcifications in a thymoma – whether benign or invasive – can naturally also be recognized by

means of CT. They can be expected in about 25% of cases (Fig. 8.22). CT shows a higher sensitivity than the conventional procedures. BARAT et al. (1988) reported a case where the calcification was only visible on CT. ELLIS et al. (1988) found calcifications in 12% of thymomas using CT, while conventional chest radiography showed them in only 4% of the patients.

Invasive thymomas can not only infiltrate all neighboring organs in the mediastinum, as described, but also metastasize hematogenously or lymphogenously. This has been reported by LIVESAY et al. (1979), MCLOUD et al. (1979), ZERHOUNI et al. (1982), SCHNYDER and CANDARDJIS (1987), and others. In 70% of cases metastasis is to the pleura and pericardium, in 20% to the brachiocephalic vein, the pulmonary artery, and the pulmonary vein (SCHNYDER and CANDARDJIS 1987).

KOROBKIN and CASANO (1989) have reported a case in which there was invasion of the superior vena cava with extension into the right atrium. Following intravenous injection of water-soluble contrast medium, the tumor in the superior vena cava and right atrium appeared on CT as an inhomogeneous mass surrounded by contrast medium and blood.

Computed tomography is not always successful in identifying an invasive thymoma. Although in the cases studied by WALTER (1988) no thymoma histologically confirmed as showing invasive growth was falsely interpreted as noninvasive on the basis of CT, it must be remembered that a local infiltrative growth into the neighboring organs on the cranial or caudal circumference (i.e., pericardium and heart) can be missed on axial CT scans. KEEN and LIBSHITZ reported 92.9% accuracy in the diagnosis of invasive growth, while GÖRICH et al. (1988) reported only 80% accuracy. Ten percent of malignant thymomas were not recognized by SCHNYDER and CANDARDJIS (1987) as showing invasive growth.

When there is a tentative diagnosis of thymoma, CT should cover the whole thorax since the metastases are most often located in the pleura (WILKINS et al. 1966; MINK et al. 1978; WALTER 1982, 1988). Pleural metastases are more easily recognized on CT scans (Fig. 8.18) than on chest radiographs in two planes (MUHM et al. 1977; SCHANER et al. 1978; LIVESAY et al. 1979; KEESEY et al. 1980; ZERHOUNI et al. 1982; McCREA and MASLER 1982). ZERHOUNI et al. (1982) examined this question in detail and found a clear superiority of CT in the various pleural regions.

Computed tomography revealed metastases in analogy with the pathoanatomic findings. BARON et al. (1982) found metastases in the lung, and metastases in the pericardium were also correctly recognized by means of CT (ZERHOUNI et al. 1982).

The rare intrapulmonary thymoma can be seen on CT scans as a clearly outlined tumor of homogeneous density (GREEN et al. 1987). Because of the lack of experience of CT display, due to calcifications and reaction with a contrast medium, no competent statement is yet possible. GREEN et al. (1987) give no indications.

8.2.2.3.4 Magnetic Resonance Imaging

W. R. WEBB and G. DE GEER

Isolated cases of thymoma diagnosed using magnetic resonance imaging (MRI) have been reported (ROSS et al. 1984; GAMSU et al. 1984; DE GEER et al. 1986; BATRA et al. 1987; SIEGEL et al. 1989). Generally speaking, MRI has had little to add to CT in the diagnosis and evaluation of this lesion. On MRI, as on CT, the diagnosis of thymoma is based on the presence of a discrete thymic mass, nodularity, or focal thymic enlargement.

Although thymoma does not appear to have distinctive MRI characteristics and cannot be consistently distinguished from normal or hyperplastic thymus on the basis of MRI intensity alone, there is a tendency for tumors to be more inhomogeneous than normal thymus or thymic hyperplasia on both T1- and T2-weighted images (GAMSU et al. 1984). In one patient (DE GEER et al. 1986), T1 values ranged from 504 to 1846 in different parts of the tumor, while T2 values ranged from 36 to 66 ms; the long T1 and T2 values could reflect areas of cystic degeneration. One other reported thymoma had T1 and T2 values of 298 and 40 respectively (ROSS et al. 1984). This T1 value is very low, in our experience, and may reflect some volume averaging of tumor with mediastinal fat. In other cases reported, thymomas have appeared more intense than muscle, and less intense than fat, on T1-weighted images (GAMSU et al. 1984; BATRA et al. 1987; SIEGEL et al. 1989). On T2-weighted images, they increase in intensity, becoming nearly equal to fat in intensity. Calcification within a thymoma cannot be detected using MRI, and appears as low intensity on all sequences (GAMSU et al. 1984; BATRA et al. 1987).

Potentially, MRI could be of value in the diagnosis of vascular or pericardial invasion by thymoma (Figs. 8.23, 8.24) but this has not been studied in a significant number of patients. Differentiation between mediastinal masses and vessels, and vascular invasion, generally speaking, is better shown using MRI than CT. In one patient with thymoma invading lung, both CT and MRI probably showed tumor strands extending into the lung parenchyma (BATRA et al. 1987).

Postradiation Changes. In patients who have received mediastinal radiation therapy for thymoma or other thymic tumors, differentiation of radiation-induced fibrosis and recurrent tumor can be difficult using CT. Often in such cases, the presence of recurrent tumor is usually first suspected because of a change in the appearance of mediastinal contours on plain radiographs or CT, but the recurrent tumor itself cannot usually be localized within the larger abnormal area. Since biopsy confirmation of recurrent tumor is usually required before beginning additional treatment, localization of areas which are suspicious for recurrent tumor can be important.

It has been reported that recurrent tumor can be distinguished from post-treatment radiation fibrosis by using T2-weighted MRI (Fig. 8.25). In 12 patients studied by GLAZER et al. (1985) post-treatment fibrosis had a low signal intensity on both T1- and T2-weighted images, while tumor showed relatively increased intensity on T2-weighted sequences. In their study, however, differentiation was difficult in patients who had recently completed treatment or had inflammatory disease. In several patients we have studied, T2-weighted MRI appeared to distinguish fibrosis from recurrent tumor, but this differentiation was not always possible. In one patient we have studied

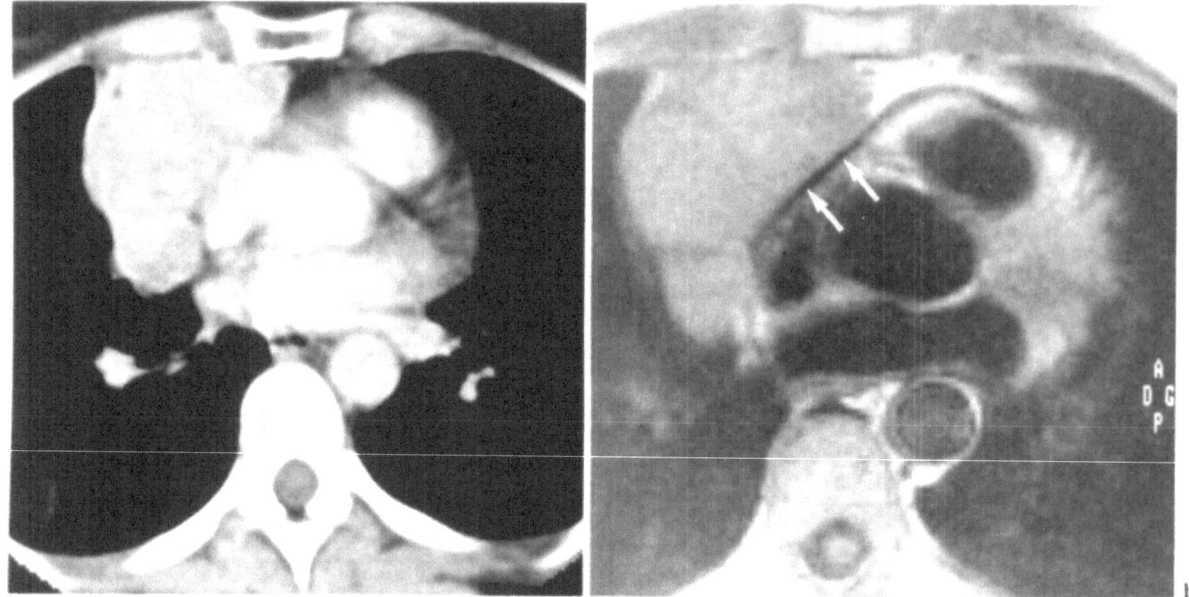

Fig. 8.23 a, b. Noninvasive thymoma. **a** On a contrast-enhanced CT scan the large thymic mass is clearly seen. **b** On T1-weighted MRI, the thymic mass is clearly distinguished from the normal fluid-filled pericardium *(arrows)*. There is no evidence of pericardial invasion or effusion

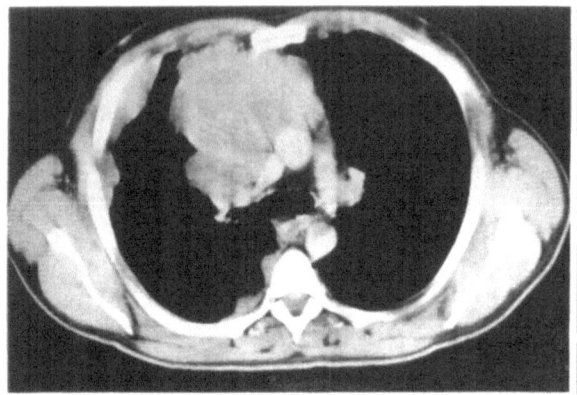

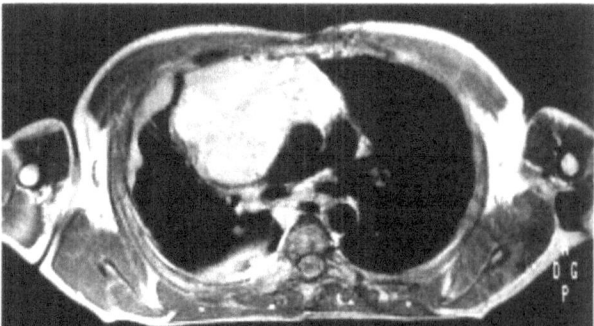

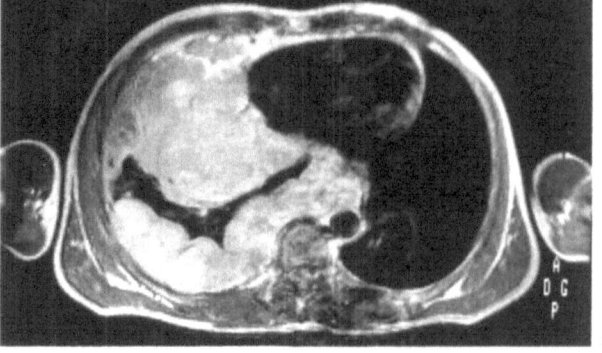

Fig. 8.24 a–c. Invasive thymoma. **a** Contrast-enhanced CT shows the large, lobulated thymoma. There is marked displacement of the mediastinal vessels. Right pleural masses represent pleural metastases occurring because of direct invasion of the pleural space. **b** TR/TE 1500/30 MRI clearly shows the relationship of the mass to the great vessels. The pleural masses are visible as well. **c** MRI at a lower level shows large lobulated pleural metastases occupying the right hemithorax

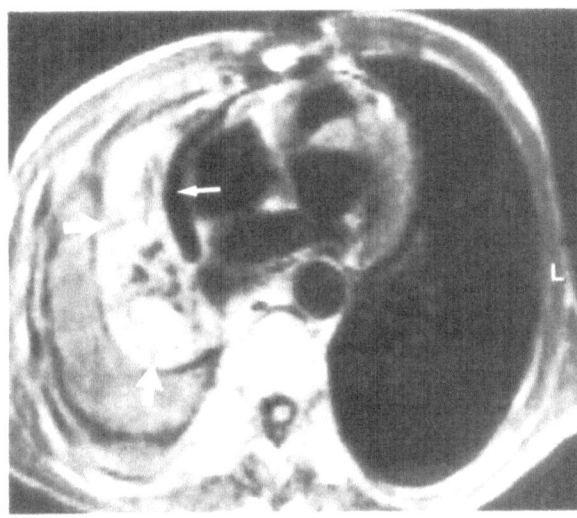 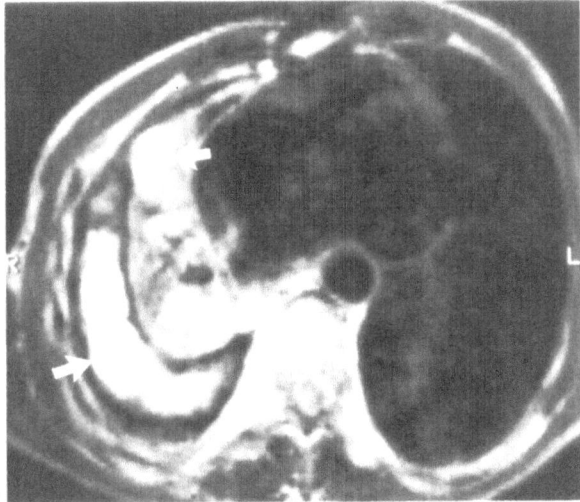

Fig. 8.25 a, b. Recurrent thymoma after radiation. **a** T1-weighted image. The collapsed and fibrotic lung *(large arrows)* lies adjacent to a collection of pleural or pericardial fluid medially *(small arrow)*. A fluid collection or mass is seen lateral to the lung, in the pleural space. **b** With T2 weighting, high intensity areas *(arrows)* within the fibrotic lung and pleural space represent recurrent tumor. This was confirmed at biopsy

with recurrent thymoma following irradiation and surgery, tumor within the irradiated lung and pleural space was clearly distinguished from fibrosis using T2-weighted images. On T1-weighted images, tumor was very similar in intensity to fibrotic lung and pleural thickening.

8.2.2.3.5 Nuclear Medicine

E. WALTER

Nuclear medical examinations were carried out with 67 gallium citrate and 75 selenium methionine. Unequivocal results cannot be expected since both false-positive and false-negative results are reported (detailed literature in KEESEY et al. 1980; MIN et al. 1978). For instance lymphoma, parathyroid, and thyroid show an uptake of selenium methionine (literature in TOOLE and WITCOFSKI 1960). A true-positive result can be exptected in 82% of cases (TEATES et al. 1978). JIMENEZ-HEFFERNAN et al. (1989) describe the uptake of ^{99m}Tc sodium pertechnetate in a mediastinal epithelial malignant thymoma. The application of ^{131}I only showed an uptake in the thyroid. After removal of the thymic carcinoma, no ^{99m}Tc storage could be found.

8.2.2.3.6 Other Methods

Since the introduction of CT other methods which were previously often used to diagnose a tumor in the mediastinum have essentially become superfluous, although some are occasionally used for supplementary diagnostics. These are reported here in order to give a complete record.

Arteriography. Selective arteriography can distinguish between cystic and solid tumors (Fig. 8.26).

BOIJSEN and REUTER (1966) reported that a displacement of the thymic artery is characteristic of thymoma. The artery originates from the internal mammary artery, approximately 5–10 cm away from its junction with the subclavian artery. In their experience thymomas showed only moderate vascularization; few tumor vessels could be seen. However, GÖTHLIN et al. (1977) described moderate vascularization of the capsule with variable vascularization of the thymoma itself. They described pathologic results as: vessel dislocation, notched vessels, vessel stenosis, hypervascularization, shunts between artery and vein, and tumor coloring.

GÖTHLIN et al. (1977) reported neoformation of vessels in benign and malignant tumors; wide vessels were, however, mainly seen in thymic carcinoma. DÜX (1977) maintained that the differentiation of benign from malignant forms of thymoma is angiographically possible. His experiences showed that whereas benign thymomas have few blood vessels, malignant forms show hyper- and neo-vascularization. DÜX (1977) also saw as an advantage of the selective demonstration the possibility of

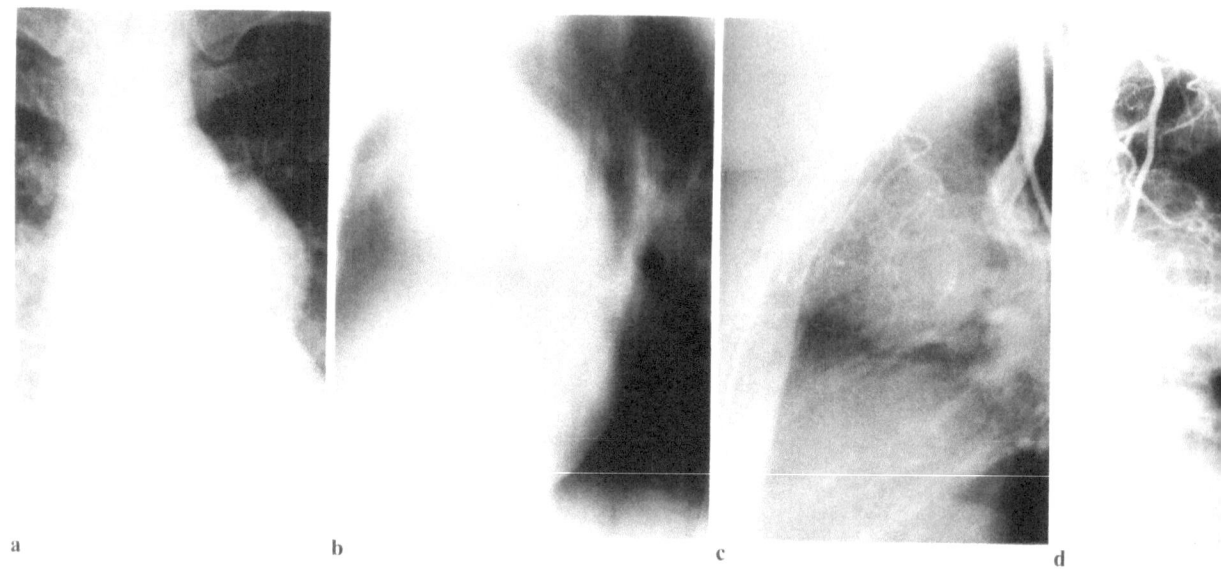

a   b   c   d

Fig. 8.26 a–d. 58-year-old woman with thymoma; no clinical signs of myasthenia gravis pseudoparalytica. **a** Posteroanterior chest radiograph showing a mass in the mediastinum with deformation of the left mediastinal contour. **b** Conventional tomography, lateral projection: polycyclic tumor which can be more easily distinguished than on the plain chest radiograph. There is no calcification within the tumor. **c,d** Arteriography shows homogeneously distributed vascularization with no criteria of malignancy. (Courtesy of Prof. Dr. DÜX, Mönchengladbach, FRG)

tumor embolism, which can lead to a reduction in tumor size.

An arteriographic examination, nowadays by means of DSA, permits differentiation against an aneurysm. CT with contrast medium gives the same results.

Finally, renal arteriography should be mentioned. Renal metastasis of a spindle cell thymoma has been seen. Angiography showed an unspecific tumor not supplied with blood vessels; this is a picture similar to that shown by malignant lymphoma of the kidney (HIETALA et al. 1978).

Phlebography. Phlebography used to be recommended as a further method of showing the thymus (KREEL 1967; YUNE and KLATTE 1970). Obliteration of vessels within the tumor, stenosis, "corkscrew" vessels, and sudden changes in vessel diameter were seen as characteristic of a thymic neoplasm. Phlebography is still sometimes used for differential diagnosis against a venous aneurysm. Of more importance is phlebography of the vena cava (Fig. 8.27) when the tumor causes stenosis or thrombotic occlusion of the upper vena cava and thus an increase in JVP.

Esophagography. Even today esophagography is required when there is difficulty in swallowing due to a thymoma, especially where there is esophageal displacement or infiltration by a thymoma in the neck or a dystopic position in the middle or posterior mediastinum. When a thymoma is positioned in the anterior mediastinum, as is usually the case, a disturbance of the esophagus is generally not to be expected.

Intravenous Urography. The demonstration of a renal metastasis of a thymoma by means of intravenous urography, with ventral displacement of the kidneys, is a rarity. Retrograde pyelography has been reported to show filling defects due to blood clots (HIETALA et al. 1978).

Kymography. Kymography used to be used to differentiate against diseases of the heart (LISSNER 1959). The method is no longer employed.

Pneumomediastinography. Pneumomediastinography was able to show the size, configuration, and relation of the thymus to the other mediastinal structures. Noninvasive thymoma of a certain size could be seen due to deformation of the thymus (MACARINI and OLIVA 1955). Small thymomas in a relatively large thymus could not be seen (HARE and ANDREWS 1970). Differentiation between a noninvasive tumor, a thymic cyst, and thymic tumors of a different pathoanatomic configuration was not possible. Where the thymus could not be separated from other mediastinal tissue an invasive growth had to be assumed although differen-

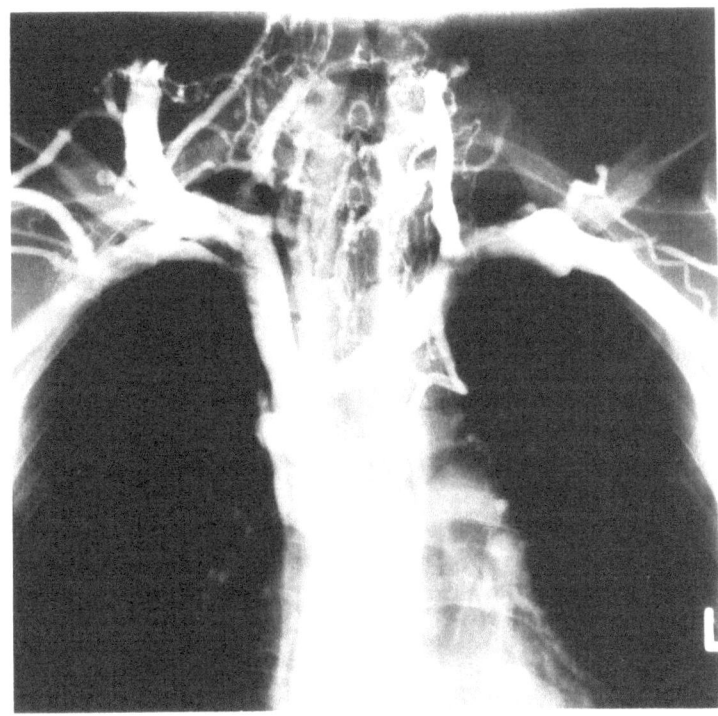

Fig. 8.27. Venacavography in a patient with invasive epithelial thymoma, illustrating stenosis of the superior vena cava and the left brachiocephalic vein. Raised JVP

tial diagnosis against adhesive lesions was not possible.

8.2.2.4 Differential Diagnosis

In cases of noninvasive thymoma the differential diagnostic possibilities are a solitary lymphoma (Fig. 8.28) and a solitary metastasis in a lymph node. In all three tumor forms the attenuation values lie between approximately 30 and 50 HU (ALCORN et al. 1977; WALTER 1982). Thus the differential diagnosis can be difficult. Contrast medium administration provides no further information (WALTER 1982). Calcifications are only to be found in thymoma, occurring in about 25% of cases (KEMP HARPER and GUYER 1965; DÜX 1977; KRAUS et al. 1970; OLIVA 1973); this is also true of cystic degeneration.

Where there are no such differential diagnostic indications neither conventional radiographic methods nor CT can distinguish a thymoma from a malignant solitary lymphoma. In such cases the diagnosis must be achieved with the help of the clinical symptoms, whether it be through the demonstration of antibodies against acetylcholine receptors (FUJII et al. 1985), the clinical picture of myasthenia gravis pseudoparalytica, or proof of other immune disorders such as pure red cell aplasia, dysgammaglobulinemia, or lupus erythematosus (WALTER and HÜBENER 1980). The use of antikeratin antiserum helps when diagnosis on the basis of the microscopic preparation is difficult (BATTIFORA et al. 1980).

Differentiation between a thymoma and a carcinoid of the thymus can also prove difficult. Calcifications are to be found in both tumors; cystic degeneration, however, is only seen in thymomas. Since in nuclear medicine no uptake of ^{131}I-MIBG can be expected in carcinoids, the clinical symptoms must assist in the differential diagnosis. Carcinoids are often hormone active (see sect. 8.3). Where there are no such indications a thymoma cannot be distinguished from a carcinoid.

Similar problems are encountered with germinal tumors. On conventional radiography and CT the appearance of large invasive thymomas can be similar to that of a seminoma of the thorax. Cystic degeneration and calcifications are found in both tumors. Thus once again the clinical symptoms must be taken into account.

Thymogenic cysts can generally be easily distinguished from a thymoma that has undergone cystic degeneration since, unlike thymomas, thymogenic cysts usually show a distinct wall of only 1–2 mm thickness. Sometimes the thymogenic cysts are ac-

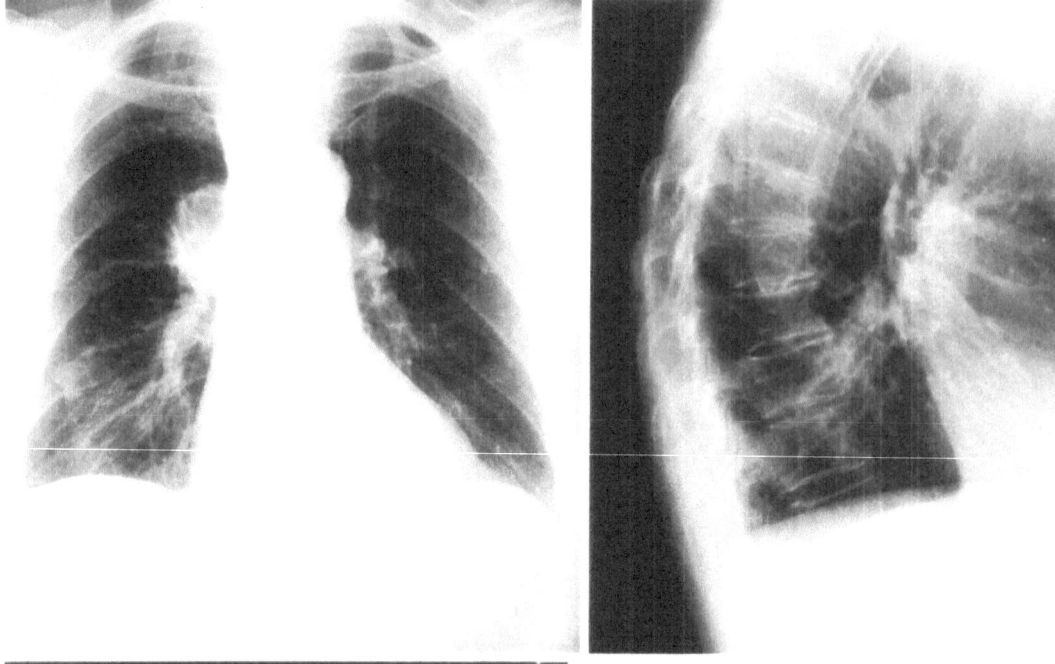

a

b

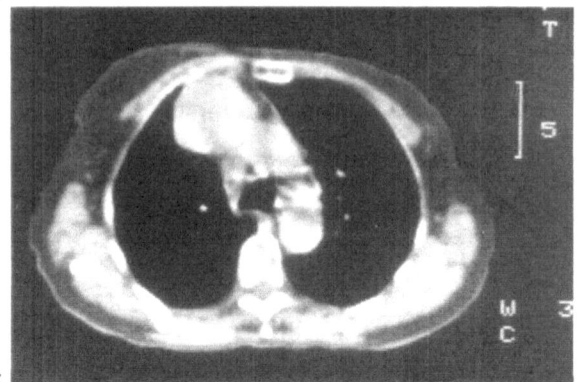

c

Fig. 8.28 a–c. Histologically confirmed isolated non-Hodgkin's lymphoma of the mediastinum. Neither conventional procedures nor CT permits differential diagnosis against an encapsulated thymoma

companied by thymic remains. An irregular border of a thickness greater than 2 mm indicates a thymoma with cystic degeneration.

Where there is a dystopic position of the thymoma within the thorax, the appearance on chest radiographs in two planes means that a pericardial cyst must also be considered. A solid thymoma shows higher attenuation values on CT than does a cyst (5–15 HU). Compared to the thymoma with cystic degeneration the pericardial cyst shows a very thin wall. In addition pericardial cysts show no calcifications or necrotic areas. According to KAPLAN et al. (1988), the application of 67 gallium citrate can prove helpful: an uptake was observed in the thymoma 24 h following isotope application.

The differential diagnosis between a thymoma, hyperplasia of the thymus, and normal thymus or between a thymoma within hyperplasia of the thy-

mus and a normal thymus can also be difficult using CT (FON et al. 1982; BROWN et al. 1983). A normal or hyperplastic thymus tends to be of symmetric configuration on CT scans while thymomas usually involve unilateral enlargement of the affected lobe. One exception to this rule was described by THOMAS and GUPTA (1988), who found enlargement of one lobe in a case in which the thymus showed a normal histologic appearance.

Solid tissue of oval configuration indicates a thymoma in patients over 40 years of age (MOORE et al. 1983). The differential diagnosis in patients aged between 20 and 40 can prove difficult (thymomas are extremeley rare before the age of 20). Where there is inhomogeneous involution of the organ, remains of the thymus with a relatively low fatty content can be seen as oval or round formations within one thymic lobe and thus can be confused with a thymoma. Irregularities in the contour of the border, and especially a local buckling, should be regarded as indicators of the presence of a thymoma (JANSSEN et al. 1983; LUPI et al. 1988). ELLIS et al. (1988) propose the following criteria for distinguishing thymomas from hyperplastic or normal thymus:

1. A significant displacement in the area of the anterior mediastinum indicates a thymoma.
2. Patients under 20 years of age have a thymoma when a very large mass or an unusual buckling of the surface of the thymus can be seen.
3. Patients between 20 and 40 have a thymoma when a mass with convex edges is observed within the remains of the thymus.

Where differential diagnosis is not possible, a fine needle biopsy is helpful (SHERMAN and BLACK-SCHAFFER 1990). This can be performed under fluoroscopic (ROSENBERG and ADLER 1978; PAK et al. 1982; SAJJAD et al. 1982; DAHLGREN et al. 1983; MILLAR et al. 1987) or CT (BETTENDORF and BAUER 1981) guidance. ROSENBERG and ADLER (1978) obtained the cytologic diagnosis of thymoma in 15 of 18 patients (83.3%) by means of fine needle biopsy. MILLAR et al. (1987) advise that the clinical indications should support cytologic diagnosis.

According to BETTENDORF and BAUER (1981) contraindications to perthoracic biopsy are: hemorrhagic diathesis, aneurysms, struma, hernia, and echinococcosis. Pneumothorax was described as a complication.

8.2.2.5 Relative Value of the Imaging Procedures

The conventional chest radiograph in two planes is still one of the most important methods in the diagnosis of a thymoma. This is true even though a thymoma, which can weigh anything between 2 and 175 g (ELLIS et al. 1988), cannot be recognized in the posteroanterior plane in 12%–31% of cases [ELLIS et al. (1988): in 50%] because it is projected in the mediastinal shadow.
The lateral view and especially oblique views are more diagnostically accurate. The accuracy of diagnosis in the lateral view is reported to be more than 90%, and oblique views are always of assistance (ELLIS et al. 1988). Approximately 6% of thymomas, however, are missed on chest radiographs in two planes (BROWN et al. 1980).
Conventional tomography is of lesser value. There is no improvement over the results with the

Table 8.7. Comparison of the diagnostic efficacy of chest radiography in two planes and CT in respect of thymomas

Author	No. of cases	Sensitivity	Specificity	Accuracy
1. Chest radiography in two planes				
MOORE et al. (1982)	4	75%	84.2	82.6
2. Computed tomography				
MOORE et al. (1982)	4	100%	89.5%	91.3%
WALTER (1988)	16	100%	87.5%	92.9%
CHEN et al. (1988)	32	97.1%	97.1%	97.1%
ELLIS et al. (1988)	26	85%	98.7%	95.8%

ordinary chest radiograph (MOORE et al. 1982). It is only useful in showing tracheobronchial stenosis or displacement by the thymoma. However, these can also be seen on CT scans.
The remaining radiologic methods described have, for the most part, no further or little value. This is also true for nuclear medicine owing to its poor diagnostic accuracy.
It is generally agreed today that, inspite of the described shortcomings, CT is superior to all conventional procedures in the diagnosis of a thymoma and the depiction of its relationship to the neighboring organs (MINK et al. 1978; LIVESAY et al. 1979; AITA and WANAMAKER 1979; FON et al. 1982; SIEGEL et al. 1989; McLOUD et al. 1979). It is thus in second place (behind chest radiography in two planes) in the diagnostic order in adults; only in children is ultrasonography placed before CT.
The diagnostic value of the chest radiograph in two planes and of CT is illustrated in Table 8.7, which clearly shows the superiority of CT.
A rational procedural sequence in the diagnosis of thymoma seems to be chest radiography in two planes (soft lateral view), possibly supplemented by oblique views, followed by CT. Only BROWN et al. (1980) recommend fluoroscopy before CT when the chest radiograph in two planes is normal. The value of MRI seems to be limited. BATRA et al. (1987) show that MRI gives no further information in displaying the tumor than does CT.

8.2.2.6 Therapy and Prognosis

When the thymoma is seen to be well encapsulated on CT, i.e., when it is probably benign, surgical extirpation is the treatment of choice. The rate of recurrence following complete tumor removal is reported to be less than 2% (FECHNER 1969; LeGOLVAN and ABELL 1977; BARON et al. 1982). FUJIMURA et al (1987) followed 31 patients commencing in 1965 and had observed no recurrences up until the time of publication.

Where there is invasive growth, i. e., a malignant tumor, various treatment modalities must be taken into account:

Malignant thymomas are taken to be radiosensitive (KERSH et al. 1985; KRÜGER et al. 1988). After as little as 25 Gy radiotherapy, complete remission is thought to be possible (GÖLDEL et al. 1987). However, KRÜGER et al. (1988) reported two cases that could not be controlled with 30 Gy. Nowadays most authors recommend the application of 40–50 Gy. The radiation field should cover not just the region of the tumor itself but also the area containing the supraclavicular lymph nodes, as the experiences of CHAHINIAN et al. (1981) show that in 18% of cases recurrences arise from there.

Side-effects of radiotherapy are rare. The application of 50 Gy is generally well tolerated (KRÜGER et al. 1988). These authors reported temporary esophagitis in three cases; chronic secondary damage was not seen. Pericarditis and pneumonitis can be expected when 45–65 Gy is applied (ARRIAGADA et al. 1984).

The majority of authors today are of the opinion that when a malignant, i. e., invasive tumor is present, radiotherapy should be combined with surgery (HARA et al. 1980; MONDEN et al. 1985; KRÜGER et al. 1988; NAKAHARA et al. 1988).

Radical tumor removal should be attempted, i. e., when there is infiltration of neighboring organs the infiltrated tissue, such as lung, pleura, superior vena cava, or aorta, should be removed, possibly to be followed by plastic reconstruction (NAKAHARA et al. 1988). HARA et al. (1980) recommend postoperative radiotherapy with various doses, i. e., 40 Gy when the tumor can be completely removed and 60–80 Gy when radical removal has been impossible. MONDEN et al. (1985) advise a dose of 40–65 Gy following radical surgery, and NAKAHARA et al. (1988), 50 Gy. The value of radical surgery before radiation treatment is illustrated by the data collected by KRÜGER et al. (1988) for stage III tumors: When there was merely a tumor biopsy and radiotherapy the tumor was brought under control in only 25% of cases; with subtotal resection and radiotherapy this figure reached 86%, and with radical surgery and radiotherapy, 100%. The experiences of NAKAHARA et al. (1988) with 35 patients with stage III tumors are in full agreement: they observed a 5-year survival rate of 100% and a 10-year survival rate of 94.7%, and thus a prognosis similar to that found by various authors for thymoma in stages I and II.

Chemotherapeutic agents are mainly used in stage IV. GÖLDEL et al. (1987) observed remission of a recurrence of a thymoma after six COP cycles. The value of chemotherapy has been reported on by various authors. Complete or partial remission of malignant thymoma upon initial treatment has been reported in 76% of patients, while in patients treated for recurrences the figure is 50%; various chemotherapeutic regimes have been used (COPP, BAPP, COP/CCNU, ADOC, cisplatin/VP 16). DY et al. (1988) report good therapeutic results in four cases of thymic carcinoma. Good tumor regression was achieved with a combination of the chemotherapeutic agents cisplatin, vinblastin, and bleomycin.

If radiotherapy and chemotherapy fail to have any effect, the daily administration of glucocorticoids can be tried (TANDAN et al. 1990).

It is difficult to provide prognostic data for general use as the data are based on different therapeutic methods. However, it is certain that:

1. The prognosis is generally worse when the thymoma is combined with myasthenia gravis or another parathymic syndrome (COHEN et al. 1988; LEWIS et al. 1987; ARAKAWA et al. 1990). LEWIS et al. (1987) report the following survival rates: thymoma combined with myasthenia: 5 year = 61%, 10 year = 49%; thymoma without myasthenia: 5 year = 71%, 10 year = 55%. A remission of the myasthenia gravis after thymectomy can be expected in 20%–30% of cases (COHEN et al. 1988).

2. Patients with an invasive thymoma have a worse prognosis than patients with a noninvasive thymoma. LEWIS et al. (1988) reported the 5-year survival rate for patients with invasive tumors to be 50%, and the 10-year survival rate, 30%; the corresponding rates for noninvasive tumors were 75% and 63% respectively.

The survival rate irrespective of accompanying symptoms or invasive or noninvasive growth is reported as 65% at 5 years and 53% at 10 years (LEWIS et al. 1988).

SPÄTH et al. (1987) described the survival rate as seen from the surgical side, whereby no distinction was drawn between invasive and noninvasive thymomas. Following a successful operation 78.5% of patients survived 5 years and 71.4%, 10 years. Where only palliative surgery was possible only 20% survived 5 and 10 years. The study showed a combined 5-year survival rate of 65.2% and a combined 10-year rate of 59.8%.

References

Ackland SP, Bur ME, Adler SS, Robertson M, Baron JM (1988) White blood cell aplasia associated with thymoma. Am J Clin Pathol 89: 260

Agarwal MB, Mehta BC (1980) Pure red cell aplasia with thymoma. J Assoc Physicians India 28: 137

Aita JF, Wanamaker WM (1979) Body computerized tomography and the thymus. Arch Neurol 36: 20

Alcorn FS, Mategrano VC, Petasnick JP, Clark JW (1977) Contributions of computed tomography in the staging and management of malignant lymphoma. Radiology 125: 717

Arakawa A, Yasunaga T, Saitoh Y et al. (1990) Radiation therapy of invasive thymoma. Int J Radiat Oncol Biol Phys 18: 529

Arriagada R, Bretel JJ, Caillaud JM et al. (1984) Invasive carcinoma of the thymus. A multicenter retrospective review of 56 cases. Eur J Cancer Clin Oncol 20: 69

Asamura H, Morinaga S, Shimosato Y (1988) Thymoma displaying endobronchial polypoid growth. Chest 94: 647

Bailey RO, Dunn HG, Rubin AM, Ritaccio AL (1988) Myasthenia gravis with thymoma and pure red blood cell aplasia. Am J Clin Pathol 89: 687

Barat M, Rybak LP, Dietrich J (1988) Metastatic thymoma to the head and neck. Laryngoscope 98: 418

Barbieri PL, Lentinis AH (1948) XV Congr Naz Radiol (cited by Cocchi 1959). Cortina 593

Barnes RDS, O'Gorman P (1962) Two cases of aplastic anaemia associated with tumours of the thymus. J Clin Pathol 15: 264

Baron RL, Lee JKT, Sagel SS, Levitt RG (1982) Computed tomography of the abnormal thymus. Radiology 142: 127

Batata MA, Martini N, Huvos AG, Aguilar RI, Beattie EJ (1974) Thymomas: clinicopathologic features, therapy and prognosis. Cancer 34: 389

Batra P, Herrmann C Jr, Mulder D (1987) Mediastinal imaging in myasthenia gravis: correlation of chest radiography, CT, MR, and surgical findings. AJR 148: 515

Battifora H, Su T-T, Bahu RM, Rao S (1980) The use of antikeratin antiserum as a diagnostic tool: thymoma versus lymphoma. Hum Pathol 11: 635

Ben-Shahar M, Rosenblatt E, Green J, Cohen I (1987) Case report: malignant thymoma associated with progressive systemic sclerosis. Am J Med Sci 294: 262

Bergh NP, Gatzinsky P, Larsson S, Lundin P, Ridell B (1978) Tumors of the thymus and thymic region: I. Clinicopathological studies on thymomas. Ann Thorac Surg 25: 91

Bernatz PE, Harrison EG, Clagett OT (1961) Thymoma: a clinicopathologic study. J Thorac Cardiovasc Surg 42: 424

Bettendorf U, Bauer K-H (1981) Thymomdiagnostik unter besonderer Berücksichtigung der computertomographisch gesteuerten perthorakalen Biopsie. Dtsch Med Wochenschr 106: 84

Blades B (1946) Mediastinal tumors. Report of cases treated at army thoracic surgery centers in the United States. Ann Surg 123: 749

Boijsen E, Reuter SR (1966) Subclavian and internal mammary angiography in the evaluation of anterior mediastinal masses. AJR 98: 447

Bonduelle M, Bordet F, Bouygues P, Charles F (1955) Un cas de polymyosite avec thymome. Verification anatomique. Rev Neurol (Paris) 92: 551

Bowie PR, Teixeira OHP, Carpenter B (1979) Malignant thymoma in a nine-year-old boy presenting with pleuropericardial effusion. J Thorac Cardiovasc Surg 77: 777

Braitman H, Herrmann C, Mulder DG (1971) Surgery for thymic tumors. Arch Surg 103: 14

Brink JA, DeLuca SA (1987) Thymoma. Am Fam Physician 36: 125

Brown LR, Muhm JR, Gray JE (1980) Radiographic detection of thymoma. AJR 134: 1181

Brown LR, Muhm JR, Sheedy PF, Unni KK, Bernatz PE, Hermann RC (1983) The value of computed tomography in myasthenia gravis. AJR 140: 31

Canedo MI, Otken L, Stefadouros MA (1977) Echocardiographic features of cardiac compression by a thymoma simulating cardiac tamponade and obstruction of the superior vena cava. Br Heart J 39: 1038

Castleman B (1966) The pathology of the thymus gland in myasthenia gravis. Ann NJ Acad Sci 135: 496

Castleman B, Norris EH (1959) The pathology of the thymus in myasthenia gravis: a study of 35 cases. Medicine (Baltimore) 28: 27

Chahinian AP, Bhardwaj S, Meyer RJ, Jaffrey IS, Kirschner PA, Holland JF (1981) Treatment of invasive or metastatic thymoma: report of eleven cases. Cancer 47: 1752

Chatten J, Katz SM (1976) Thymoma in a 12-year-old boy. Cancer 37: 953

Chen J, Weisbrod GL, Herman SJ (1988) Computed tomography and pathologic correlations of thymic lesions. J Thorac Imag 3: 61

Clark DA, Dessypris EN, Krantz SB (1984) Studies on pure red cell aplasia. Results of immunosuppressive treatment of 37 patients. Blood 63: 277

Cocchi U (1959) Röntgendiagnostik und Strahlentherapie des Thymus. Strahlentherapie (Sonderbd) 109: 426

Cohen II, Templeton A, Philips AK (1988) Tumors of the thymus. Med Pediatr Oncol 16: 135

Cooper GN, Narodick BG (1972) Posterior mediastinal thymoma. Case report. J Thorac Cardiovasc Surg 63: 561

Crane AR, Carrigan PT (1953) Primary subpleural intrapulmonic thymoma. J Thorac Surg 25: 600

Cruz PD, Coldiron BM, Sontheimer RD (1987) Concurrent features of cutaneous lupus erythematosus and pemphigus erythematosus following myasthenia gravis and thymoma. J Am Acad Dermatol 16: 472

Dahlgren S, Sandstedt B, Sundström C (1983) Fine needle aspiration cytology in thymic tumors. Acta Cytol 27: 1

de Geer G, Webb WR, Gamsu G (1986) Normal thymus: assessment with MR and CT. Radiology 158: 313

Dewes W, Schrappe-Bächer M, Focke-Wenzel EK, Schmitz-Dräger H-G (1986) Zur Röntgendiagnostik invasiver Thymome. ROFO 144: 388

Dewes W, Chandler WF, Gormanns R, Ebhardt G (1987) Brain metastasis of an invasive thymoma. Neurosurgery 20: 484

Düx A (1977) Differentialdiagnose pathologischer Mediastinalprozesse. In: Teschendorf W, Anacker H, Thurn P (eds) Röntgenologische Differentialdiagnostik, vol I, 2, 5th edn. Thieme, Stuttgart

Dy C, Calvo FA, Mindán JP et al. (1988) Undifferentiated epithelial-rich invasive malignant thymoma: complete response to cisplatin, vinblastine, and bleomycin therapy. J Clin Oncol 6: 536

Ellis K, Gregg HG (1964) Thymomas: roentgen considerations. AJR 91: 105

Ellis K, Austin JHM, Jaretzki A (1988) Radiologic detection of thymoma in patients with myasthenia gravis. AJR 151: 873

Erslev AJ (1983) Pure red cell aplasia. In: Williams WJ, Beutler E, Erslev AJ, Lichtman MA (eds) Hematology. McGraw-Hill, New York, p 409

Fechner RE (1969) Recurrence of noninvasive thymomas. Report of four cases and review of literature. Cancer 23: 1423

Fischer K, Mertens HG, Schimrigk K (1965) Ein Beitrag zur Immunpathologie bei Myasthenia gravis. Dtsch Med Wochenschr 90: 1760

Fon GT, Bein ME, Mancuso AA, Keesey JC, Lupetin AR, Wong WS (1982) Computed tomography of the anterior mediastinum in myasthenia gravis. A radiologic-pathologic correlative study. Radiology 142: 135

Fujii Y, Monden Y, Hashimoto J, Nakahara K, Kawashima Y (1985) Acetylcholine receptor antibody-producing cells in thymus and lymph nodes in myasthenia gravis. Clin Immunol Immunopathol 34: 141

Fujimura S, Kondo T, Handa M, Shiraishi Y, Tamahashi N, Nakada T (1987) Results of surgical treatment for thymoma based on 66 patients. J Thorac Cardiovasc Surg 93: 708

Fukayama M, Maeda Y, Funata N, Koike M, Saito K, Sakai T, Ikeda T (1988) Pulmonary and pleural thymoma: diagnostic application of lymphocyte markers to the thymoma of unusual site. Am J Clin Pathol 89: 617

Gamsu G, Stark DD, Webb WR et al. (1984) Magnetic resonance imaging of benign mediastinal masses. Radiology 151: 709

Gibson LE, Muller SA (1987) Dermatologic disorders in patients with thymoma. Acta Derm Venereol (Stockh) 67: 351

Glazer HS, Lee JKT, Levitt RG et al. (1985) Radiation fibrosis: differentiation from recurrent tumor by MR imaging. Radiology 156: 721

Göldel N, Frederik A, Böning L, Wilmanns W (1987) Erfolgreiche Chemotherapie bei metastasiertem malignem Thymom. Dtsch Med Wochenschr 112: 1418

Goldman AJ, Herrmann C, Keesey JC, Mulder DG, Brown WJ (1975) Myasthenia gravis and invasive thymoma: a 20-year experience. Neurology 25: 1021

Good CA (1947) Roentgenologic findings in myasthenia gravis associated with thymic tumor. AJR 57: 305

Görich J, Müller M, Beyer-Enke SA, Zuna I, Probst G, van Kaick G (1988) Computertomographische Befunde bei 36 Patienten mit Raumforderungen des Thymus. ROFO 149: 466

Görich J, Beyer-Enke SA, Schmitteckert H, Flentje M, van Kaick G (1989) Pleural metastasis of malignant thymoma. A pitfall in the CT diagnosis of pleural mesothelioma. Comput Med Imag Graph 13: 169

Göthlin J, Jonsson K, Lunderquist A, Rausing A, Alburquerque LM (1977) The angiographic appearance of thymic tumors. Radiology 124: 47

Gough JH, Gold RG, Gibson RV (1967) Acquired pulmonary stenosis and pulmonary artery compression. Thorax 22: 358

Gravanis MB (1968) Metastasizing thymoma. Report of a case and review of the literature. Am J Clin Pathol 49: 690

Gray GF, Gutowski WT (1979) Thymoma. A clinicopathologic study of 54 cases. Am J Surg Pathol 3: 235

Green WR, Pressoir R, Gumbs RV, Warner O, Naab T, Qayumi M (1987) Intrapulmonary thymoma. Arch Pathol Lab Med 111: 1074

Gremmel H, Vieten H (1961) A propos de l'etude clinique et radiologique de tumeurs du thymus. Ann Radiol 4: 669

Grips KH, Ochs H, Otten H, Labedzki L, Tantow J (1976) Aplastische Anämie und Thymom. Dtsch Med Wochenschr 101: 1389

Gulya D, Khaidarly I (1968) A case of benign thymoma of the lung. Grudn Khir 10: 1145

Haller JA, Mazur DO, Morgan WW (1969) Diagnosis and management of mediastinal masses in children. J Thorac Cardiovasc Surg 59: 385

Hara N, Yoshida T, Furukawa T, Inokuchi K (1980) Thymoma: clinicopathologic features, therapy, and prognosis. Jpn J Surg 10: 232

Hare WSC, Andrews JT (1970) The occult thymoma: radiological and radioisotopic aids to diagnosis. Aust Ann Med 1: 30

Hasner E, Westengård E (1963) Thymomas. Acta Chir Scand 126: 58

Hasse W (1968) Die Geschwülste des Mediastinums im Kindesalter. Langenbecks Arch Chir 322: 1236

Hasse W, Waldschmidt J (1967) Mediastinaltumoren im Kindesalter. Zentralbl Chir 92: 573

Hecker WC, Rüter E, Vogt-Moykopf I (1967) Beitrag zur Klinik kindlicher Mediastinaltumoren. Analyse von 59 Fällen. Thoraxchirurgie 15: 392

Heilmann HP (1975) Das Thymom, Diagnostik und Therapie. In: Frommhold W, Gerhardt P (eds) Klinisch-radiologisches Seminar, vol 4. Erkrankungen des Mediastinums. Thieme, Stuttgart

Hietala S-O, Hazra TA, Texter JH (1978) Malignant thymoma with renal metastases. Acta Radiol Diagn 19: 337

Hirst E, Robertson TI (1967) The syndrome of thymoma and erythroblastopenic anemia. Medicine 46: 225

Hofmann W, Möller P, Manke H-G, Otto FH (1985) Thymoma. A clinicopathologic study of 98 cases with special reference to three unusual cases. Pathol Res Pract 179: 337

Horanyi VJ, Korenyi K (1955) Intrapulmonary thymoma in children. Thoraxchir Vasc Chir 3: 245

Ingenito GG, Berger JR, David NJ, Norenberg MD (1990) Limbic encephalitis associated with thymoma. Neurology 40: 382

Insler MS, Shelin RG (1987) Sjörgen's syndrome and thymoma. Am J Ophthalmol 104: 90

Janssen RS, Kaye AD, Lisak RP et al. (1983) Radiologic evaluation of the mediastinum in myasthenia gravis. Neurology 33: 534

Jimenez-Heffernan A, Pineda-Albornoz A, Maranon-Lopez J, Rodriguez-Quesada B (1989) Mediastinal uptake of Tc-99m pertechnetate in a thymoma. Clin Nucl Med 14: 375

Jose B, Yu AT, Morgan TF, Glicksman AS (1980) Malignant thymoma with extrathoracic metastasis: a case report and review of literature. J Surg Oncol 15: 259

Jose CC, John S, Singh AD (1988) Extrathoracic metastatic thymoma. A case report. Australas Radiol 32: 500

Juarbe C, Conley JJ, Gillooley JF, Angel MF (1989) Metastatic cervical thymoma. Otolaryngol Head Neck Surg 100: 232

Kalish PE (1963) Primary intrapulmonary thymoma. NY State J Med 63: 1705

Kaplan IL, Swayne LC, Widmann WD, Wolff M (1988) Case report. CT demonstration of "ectopic" thymoma. J Comput Assist Tomogr 12: 1037

Katz JH (1953) Malignant thymoma in myasthenia gravis.

Report of an unusual case with a brief discussion of the role of the thymus in the disease. N Engl J Med 248: 1059

Kaung DT, Cech RF, Peterson RF (1968) Benign thymoma and erythroid hypoplasia. Thirteen-year "cure" following thymectomy. Cancer 22: 445

Keen SJ, Libshitz HI (1987) Thymic lesions. Experience with computed tomography in 24 patients. Cancer 59: 1520

Keesey J, Bein M, Mink J et al. (1980) Detection of thymoma in myasthenia gravis. Neurology 30: 233

Kemp Harper RA, Guyer PB (1965) The radiological features of thymic tumours: a review of sixty-five cases. Clin Radiol 16: 97

Kersh CR, Eisert DR, Hazra TA (1985) Malignant thymoma: role of radiation therapy in management. Radiology 156: 207

Keynes GL (1949) The results of thymectomy in myasthenia gravis. Br Med J 2: 611

King RM, Telander RL, Smithson WA, Banks PM, Mao-Tang H (1982) Primary mediastinal tumors in children. J Pediatr Surg 17: 512

Klein JJ, Gottlieb AJ, Mones RJ, Appel SH, Osserman KE (1964) Thymoma and polymyositis. Onset of myasthenia gravis after thymectomy: report of two cases. Arch Intern Med 113: 192

Korobkin M, Casano VA (1989) Intracaval and intracardiac extension of malignant thymoma: CT diagnosis. J Comput Assist Tomogr 13: 348

Kraus R, Klemencic J, Keller R (1970) Erkrankungen und Tumoren des Mediastinums. In: Diethelm L, Ohlsson O, Strnad F, Vieten H, Zuppinger A (eds) Röntgendiagnostik der oberen Speise- und Atemwege, der Atemorgane und des Mediastinums. Springer, Berlin Heidelberg New York (Handbuch der medizinischen Radiologie, vol IX/6, p 193)

Kreel L (1967) Selective thymic venography. New method for visualization of the thymus. Br Med J 1: 406

Krüger JB, Sagerman RH, King GA (1988) Stage III thymoma: results of postoperative radiation therapy. Radiology 168: 855

Kung I, Loke SL, So SY, Lam WK, Mok CK, Khin MA (1985) Intrapulmonary thymoma: report of two cases. Thorax 40: 471

Langston JD, Wagman GF, Dickenman RC (1959) Granulomatous myocarditis and myositis associated with thymoma. AMA Arch Pathol 68: 367

Larsson O (1963) Thymoma and systemic lupus erythematosus in the same patient. Lancet 28: 665

LeGolvan DP, Abell MR (1977) Thymomas. Cancer 39: 2142

Leipner N, Cremer H, Engel C (1982) Thymome – klinisch-pathologische Aspekte. Onkologie 5: 196

Lennert KA, Hepp G (1968) Zur Klinik der Thymustumoren. Dtsch Med Wochenschr 93: 1649

Levasseur P, Kaswin R, Rojas-Miranda A, N'Guimbous JF, Merlier M, Le Brigand H (1976) Profil des tumeurs chirurgicales du mediastin. A propos d'une serie de 742 opérés. Nouv Press Med 42: 2857

Lewis JE, Wick MR, Scheithauer BW, Bernatz PE, Taylor WF (1987) Thymoma. A clinicopathologic review. Cancer 60: 2727

Lissner J (1959) Der Wert des Pneumomediastiums bei der Differentialdiagnose mediastinaler Erkrankungen. ROFO 91: 445

Littler WA, Meade JB, Hamilton DI (1970) Acquired pulmonary stenosis. Thorax 25: 465

Livesay JJ, Mink JH, Fee HJ, Bein ME, Sample WF, Mulder DG (1979) The use of computed tomography to evaluate suspected mediastinal tumors. Ann Thorac Surg 27: 305

Lupi L, Bighi S, Limone GL, Cervi PM (1988) Radiographic and computed tomographic detection of thymoma in patients with myasthenia gravis. Diagn Radiol 13: 17

Lyonnais J (1988) Thymoma and pancytopenia. Am J Hematol 28: 195

Macarini N, Oliva L (1955) L'insufflatione del mediastino anteriore e posteriore nella patologia. Minerva Med 46: 781

Martinez AC (1987) Thymoma without myasthenia gravis. Electrophysiological study after thymectomy. J Neurol Neurosurg Psychiatry 50: 501

Masaoka A, Hashimoto T, Shibata K, Yamakawa Y, Nakamae K, Iizuka M (1989) Thymomas associated with pure red cell aplasia. Histologic and follow-up studies. Cancer 64: 1872

McArdle JP, Millingen KS (1988) Case report: limbic encephalitis associated with malignant thymoma. Pathology 20: 292

McBurney RP, Clagett OT, McDonald JR (1951) Primary intrapulmonary neoplasm (thymoma?) associated with myasthenia gravis. Report of case. Proc Staff Meet Mayo Clin 26: 345

McCrea ES, Maslar JA (1982) Thymoma with distant intrathoracic implants, with CT confirmation. Cancer 50: 1612

McLoud TC, Wittenberg J, Ferrucci JT (1979) Computed tomography of the thorax and standard radiographic evaluation of the chest: a comparative study. J Comput Assist Tomogr 3: 170

Meigs AV, de Schweinitz GE (1984) Round-celled sarcoma of the anterior mediastinum: extensive metastasis, including the brain, both choroid coats, oculo-motor and optic nerves and external ocular muscles. Am J Med Sci 108: 193

Mendelow H, Jenkins G (1934) Studies in myasthenia gravis: cardiac and associated pathology. J Mt Sinai Hosp 21: 218

Millar J, Allen R, Wakefield JSJ, Buchanan AJ, Gupta RK (1987) Diagnosis of thymoma by fine-needle aspiration cytology: light and electron microscopic study of a case. Diagn Cytopathol 3: 166

Miller JH (ed) (1985) Imaging in pediatric oncology. Williams and Wilkins, Baltimore, p 152

Min K-W, Waddell CC, Pircher FJ, Granville GE, Gyorkey F (1978) Selective uptake of 75-Se-Selenomethionine by thymoma with pure red cell aplasia. Cancer 41: 1323

Mink JH, Bein ME, Sukov R, Herrmann C, Winter J, Sample WF, Mulder D (1978) Computed tomography of the anterior mediastinum in patients with myasthenia gravis and suspected thymoma. AJR 130: 239

Monden Y, Nakahara K, Iioka S et al. (1985) Recurrence of thymoma: clinicopathological features, therapy and prognosis. Ann Thorac Surg 39: 165

Moore AV, Korobkin M, Powers B et al. (1982) Thymoma detection by mediastinal CT: patients with myasthenia gravis. AJR 138: 217

Moore AV, Korobkin M, Olanow W, Heaston DK, Ram PC, Dunnick NR, Silverman PM (1983) Age-related changes in the thymus gland: CT-pathologic correlation. AJR 141: 241

Moskowitz PS, Noon MA, McAlister WH, Mark JBD (1980) Thymic cyst hemorrhage: a cause of acute, symptomatic mediastinal widening in children with aplastic anemia. AJR 134: 832

Muhm JR, Brown LR, Crowe JK (1977) Detection of pulmonary nodules by computed tomography. AJR 128: 267

Nakahara K, Ohno K, Hashimoto J et al. (1988) Thymoma: results with complete resection and adjuvant postoperative irradiation in 141 consecutive patients. J Thorac Cardiovasc Surg 95: 1041

Nickels J, Franssila K (1976) Thymoma metastasizing to extrathoracic sites. A case report. Acta Pathol Microbiol Scand [Sect A] 84: 331

Nishimura T, Kondo M, Miyazaki S, Mochizuki T, Umadome H, Shimono Y (1982) Two-dimensional echocardiographic findings of cardiovascular involvement by invasive thymoma. Chest 81: 752

Oda K, Miyasaki K, Ohta M, Shibasaki H (1987) A case of myasthenia gravis associated with thymoma, multiple schwannomas and monoclonal IgA gammopathy. Jpn J Med 26: 223

Oliva L (1973) Erkrankungen des Mediastinums. In: Schinz HR, Baensch WE, Frommhold W, Glauner R, Uehlinger JE, Wellauer J (eds) Pleura, Mediastinum und Lunge. Thieme, Stuttgart (Lehrbuch der Röntgendiagnostik, vol IV/2, 6th edn)

Oppermann HC, Brandeis WE (1975) Konnatales Thymom. Z Kinderchir 16: 366

Oppermann HC, Willich E (1978) Zur Röntgendiagnostik und Differentialdiagnose der Mediastinaltumoren im Kindesalter. Radiologe 18: 218

Oppermann HC, Ulmer HE, Vogt-Moykopf J (1977) Thymom: seltene Ursache einer akuten respiratorischen Insuffizienz im Kindesalter. Z Kinderchir 21: 178

Or R, Raz I, Raveh D, Lichovitzki G, Kleinman Y (1987) Thymoma presenting as a superior vena cava syndrome: remission following therapy. Klin Wochenschr 65: 617

Otto HF (1984) Pathologie des Thymus. In: Doerr W, Seifert G (eds) Spezielle pathologische Anatomie, vol 17. Springer, Berlin Heidelberg New York

Otto HF, Hüsselmann H (1978) Klinisch-pathologische Studie zur Klassifikation und Prognose von Thymustumoren. Z Krebsforsch 91: 81

Pak HY, Yokota SB, Friedberg HA (1982) Thymoma diagnosed by transthoracic fine needle aspiration. Acta Cytol 26: 210

Papliński Z, Szyszko J (1967) Intrapulmonary thymoma. Polski Przegl Chir 39: 343

Pokorny WJ, Sherman JO (1974) Mediastinal masses in infants and children. J Thorac Cardiovasc Surg 68: 869

Pugatch RD, Faling LJ (1981) Computed tomography of the thorax: a status report. Chest 80: 618

Rachmaninoff N, Fentress V (1964) Thymoma with metastasis to the brain. Am J Clin Pathol 41: 618

Ridenhour CE, Henzel JH, DeWeese MS, Kerr SE (1970) Thymoma arising from undescended cervical thymus. Surgery 67: 614

Rogers BHG, Manaligod JR, Blazek WV (1968) Thymoma associated with pancytopenia and hypogammaglobulinemia. Report of a case and review of the literature. Am J Med 44: 154

Rosai JG, Levine D (1976) Tumors of the thymus. Atlas of tumor pathology, second series, fascicle 13, Armed Forces Institute of Pathology, Washington/DC, p 1

Rosenberg JC (1985) Neoplasms of the mediastinum. In:

De Vita VT, Hellman S, Rosenberg SA (eds) Cancer. Principles and practice of oncology, 2nd edn. Lippincott, Philadelphia

Rosenberger A, Adler O (1978) Fine needle aspiration biopsy in the diagnosis of mediastinal lesions. AJR 131: 239

Rosenthal T, Hertz M, Samra Y, Shahin N (1974) Thymoma: clinical and additional radiologic signs. Chest 65: 428

Ross JS, O'Donovan PB, Novoa R et al. (1984) Magnetic resonance of the chest: initial experience with imaging and in vivo T1 and T2 calculations. Radiology 152: 95

Rothberg MS, Eisenbud L, Griboff S (1989) Chronic mucocutaneous candidiasis-thymoma syndrome. A case report. Oral Surg Oral Med Oral Pathol 68: 411

Rundle LG, Sparks FP (1963) Thymoma and dermatomyositis. Arch Pathol 75: 64

Sajjad SM, Lukeman JM, Llamas L, Fernandez T (1982) Needle biopsy diagnosis of thymoma: a case report. Acta Cytol (Baltimore) 26: 503

Salyer WR, Eggleston JC (1976) Thymoma. A clinical and pathological study of 65 cases. Cancer 37: 229

Sanders DB, Ignatiadis PD, Sweet DE (1976) Thymoma with distant metastases. Trans Am Neurol Assoc 101: 286

Scatarige JC, Fishman EK, Zerhouni EA, Siegelman SS (1985) Transdiaphragmatic extension of invasive thymoma. AJR 144: 31

Schaner EG, Chang AE, Doppman JL, Conkle DM, Flye WM, Rosenberg SA (1978) Comparison of computed and conventional whole lung tomography in detecting pulmonary nodules: a prospective radiologic-pathologic study. AJR 131: 51

Schmid JR, Kiely JM, Harrison EG, Bayrd ED, Pease GL (1965) Thymoma associated with pure red-cell agenesis. Cancer 18: 216

Schnyder P, Candardjis G (1987) Computed tomography of thymic abnormalities. Eur J Radiol 7: 107

Schweisguth O, Chapuis Y (1962) Le diagnostic radiologique des tumeurs médiastinales de l'enfant. Ann Radiol (Paris) 5: 603

Seybold WD, McDonald JR, Clagett OT, Good CA (1950) Tumors of the thymus. J Thorac Surg 20: 195

Shaver VC, Bailey WR Jr, Marrangoni AG (1965) Acquired pulmonic stenosis due to external cardiac compression. Am J Cardiol 16: 256

Sherman ME, Black-Schaffer S (1990) Diagnosis of thymoma by needle biopsy. Acta Cytol 34: 63

Siegel MJ, Glazer HS, Wiener JI, Molina PL (1989) Normal and abnormal thymus in childhood: MR imaging. Radiology 172: 367

Silverman NA, Sabiston DC Jr (1977) Primary tumors and cysts of the mediastinum. Curr Probl Cancer 2: 1

Soorae AS, Stevenson HM (1980) Cystic thymoma simulating pulmonary stenosis. Br J Dis Chest 74: 193

Souadjian JV, Enriquez P, Silverstein MN, Pépin J-M (1974) The spectrum of diseases associated with thymoma. Arch Intern Med 134: 374

Spahr J, Frable WJ (1981) Pulmonary cytopathology of an invasive thymoma. Acta Cytol 25: 163

Späth G, Inniger R, Huth C, Laberke HG, Hoffmeister HE (1987) Thymome – eine retrospektive Studie über 48 Fälle. Chirurg 58: 529

Stevens MJ, Biggs BJ (1989) Metastatic thymoma: case report. Australas Radiol 33: 168

Stillman MA, Baer RL (1972) Pemphigus and thymoma. Acta Derm Venereol (Stockh) 52: 393

Talerman A, Amigo A (1968) Thymoma associated with

aregenerative and aplastic anemia in a five-year-old child. Cancer 21: 1212

Tandan R, Taylor R, DiCostanzo DP, Sharma K, Fries T, Roberts J (1990) Metastasizing thymoma and myasthenia gravis. Favorable response to glucocorticoids after failed chemotherapy and radiation therapy. Cancer 65: 1286

Teates CD, Bray S, Williamson BRJ (1978) Tumor detection with 67 gallium citrate: a literature survey (1970–1978). Clin Nucl Med 3: 456

Thies E, Thies E (1972) Tumoren des Thymus. Bruns' Beitr Klin Chir 219: 619

Thomas CV, Manivel JC (1987) Thymic carcinoma and aplastic anemia: report of a previously undocumented association. Am J Hematol 25: 333

Thomas NB, Gupta SC (1988) Unilobar enlargement of normal thymus gland causing mass effect. Br J Radiol 61: 244

Thorburn JD, Stephens B, Grimes OF (1952) Benign thymoma in the hilus of the lung. J Thorac Surg 24: 540

Thorlacius S, Aarli JA, Riise T, Matre R, Johnsen HJ (1989) Associated disorders in myasthenia gravis: autoimmune diseases and their relation to thymectomy. Acta Neurol Scand 80: 290

Toole JF, Witcofski R (1966) Selenmethionine Se 75 scan for thymoma. JAMA 198: 1219

Venegas RJ, Sun NCJ (1988) Cardiac tamponade as a presentation of malignant thymoma. Acta Cytol 32: 257

Wadon A (1934) Thymoma intratracheale. Central All Path Pathol Anat 60: 308

Walter E (1982) Computertomographische Diagnostik des Thymus. In: Lissner J, Doppman JL (eds) CT 82. Internationales Computertomographie Symposium, Seefeld/Tirol. Schnetztor, Konstanz

Walter E (1988) Erkrankungen und Tumoren des Thymus im Erwachsenenalter. In: Diethelm L, Heuck F, Olsson O, Strnad F, Vieten H, Zuppinger A (eds) Röntgendiagnostik der oberen Speise- und Atemwege und des Mediastinums. Springer, Berlin Heidelberg New York (Handbuch der medizinischen Radiologie, vol IX, part 5c)

Walter E, Hübener K-H (1980) Computertomographische Charakteristika raumfordernder Prozesse im vorderen Mediastinum und ihre Differentialdiagnose. ROFO 133: 391

Wechsler AS, Olanow CW (1980) Myasthenia gravis. Surg Clin North Am 60: 931

Wernecke K, Peters PE, Galanski M (1986) Mediastinal tumors: evaluation with suprasternal sonography. Radiology 159: 405

Wernitz C (1976) Großes gutartiges Thymom bei einem 6 Jahre alten Kind. ROFO 125: 85

Wick MR, Nichols WC, Ingle JN, Bruckman JE, Okazaki H (1981) Malignant, predominantly lymphocytic thymoma with central and peripheral nervous system metastases. Cancer 47: 2036

Wilkins EW, Edmunds LH, Castleman B (1966) Cases of thymoma at the Massachusetts General Hospital. J Thorac Cardiovasc Surg 52: 322

Willich E (1970) Röntgendiagnostik der Mediastinaltumoren im Kindesalter. Pädiatr Prax 9: 79

Willich E (1988) Bildgebende Diagnostik des Thymus vom Wachstums- bis ins Erwachsenenalter. In: Diethelm L, Heuck F, Olsson O, Strnad F, Vieten H, Zuppinger A (eds) Röntgendiagnostik der oberen Speise- und Atemwege und des Mediastinums. Springer, Berlin Heidelberg New York (Handbuch der medizinischen Radiologie, vol IX, part 5c)

Willnow U, Tischer W (1973) Thymusgeschwülste im Kindesalter. Zentralbl Chir 98: 581

Yeoh CB, Ford JM, Lattes R, Wylie RH (1966) Intrapulmonary thymoma. J Thorac Cardiovasc Surg 51: 131

Yune HY, Klatte EC (1970) Thymic venography. Radiology 96: 521

Zeok JV, Todd EP, Dillon M, DeSimone P, Utley JR (1979) The role of thymectomy in red cell aplasia. Ann Thorac Surg 28: 257

Zerhouni EA, Scott WW, Baker RR, Wharam MD, Siegelman SS (1982) Invasive thymomas: diagnosis and evaluation by computed tomography. J Comput Assist Tomogr 6: 92

8.2.3 Carcinoma of the Thymus

8.2.3.1 Occurrence and Clinical Symptoms

8.2.3.1.1 Occurrence

Squamous cell carcinoma is one of the rarer primary tumors of the thymus. Other rare tumors reported are clear cell carcinoma (SNOVER et al. 1982; WOLFE et al. 1983; CHEN 1984; STEPHENS et al. 1987), small cell carcinoma (ROSAI 1976; COHEN et al. 1988; DÖRMANN 1989), basaloid carcinoma (SNOVER et al. 1982), undifferentiated lymphoepithelioma-like carcinoma (HARTMANN et al. 1990), and sarcomatoid tumors (SNOVER et al. 1982).

Squamous cell carcinoma as a primary carcinoma of the thymus was first recognized and described by CASTLEMAN (1955) and FRANK et al. (1956).

In a study of 148 tumors of the mediastinum, SHIMOSATO et al. (1977) found eight primary squamous cell carcinomas of the thymus, and according to MORINAGA et al. (1987) only 30 such malignant growths have been reported. If one compiles all the data in the literature (FRANK et al. 1956; WATSON et al. 1968; SHIMOSATO et al. 1977; MORINAGA et al. 1987; JONES et al. 1987; DIMARIO et al. 1988; SATO et al. 1986; SNOVER et al. 1982; COHEN et al. 1988), it is seen that of 19 patients with primary thymic carcinomas of squamous cell character, 13 were men and six women; thus a male to female ratio of 2:1 can be assumed. The ages of these patients ranged from 20 years (WATSON et al. 1968) to 66 years (FRANK et al. 1956), giving an average age of 51 years although the majority of patients (70%) were in their 5th or 6th decade.

Squamous cell carcinoma of the thymus cannot be distinguished macroscopically from invasive thymoma. The histologic differences may be so small that differentiation between squamous cell carcinoma and thymoma may be difficult (DiMA-RIO et al. 1988).

Histologically the malignoma consists of squamous cells – occasionally producing keratin – and fibrous tissue, features of a thymoma may be present (MORINAGA et al. 1987, DiMARIO et al. 1988). The tumor has a poor supply of blood vessels and necrotic areas can be seen although the tendency to necrosis is greater in squamous cell carcinoma of the thymus than in that of the lung. Cystic colliquation and calcifications are frequent (FRANK et al. 1956). Normal thymic tissue can be found histologically at the edge of the tumor (DiMARIO et al. 1988) or the whole thymus can be covered by malignant growth (FRANK et al. 1956).

The tumor can spread within the thymus capsule, in which case no infiltration of the neighboring organs can be seen (SHIMOSATO et al. 1977). However, the tumor tends toward both infiltrative growth in the surrounding area and the formation of metastases. There have been reports of infiltration of the fatty tissue surrounding the tumor in the anterior mediastinum, especially in the retrosternal space (FRANK et al. 1956), of the lungs, of the vagal and phrenic nerves (SHIMOSATO et al. 1977; MORINAGA et al. 1987), of the pericardium, myocardium, and pleura (MORINAGA et al. 1987; DiMARIO et al. 1988), and of the regional lymph nodes. Metastases are mainly found in the lymph nodes, liver, peritoneum, and bones (SHIMOSATO et al. 1977), as well as the pleura and diaphragm (MORINAGA et al. 1987).

There are various theories as to the histogenesis of the malignancies. MAEZAWA et al. (1974) and WICK et al. (1982) are of the opinion that squamous cell carcinoma of the thymus originates from aberrant cells during the development of the branchial cleft. FISCHER (1964) believed that Hassall's corpuscles are responsible for the genesis of the tumor. MORINAGA et al. (1987) suspect [like SHIMO-SATO et al. (1977)] that the tumor originates in the thymus and is a variation on thymus cells, since they observed a mixed growth of squamous cell carcinoma and lymphoepithelial thymoma.

8.2.3.1.2 Clinical Symptoms

The main clinical symptom shown by squamous cell carcinoma is chest pain (SHIMOSATO et al. 1977; JONES et al. 1987; SNOVER et al. 1982; and others) radiating into the neck or shoulder or between the shoulder blades (SHIMOSATO et al. 1977; MORINAGA et al. 1987). General symptoms such as tiredness,

loss of weight, dyspnea, and cough, possibly with purulent phlegm, are also to be seen (SHIMOSATO et al. 1977 and others).

Concomitant illnesses are rare; only DiMARIO et al. (1988) have reported myasthenia as a concomitant disease.

8.2.3.2 Diagnosis with Imaging Procedures

8.2.3.2.1 Conventional Radiology

Radiologic results have been reported by FRANK et al. (1956), JONES et al. (1987), and MORINAGA et al. (1987); the other reports are essentially limited to pathoanatomic descriptions.

Chest radiography in two planes shows widening of the mediastinum on one or both sides due to displacement by the tumor in the anterior superior mediastinum. The tumor lies – in correspondence with the usual position of the thymus – ventral to the ascending thoracic aorta, i.e., retrosternally. The tumor usually has a polycyclic border easily distinguished from the lung. Thus the radiographic appearance is similar to that of a thymoma, a lymph node conglomerate tumor, or a similar growth in the anterior mediastinum.

Conventional tomography can show stenosis of the trachea due to the tumor growth in the superior mediastinum (SHIMOSATO et al. 1977) but this can also be seen with CT. Conventional tomography yields no information over and above that provided by CT.

No arteriographic results are reported. Angiography is possibly of use in demonstrating tumor-induced compression of the pulmonary artery or vein, as described by MORINAGA et al. (1987), and infiltration of the superior vena cava (SHIMOSATO et al. 1977).

8.2.3.2.2 Ultrasonography

No results have yet been reported.

8.2.3.2.3 Computed Tomography

Only JONES et al. (1987), DiMARIO et al. (1988), and MORINAGA et al. (1987) have reported CT results. They all describe large lobulated tumors in the anterior superior mediastinum. In keeping with its malignant character, the tumor shows its infiltrating growth in the form of blurred edges. Infiltrations of the great vessels and pericardium have been reported. The CT appearance is similar to that seen with an invasive thymoma. Clear demarcation of the carcinoma within the mediastinum is possible when it has not broken through the thymus capsule (SHIMOSATO et al. 1977).

8.2.3.2.4 Magnetic Resonance Imaging

No results are available.

8.2.3.2.5 Nuclear Medicine

No results are available.

8.2.3.3 Differential Diagnosis

It is difficult to make pronouncements regarding differential diagnosis against tumors of other histologic type on the basis of the limited radiologic results so far available. It can be assumed, however, that differentiation between squamous cell carcinoma and other tumors in the anterior mediastinum, such as an invasive thymoma, a thoracic seminoma, or a lymph node conglomerate tumor, will not be possible radiologically.

8.2.3.4 Relative Value of the Imaging Procedures

Chest radiography in two planes remains the basis of all diagnostics. Conventional tomography provides no further information. CT should immediately follow the chest radiograph; it can show the demarcation of the tumor, its size, and its relation to neighboring organs in the mediastinum, i.e., it answers all questions as to the operability of the tumor. The value of ultrasonography and MRI cannot be evaluated owing to the lack of reports on their use.

8.2.3.5 Therapy and Prognosis

Extirpation and postoperative radiotherapy with occasional chemotherapy are recommended. Use of radiotherapy on its own was reported by SHIMOSATO et al. (1977). The tumor disappeared completely following the application of 60 Gy, but the patient died a year later owing to metastases. According to a literature review by DiMARIO et al.

(1988) the prognosis is poor: the 10-year survival rate is below 50% and the 5-year recurrence rate is ca. 22%.

References

Castleman B (1955) Tumors of the thymus gland. In: Atlas of tumor pathology, section 5 fascicle 19. AFIP, Washington, DC

Chen KTK (1984) Squamous carcinoma of the thymus. J Surg Oncol 25: 61

Cohen II, Templeton A, Philips AK (1988) Tumors of the thymus. Med Pediatr Oncol 16: 135

DiMario FJ, Lisak RP, Kornstein MJ, Brooks JJ (1988) Myasthenia gravis and primary squamous cell carcinoma of the thymus: a case report. Neurology 38: 580

Dörmann MR (1989) Kleinzelliges Thymuscarcinom und Osteomyelosklerose. Klinikarzt 18: 614

Fisher ER (1964) Pathology of the thymus and its relation to human disease: the thymus in immunology. Hoeber, New York, pp 676–729

Frank HA, Reiner L, Fleischner FG (1956) Co-occurrence of large leiomyoma of the esophagus and squamous-cell carcinoma of the thymus. Report of a case, with roentgenologic, pathological and clinical discussion. N Engl J Med 255: 159

Hartmann CA, Roth C, Minck C, Niedobitek G (1990) Thymic carcinoma. Report of five cases and review of the literature. J Cancer Res Clin Oncol 116: 69

Jones GW, Laukkanen E, Miller RR (1987) Well-differentiated squamous cell carcinoma of the thymus. Can Med Assoc J 137: 43

Kuo TT, Chang JP, Lin FJ, Wu WC, Chang CH (1990) Thymic carcinomas: histopathological varieties and immunohistochemical study. Am J Surg Pathol 14: 24

Maezawa M, Mikami J, Ooami H (1974) An autopsy case of squamous cell carcinoma of possile thymic origin. Lung Cancer 14: 91

Morinaga S, Sato Y, Shimosato Y, Sinkai T, Tsuchiya R (1987) Multiple thymic squamous cell carcinomas associated with mixed type thymoma. Am J Surg Pathol 11: 982

Rosai J, Levine G, Weber WR, Higa E (1976) Carcinoid tumors and oat cell carcinomata of the thymus. Pathol Annu 11: 201

Sato Y, Watanabe S, Mukai K, Kodama T, Upton MP, Goto M, Shimosato Y (1986) An immunohistochemical study of thymic epithelial tumors. Am J Surg Pathol 10: 862

Shimosato Y, Kameya T, Nagai K, Suemasu K (1977) Squamous cell carcinoma of the thymus. An analysis of eight cases. Am J Surg Pathol 1: 109

Snover DC, Levine GD, Rosai J (1982) Thymic carcinoma. Five distinctive histological variants. Am J Surg Pathol 6: 451

Stephens M, Khalil J, Gibbs AR (1987) Primary clear cell carcinoma of the thymus gland. Histopathology 11: 763

Watson RR, Weisel W, O'Connor TM (1968) Thymic neoplasm. A surgical enigma. Arch Surg 97: 230

Wick MR, Weiland LH, Scheithauer BW, Bernatz PE (1982) Primary thymic carcinomas. Am J Surg Pathol 6: 613

Wolfe JT, Wick MR, Banks PM, Scheithauer BW (1983) Clear cell carcinoma of the thymus. Mayo Clin Proc 58: 365

8.3 Carcinoid Tumors of the Thymus

8.3.1 Pathologic Features

W. J. HOFMANN and H. F. OTTO

In 1972, ROSAI and HIGA identified carcinoid tumors of the thymus as a specific entity distinctly different from thymomas. The authors proposed that the tumors, for which they suggested the term "thymic carcinoid," should be distinguished from true thymomas by virtue of the clinical, histomorphologic, immunohistologic, and ultrastructural differences between them. Ever since, "carcinoid tumors of the thymus" have been defined as a clinicopathologic entity. This tumor entity, however, is rare (ROSAI et al. 1972; OTTO and HÜSSELMANN 1976; ROSAI and LEVINE 1976; WICK et al. 1980, 1982; WICK and SCHEITHAUER 1984; OTTO 1984; WICK and ROSAI 1988; HOFMANN and OTTO 1989 a). Among the tumors of the anterior mediastinum, carcinoid tumors of the thymus represent a very small group of 2.5%–4% (WICK et al. 1980).

Carcinoid tumors of the thymus are derived from the foregut and their biologic characteristics are similar to those of other carcinoids.

Thymic carcinoids are solid, usually large, lobulated tan-gray neoplasms with focal areas of necrosis, hemorrhage, and calcification. Invasion of adjacent mediastinal blood vessels, pleura, and pericardium is apparent to the surgeon in more than 50% of cases. Thymic carcinoids are malignant tumors that in more than 30% of cases recur locally and/or metastasize widely (OTTO and HÜSSELMANN 1976; OTTO 1984; WICK and ROSAI 1988). In a study of 15 patients with thymic carcinoids followed at the Mayo Clinic, Rochester, Minnesota, for up to 25 years, WICK and co-workers (1982) reported metastasis in 73% of patients. Metastatic sites included mediastinal and cervical lymph nodes, liver, bone (usually osteoblastic), skin, and lungs. MARINO and MÜLLER-HERMELINK (1985) classify thymic carcinoids (and small cell carcinomas of the thymus/mediastinum) as neuroectodermal carcinomas.

Histologically (Table 8.8, Fig. 8.29), thymic carcinoids are composed of cords, ribbons and festoons, islands, and/or rosette-like formations composed of oval or round cells with amphophilic cytoplasm and uniform nuclei. The epithelial (or neuroectodermal) nature of these tumors is reflected by their reactivity for cytokeratin in virtually all cases (MIETTINEN 1987). Neurofilament reactivity has been reported in some thymic neuroendocrine neoplasms as well (MIETTINEN et al. 1983). Histochemically (Fig. 8.30 d), the tumor cells are nonargentaffin but argyrophil (GRIMELIUS and/or SEVIER-MUNGER stain). Formalin-induced

Table 8.8. Histochemical and immunohistologic results in respect of nine carcinoid tumors of the thymus[a] (compiled data from HERBST et al. 1987 and HOFMANN et al. 1989 b)

	Case 1	Case 2	Case 3	Case 4	Case 5	Case 6	Case 7	Case 8	Case 9
Grimelius (argyrophil)	+<<−	+<<−	−	−	+<<−	+/−	+<<−	−	+<<−
Masson-Fontana-Hamperl (argentaffin)	−	−	−	−	−	+<<−	−	−	−
Neuron-specific enolase	+/−	+/−	+	(+)	+/−	+/−	+/−	+	+
Chromogranin A	+<<−	+/−	−	−	+>>−	+/−	+/−	+<<−	+<<−
Synaptophysin	(+)	+	+	+	+	+	+	(+)	+
Neurotensin	−	−	n.d.	+<<−	n.d.	+<<−	+<<−	n.d.	n.d.
ACTH	−	−	n.d.	+<<−	n.d.	−	+>>−	n.d.	n.d.
Calcitonin	−	+>>−	n.d.	−	n.d.	−	−	n.d.	n.d.
Cholecystokinin	+<<−	−	n.d.	+<<−	n.d.	+<<−	+<<−	n.d.	n.d.

+ : all tumor cells positive
+>>− : most tumor cells positive
+/− : about half of the tumor cells positive
+<<− : few tumor cells positive
− : all tumor cells negative
( ): weak reaction
n.d.: determination was not done
[a] All investigated neoplasms were negative to antisera against calcitonin gene-related peptide (CGRP), gastrin, serotonin, somatostatin, and substance P

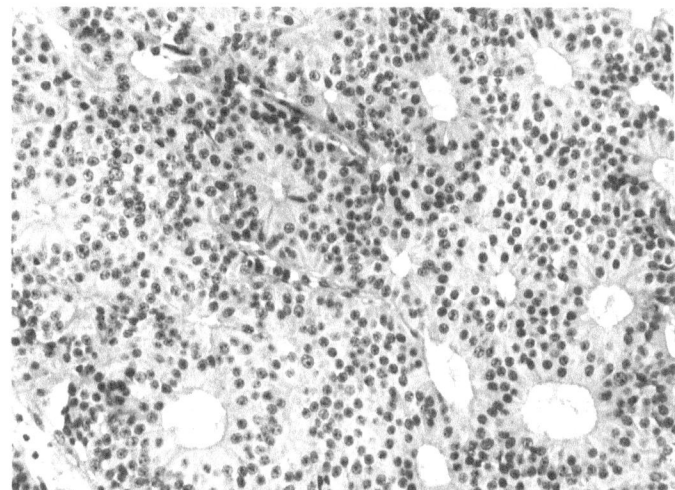

Fig.8.29 Histology of a carcinoid tumor of the thymus: relatively uniform tumor cells form solid nests and true rosettes separated by a fine fibrovascular stroma. The nuclei of the tumor cells are round to oval with evenly distributed chromatin. H&E, × 158

fluorescence and α-glycerophosphate dehydrogenase can also be demonstrated in thymic carcinoids (JUDGE et al. 1976). Ultrastructurally, the tumor cells contain membrane-bound, dense-core neurosecretory granules ranging in size from 100 to 450 μm (OTTO and HÜSSELMANN 1976; OTTO 1984).

Thymic carcinoids are able to produce α-MSH, somatostatin, parathormone, serotonin, calcitonin, met-enkephalin, leu-enkephalin, β-endorphin, cholecystokinin, and neurotensin (Table 8.8). In many cases the tumor cells contain ACTH. Some induce paraneoplastic syndromes such as Cushing's syndrome, hyperparathyroidism, or ZOLLINGER-ELLISON syndrome (ROSAI and HIGA 1972; SALYER et al. 1976; OTTO and HÜSSELMANN 1976; HERBST et al. 1987; WICK and ROSAI 1988). Sometimes they are associated with multiple endocrine neoplasia (MEN I and MEN II).

In recent years, several general immunohistochemical markers of neuroendocrine differentiation have been characterized, including neuron-specific enolase (NSE), an isoenzyme of 2-phospho-D-glycerate hydrolase, chromogranin, and synaptophysin. These markers provide useful tools for the cellular (diagnostic) characterization of the thymic neuroendocrine tumors (Table 8.8, Fig. 8.30) (HOFMANN et al. 1989b).

8.3.2 Occurrence and Clinical Symptoms

E. WALTER

8.3.2.1 Occurrence

In 85% of patients, carcinoids are found in the upper and lower bowel, in 50% of cases near the appendix (MCDONALD 1984). The remaining, much rarer, locations are the esophagus, stomach, gallbladder and biliary tract, pancreas, ovaries, testicles, lungs and bronchi, parotid, teratoma, and also the thymus (HUGHES et al. 1975; STRASBERG et al. 1979; ADOLPH et al. 1987).

Only 2.5% of the primary tumors of the thymus are carcinoids, (OTTO 1985), and only small numbers of cases are generally reported (ROSAI and HIGA 1972; HOSODA et al. 1975; ROSAI et al. 1976; SALYER et al. 1976; OTTO and HÜSSELMANN 1976; WICK and SCHEITHAUER 1984; JOSE et al. 1988; WOECKEL et al. 1990; and others). ECONOMOPOULOS et al. (1990) reported on seven patients (six men, one woman) observed over a period of 38 years (1950–1988). All in all about 100 cases have been reported (JOSE et al. 1988). The thymic carcinoid reported by WOECKEL et al. (1990) weighed 1605 g and is the largest hormone-active (calcitonin) tumor of this histology reported to date.

Patients between the ages of 9 and 87 have been affected, and there is a male to female ratio of 3:1 (OTTO 1985).

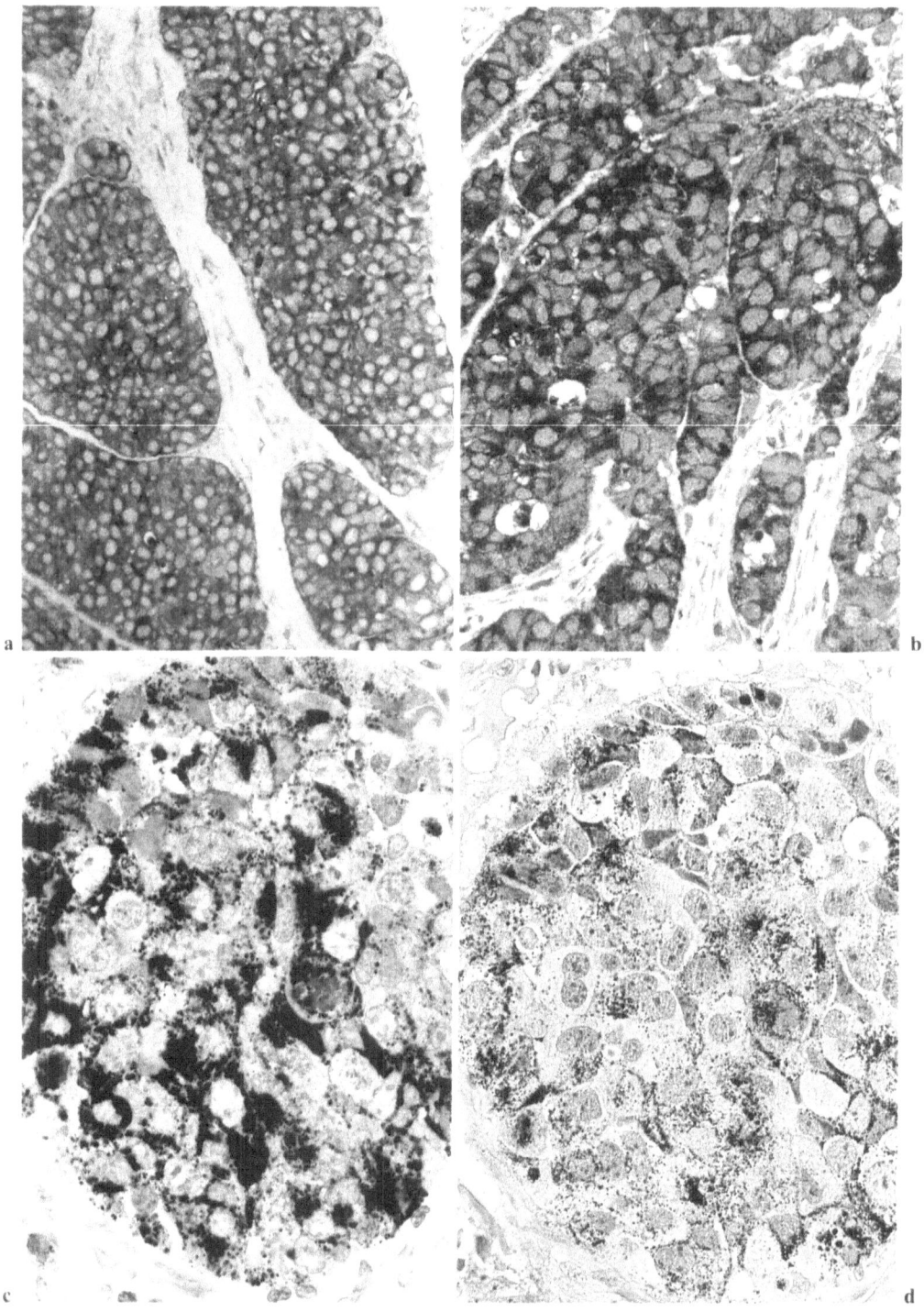

Fig. 8.30a–d. Immunohistology (**a–c**) and histochemistry (**d**) of a carcinoid tumor of the thymus. **a** All tumor cells show a broad and homogeneous expression of neuron-specific enolase (NSE). Anti-NSE, immunoperoxidase method, ×202. **b** Many tumor cells contain synaptophysin in their cytoplasm. Anti-Sy38, immunoperoxidase method, ×202. **c** A lot of tumor cells show reactivity with a monoclonal antibody to chromogranin A. Immunoperoxidase method, ×398. **d** The same tumor cells are argyrophylic, indicating the presence of neurosecretory granules. Grimelius, ×398

8.3.2.2 Clinical Symptoms

Carcinoids show no clinical symptoms in 40%–50% of patients (WICK and SCHEITHAUER 1984; WICK and ROSAI 1988), being discovered during routine chest examinations. They can, however, produce uncharacteristic symptoms due to local displacement. These symptoms are usually described as pain in the chest or back, possibly radiating into the arms or legs (HUGHES et al. 1975), dyspnea, precordial sensations, arrhythmia, compression syndrome of the superior vena cava cava (WICK and SCHEITHAUER 1984; HERBST et al. 1987), sanguineous sputum (WOECKEL et al. 1990), night sweats, poor appetite, and weight loss (MCCAUGHEY et al. 1987; COOPER et al. 1979) carcinoids of the thymus can also present clinical symptoms due to hormone production. Carcinoids of the jejunum, ileum, cecum, and colon mainly produce serotonin, which causes the typical flush symptoms as well as fibrosis of the endocardium. They also tend to produce kallikrein, enteroglucagon, and substance P (HERBST et al. 1987). Carcinoids of the thymus, like those of the lung, stomach, duodenum, and pancreas, can also produce a large number of specific exocrine hormones such as ACTH, calcitonin, cholecystokinin, antidiuretic hormone, vasoconstricting intestinal peptides, glucagon, insulin, and gastrin (PEARSE 1974; FROHMANN et al. 1980; ISENBERG et al. 1981; HERBST et al. 1987; and others). The histochemical identification of the neural peptides does not necessarily have a corresponding clinical picture (HERBST et al. 1987).

In up to 33% of the patients with a hormone-active thymic carcinoid, production of ACTH and the corresponding symptoms of Cushing's disease must be expected (WICK et al. 1980; BROWN et al. 1982; WICK and SCHEITHAUER 1984; OTTO 1984). Combination of an ATCH-producing thymic carcinoid with neoplasms of other endocrine organs such as pituitary, parathyroid, or islet cell tumors (type MEN I) is often found; thus a Zollinger-Ellison-syndrome can also indicate this syndrome (JOSE et al. 1980). In exceptional cases the thymic carcinoid can occur together with a medullary thyroid carcinoma (type MEN II) (MARCHEVSKY and DIKMAN 1979; EBERLE et al. 1982). A familial disposition to such multiple endocrinal adenopathy was reported by MANES and TAYLOR in 1973, and an autosomal dominant hereditary factor is proved (EBERLE et al. 1982).

Rare combinations are found with the Eaton-Lambert-syndrome (pseudomyasthenia) (WICK and ROSAI 1988) and with hypertrophic osteoarthropathy (ROSAI et al. 1976).

Hyperpigmentation of the skin and mucous membranes – reversible after tumor extirpation – can indicate the presence of a thymic carcinoid. This is caused by an increased corticotropin release stimulating melanocytes (BROWN et al. 1982; LIESKE et al. 1985). No connection could be found with myasthenia, hypogammaglobulinemia, or defective red cell development (DAY and GEDGAUDES 1984).

Clinical symptoms also arise as a result of tumoral spread. Thymic carcinoid is in general more malignant than thymic carcinoma, and in 50% of patients infiltration of the pleura, pericardium, and blood vessels (OTTO 1984; ROSENBERG 1985), as well as of the phrenic nerve (HUGHES et al. 1975), has already occurred at the time of discovery.

LEVINE and ROSAI (1978) found mediastinal and cervical lymph node metastases in 40% of their patients with malignant thymic carcinoids. Like thymomas, thymic carcinoids tend to give rise to pleural metastases (LEVINE and ROSAI 1976). There is a higher incidence of hematogenous dissemination with carcinoids than with thymomas; in 20%–30% of cases such dissemination is extrathoracic (WICK et al. 1980). When the infiltrating carcinoid is larger than 2 cm in diameter, distant metastases must be reckoned with in 80% of cases; they mainly occur in the liver, bones (usually osteoplastic), and lungs (NYGAARD et al. 1979), in the latter case possibly displaying calcification (ISENBERG et al. 1981). In isolated cases metastases have been reported in the spinal cord (ISENBERG et al. 1981), spleen, peritoneum, and brain (ADOLPH et al. 1987).

Late metastatic spread has been observed up to 8 years following the discovery and treatment of the primary tumor (WICK et al. 1982).

The ideal treatment is resection of the tumor. Where there is an invasive tumor which cannot be completely removed, radio- or chemotherapy is necessary. Due to the poor response of the tumor to this treatment, the prognosis must be viewed as unfavorable (WICK and ROSAI 1988). The 5-year mortality of patients with a carcinoid showing no hormone activity is 30%; if there is evidence of Cushing's disease or MEN the mortality is 65% (WICK et al. 1980).

8.3.3 Diagnosis with Imaging Procedures

8.3.3.1 Conventional Radiology

As in the case of thymoma, conventional chest radiography in two planes is of little help with the small tumors because the disease shows clinical symptoms at an early stage owing to the hormone activity. In the cases reported by Brown et al. (1982) the thymic carcinoids had a diameter of 1.5–8.5 cm. In four out of five cases the authors could not even identify the small tumors retrospectively on the chest radiograph in two planes (Brown et al. 1982). Large tumors show the characteristic picture of a space-occupying lesion in the mediastinum, such as is seen with conventional radiographic diagnosis of thymoma (Rosai and Higa 1972; Salyer et al. 1976; Deneffe and Moerman 1986; and others). The lesion, which is clearly distinguished from the lung by virtue of its well-defined smooth or polycyclic border, overlaps the edge of the mediastinum on the posteroanterior radiograph and in the lateral view is usually to be found lying retrosternally in the anterior superior mediastinum. Demarcation of the tumor within the mediastinum is not possible on conventional images (Figs. 8.31 a, 8.32 a, b).

Conventional tomography does not provide any further information (Fig. 8.31 b). Angiography of the aortic arch shows no pathologic findings (Gelfand et al. 1981; Strasberg et al. 1979).

Selective angiographic examinations of the thymus have been reported only by Düx (1977), who found a well-demarcated, hypervascular tumor (Fig. 8.31 c, d). Experiences with the examination of carcinoids of the upper bowel have shown only indirect changes to the branches of the mesenteric artery, such as are also produced by nonmalignant diseases. The tumor possibly shows a slight increase in contrast medium density in the capillary phase; pathognomonic angiographic results have not been found (Gold and Redman 1972; Seigel et al. 1980). Whether this holds true for thymic carcinoids will only be revealed by further studies.

Bony metastases are typically osteoplastic (Wick and Rosai 1988; Thomas 1968); hypertrophic osteoarthropathy (Rosai et al. 1976) can also be demonstrated radiologically.

8.3.3.2 Ultrasonography

The authors know of no publications on ultrasonographic findings in cases of thymic carcinoid.

8.3.3.3 Computed Tomography

The CT results in patients with thymic carcinoid (Fig. 8.32 c) are similar to those in patients with invasive or noninvasive thymoma. The noninvasive thymic carcinoid can be seen as a sharp-edged, solid tumor well defined against the neighboring organs; invasive tumors, by contrast, show indistinct borders. Both noninvasive and invasive tumors display attenuation values between 15 and 50 HU, i.e., there is no difference from thymomas in this respect (Brown et al. 1982; Weiss et al. 1987). On the application of a bolus of contrast medium only slight enhancement can be expected; values of 80 HU can be attained (Weiss et al. 1987). Although small, often calcified, necrotic centers are a characteristic pathoanatomic feature of thymic carcinoid (Levine and Rosai 1976), due to their size they cannot always be identified on CT scans. Brown et al. (1982) found calcifications in only one of the two carcinoids examined with CT. Cystic changes, which are often seen in thymomas, could not be seen with CT, nor would one have expected them, given the past pathoanatomic findings (Rosenberg 1985). The malignant thymic carcinoid infiltrates the neighboring organs such as the blood vessels, pleura, and pericardium. In such cases the tumor cannot be differentiated from these organs on CT scans.

8.3.3.4 Magnetic Resonance Imaging

No results have yet been reported.

8.3.3.5 Nuclear Medicine

It is a well-known fact that ^{131}I-MIBG (^{131}I-meta-iodobenzylguanidine) is stored by pheochromocytomas, neuroblastomas, and bronchial and intestinal carcinoids (Feldman et al. 1986; Adolph et al. 1987). Thymic carcinoids are similar to the latter as a result of their common neuroectodermal origins; thus it could be assumed that they would also store ^{131}I-MIBG. Mey et al. (1988) found results fitting this thesis: 24–48 h following injection of 1 mCi ^{131}I-MIBG an uptake could be seen which disappeared on resection. Adolph and associates (1987) reported differing results: while all the tumor manifestations of intestinal carcinoids examined stored the radioisotope following injection of 1.5–2 mCi ^{131}I-MIBG (maximal values reached on day 1 after injection), of six tumor manifestations

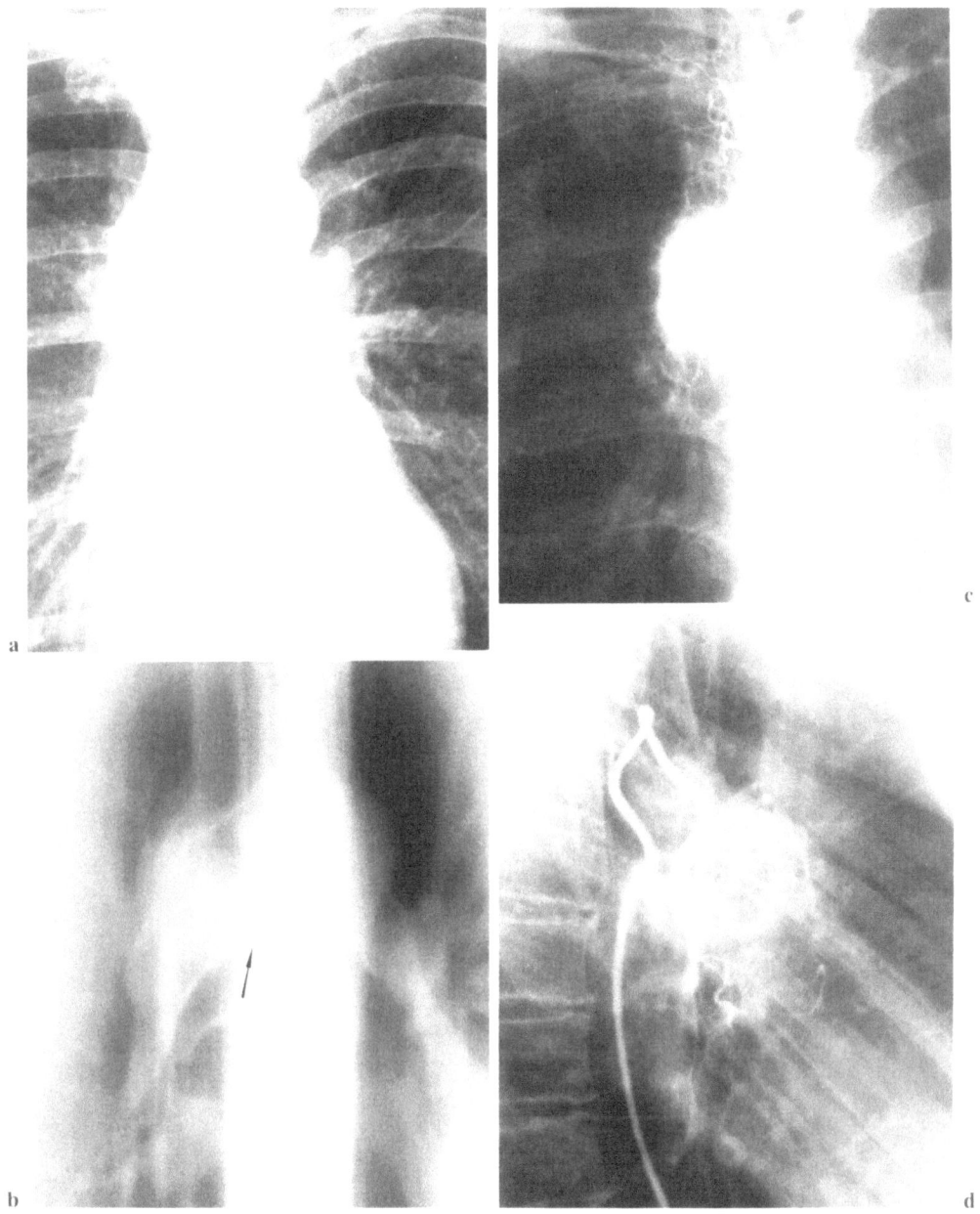

of bronchial carcinoids only four showed an increase in MIBG concentration in the tumor, and both thymic carcinoids in the series showed no radioisotope storage whatsoever.

The reason for these discrepancies must be looked for in the chemical similarity between serotonin and MIBG (ADOLPH et al. 1987). While intestinal carcinoids examined histochemically by WILANDER et al. (1985) showed serotonin production, the clinical picture of serotinin-induced carcinoid syndrome is seldom observed with thymic carci-

Fig. 8.31a–d. Thymic carcinoid. **a** Posteroanterior chest radiograph showing enlargement of the mediastinum to the right due to a radiologically uncharacteristic mass. **b** Conventional tomography: There is compression and infiltration of the right main bronchus by the tumor; today this finding can also be illustrated by CT. **c,d** Selective arteriography of the internal thoracic artery. A well-vascularized tumor is seen in the anterior mediastinum, representing thymic carcinoid, as confirmed operatively. (By courtesy of Prof. Dr. DÜX, Mönchengladbach, FRG)

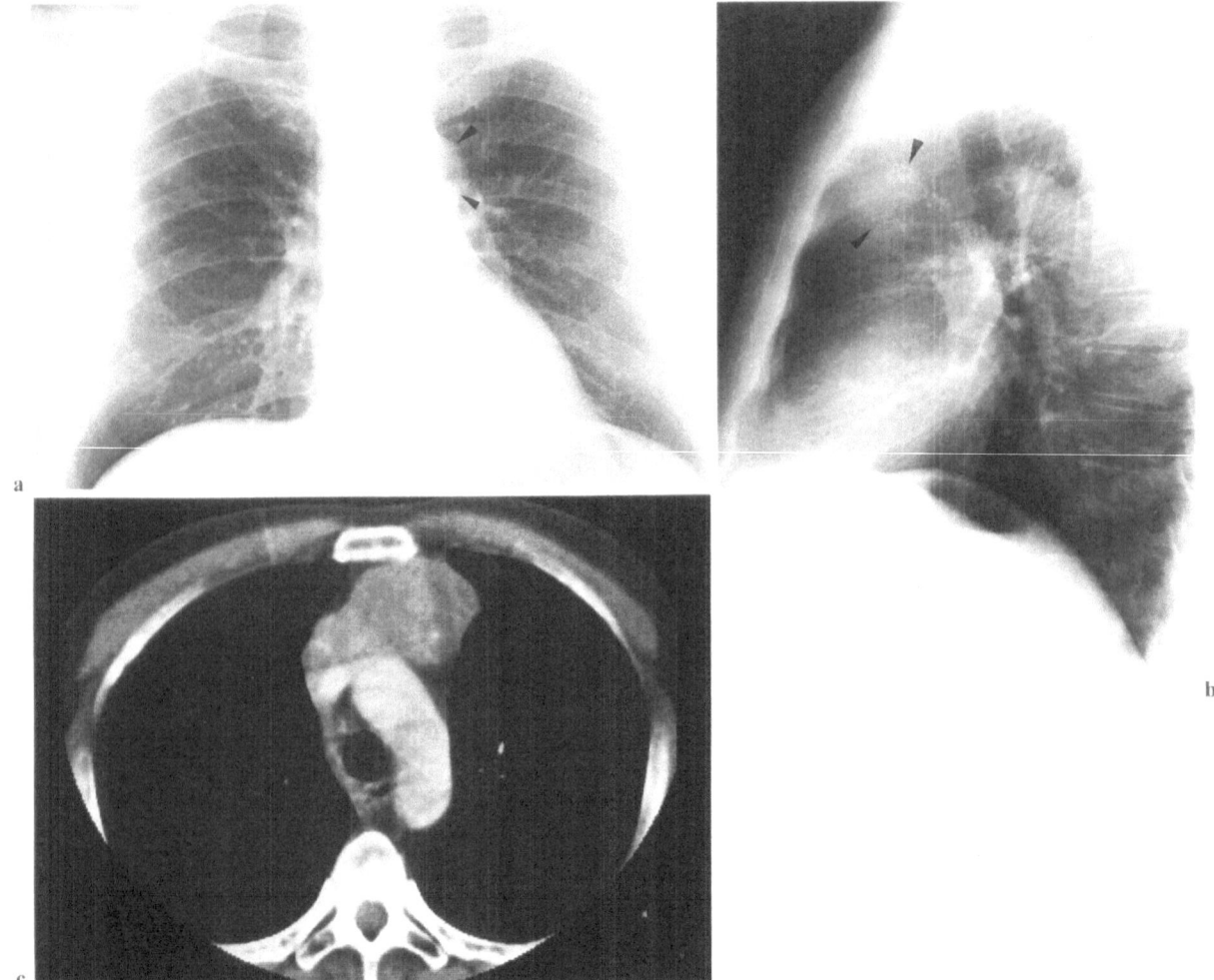

Fig. 8.32 a–c. Thymic carcinoid. **a,b** Chest radiography in two planes. A mass sharply demarcated from the lung is present in the anterior mediastinum. There are no pathognomonic findings that would allow the diagnosis of carcinoid. (Courtesy of Dr. PETZEL, Krankenhaus Stuttgart-Bad Cannstadt, FRG) **c** CT scan of the anterior mediastinum: A solid mass present in the anterior mediastinum is poorly delineated against the aortic arch, representing invasive carcinoid of the thymus. There is discreet calcification. On the CT scan, also, no findings pathognomonic for carcinoid of the thymus can be recognized. (Courtesy of Dr. KLOTT and co-workers, Stuttgart-Bad Cannstatt, FRG)

noids (ROSENBERG 1985). These only infrequently show serotonin production, which can explain the irregular storage of ^{131}I-MIBG in the tumor. Since no other nuclear medical procedures have been reported, their differential diagnostic value remains uncertain.

8.3.4 Differential Diagnosis

All solid homogeneous tumors of the anterior mediastinum must be considered in the differential diagnosis of thymic carcinoid.

Thymomas, whether invasive or noninvasive, can simulate thymic carcinoids on CT scans. Cystic degeneration, typical in thymomas, is often missing with carcinoids (COHEN et al. 1988). Calcifications, seen in approximately 25% of thymomas are seldom found in carcinoids.

Like carcinoids, the solitary lymphoma is visualized on CT scans as a discrete homogeneous dense lesion with no fatty areas so that morphologically differential diagnosis is impossible. This is also true for the thoracic seminoma.

Chest radiography, conventional tomography, and CT produce no pathognomonic evidence for thymic carcinoids. Thus the diagnosis "thymic carcinoid" cannot be achieved radiologically. Where the clinical symptoms are appropriate and a "thymoma" or solitary "lymphoma" can be seen, the presence of a thymic carcinoid can be postulated, especially as a pathognomonic uptake of ^{131}I-MIBG in a thymic carcinoid can rarely be expected.

8.3.5 Relative Value of the Imaging Procedures

Chest radiography in two planes remains the basis of all diagnostics. Conventional tomography is unnecessary. CT is, as with all mediastinal tumors, the method of choice. CT can differentiate between invasive and noninvasive growth as well as showing any infiltration of neighboring organs. Local metastases of the lymph nodes and pleura can also be seen. Thus CT is superior to conventional tomography. Although an uptake in the thymus can seldom be expected, a nuclear medical examination with ^{131}I-MIBG under thyroid blocking should be tried because if this is positive the carcinoid is proven. MRI and ultrasonographic results are not yet available, so that the value of these procedures cannot be evaluated; this is also true of arteriography.

8.3.6 Therapy and Prognosis

The therapy of choice is resection of the tumor. Radiotherapy and chemotherapy are employed especially for invasive tumors that cannot be completely resected. Due to the poor responsiveness of the tumor to radio- and chemotherapy, the prognosis is poor (WICK and ROSAI 1988). WICK et al. (1980) reported that after 5 years 30% of patients with carcinoids without hormone activity had died, while the figure for those in whom thymic carcinoids was accompanied by Cushing's disease or MEN was 65%.

References

Adolph JMG, Kimmig BN, Georgi P, zum Winkel K (1987) Carcinoid tumors: CT and I-131 meta-iodo-benzylguanidine scintigraphy. Radiology 164: 199

Brown LR, Aughenbaugh GL, Wick MR, Baker BA, Salassa RM (1982) Roentgenologic diagnosis of primary corticotropin-producing carcinoid tumors of the mediastinum. Radiology 142: 143

Cohen II, Templeton A, Philips AK (1988) Tumors of the thymus. Med Pediatr Oncol 16: 135

Cooper RB, van Way CW, Robinson WA (1979): Carcinoid tumor of the thymus. Rocky Mountain Medical J, 76: 238

Day DL, Gedgaudas E (1984) The thymus. Radiol Clin North Am 22: 519

Deneffe G, Moerman P (1986) Carcinoid tumour of the thymus: a case report. Acta Chir Belg 86: 72

Düx A (1977) Mediastinum. In: Teschendorf W, Anakker H, Thurn P (eds) Röntgenologische Differentialdiagnostik, Band I, 2. Thieme, Stuttgart, p 604

Eberle F, Martini GA, Scheuer A, Rohr G, Söhl R, Bischof W, Wahl R (1982) Thymuskarzinoid und multiple endokrine Neoplasie Typ I (MEN I). Internist 23: 718

Economopoulos GC, Lewis JW Jr, Lee MW, Silverman NA (1990) Carcinoid tumors of the thymus. Ann Thorac Surg 50: 58

Feldman JM, Blinder RA, Lucas KJ, Coleman RE (1986) Iodine-131 metaiodbenzylguanidine scintigraphy of carcinoid tumors. J Nucl Med 27: 1691

Frohman LA, Szabo M, Berelowitz M, Stachura ME (1980) Partial purification and characterization of a peptide with growth hormone-releasing activity from extrapituitary tumors in patients with acromegaly. J Clin Invest 65: 43

Gelfand ET, Basualdo CA, Callaghan JC (1981) Carcinoid tumor of the thymus associated with recurrent pericarditis. Chest 79: 350

Gold RE, Redman HC (1972) Mesenteric fibrosis simulating the angiographic appearance of ileal carcinoid tumor. Radiology 103: 85

Herbst WM, Kummer W, Hofmann W, Otto H, Heym C (1987) Carcinoid tumors of the thymus. An immunohistochemical study. Cancer 60: 2465

Hofmann WJ, Otto HF (1989a) Pathology of tumors of the thymic region. In: Martini N, Vogt-Moykopf I (eds) Thoracic surgery: frontiers and uncommon neoplasms. CT Mosby, St. Louis, pp 157–175

Hofmann WJ, Eberlein-Gonska M, Wiedenmann B, Otto HF (1989b) Histochemische und immunhistochemische Untersuchung von 8 Thymuscarcinoiden mit neuroendokrinen Zellmarkern. Eine Studie zur Evaluation unterschiedlicher diagnostischer Methoden an mediastinalen Carcinoiden. Verh Dtsch Ges Pathol 73: 517

Hosoda S, Suzuki H, Kito H et al. (1975) Argyrophilic thymic carcinoid – clinicopathologic study of four cases. Acta Pathol Jpn 25: 717

Huges JP, Ancalmo N, Leonard GL, Ochsner JL (1975) Carcinoid tumor of the thymus gland: report of a case. Thorax 30: 470

Isenberg DA, Linch D, Brenton DP, Smith JF (1981) A case of carcinoid tumour of the thymus in association with hyperparathyroidism. Clin Oncol 7: 61

Jose CC, Varghese CV, Singh AD (1988) Thymic carcinoid in a case of Zollinger Ellison syndrome. A case report. Australas Radiol 32: 408

Judge DM, Changaris DG, Harvey HR, Trapukdi S (1976) Malignant APUDoma (cardinoid) of the anterior mediastinum: simplified methods of demonstrating biogenic amines in endocrine neoplasms. Arch Pathol Lab Med 100: 491

Levine GD, Rosai J (1976) A spindle cell variant of thymic carcinoid tumor. Arch Pathol Lab Med 100: 293

Levine GD, Rosai J (1978) Thymic hyperplasia and neoplasia: a review of current concepts. Hum Pathol 9: 495

Lieske TR, Kincaid J, Sunderrajan EV (1985) Thymic carcinoid with cutaneous hyperpigmentation. Arch Intern Med 145: 361

MacDonald JS (1984) Carcinoid tumors. In: De Vita VT, Hellman S, Rosenberg SA (eds) Cancer. Lippincott, Philadelphia

Manes JL, Taylor HB (1973) Thymic carcinoid in familial multiple endocrine adenomatosis. Arch Pathol 95: 252

Marchevsky AM, Dikman SH (1979) Mediastinal carcinoid with an incomplete Sipple's syndrome. Cancer 43: 2497

Marino M, Müller-Hermelink HK (1985) Thymoma and thymic carcinoma. Virchows Arch [A] 407: 119

McCaughey ES, Walker V, Rolles CJ, Scheurmier NIM, Hale AC, Rees LH (1987) Ectopic ACTH production by a thymic carcinoid tumour. Eur J Pediatr 146: 590

Mey P, George P, Pein F, Cellier P, Minier JF (1988) Tumeur Carcinoide Thymique visualisée par I 131-MIBG. Ann Radiol 31: 181

Miettinen M (1987) Synaptophysin and neurofilament proteins as markers for neuroendocrine tumors. Arch Pathol Lab Med 111: 813

Miettinen M, Partanen S, Lehto VP, Virtanen I (1983) Mediastinal tumors: ultrastructural and immunohistochemical evaluation of intermediate filaments as diagnostic aids. Ultrastruct Pathol 4: 337

Nygaard T, Naidich P, Mendelsohn G, Hutcheon D (1979) Clinical conferences at the Johns Hopkins Hospital: "carcinoid tumor". Johns Hopkins Med J 145: 170

Otto HF (1984) Pathologie des Thymus. In: Doerr W, Seifert G (eds) Spezielle pathologische Anatomie, vol 17. Springer, Berlin Heidelberg New York

Otto HF (1985) Letters to the case. Pathol Res Pract 180: 448

Otto HF, Hüsselmann H (1976) Thymus Carcinoid. Fallbericht und Literaturübersicht. Z Krebsforsch 88: 55

Pearse AGE (1974) The APUD cell concept and its implications in pathology. Pathol Annu 9: 27

Preston Hughes J, Ancalmo N, Leonard GL, Ochsner JL (1975) Carcinoid tumour of the thymus gland: report of a case. Thorax 30: 470

Rosai J, Higa E (1972) Mediastinal endocrine neoplasm of probable thymic origin, related to carcinoid tumor. Cancer 29: 1061

Rosai J, Levine JD (1976) Tumors of the thymus. Atlas of tumour pathology, second series, fascicle 13. Armed Forces Institute of Pathology, Washington, DC

Rosai J, Higa E, Davie J (1972) Mediastinal endocrine neoplasm in patients with multiple endocrine adenomatosis. Cancer 29: 1075

Rosai J, Levine G, Weber WR, Higa E (1976) Carcinoid tumors and oat cell carcinomas of the thymus. Pathol Annu 11: 201

Rosenberg JC (1985) Neoplasms of the mediastinum. In: De Vita VT, Hellman S, Rosenberg SA (eds) Cancer. Principles and practice of oncology, 2nd edn. Lippincott, Philadelphia

Salyer WR, Salyer DC, Eggleston JC (1976) Carcinoid tumors of the thymus. Cancer 37: 958

Seigel RS, Kuhns LR, Borlaza GS, McCormick TL, Simmons JL (1980) Computed tomography and angiography in ileal carcinoid tumor and retractile mesenteritis. Radiology 134: 437

Strasberg B, Weinberger I, Kessler E, Agmon J (1979) Thymic carcinoid tumor. NY State J Med 79: 1755

Thomas BM (1968) Three unusual carcinoid tumours, with particular reference to osteoblastic bone metastases. Clin Radiol 19: 221

Weiss C, Dinkel E, Wimmer B, Schildge J, Grosser G (1987) Der Thymus im Computertomogramm. Normalbefunde und Pathologie. Radiologe 27: 414

Wick MR, Rosai J (1988) Neuroendocrine neoplasms of the thymus. Pathol Res Pract 183: 188

Wick MR, Scheithauer BW (1984) Thymic carcinoid. A histologic, immunohistochemical, and ultrastructural study of 12 cases. Cancer 53: 475

Wick MR, Scott RE, Li C-Y, Carney JA (1980) Carcinoid tumor of the thymus. A clinicopathologic report of seven cases with a review of the literature. Mayo Clin Proc 55: 246

Wick MR, Bernatz PE, Carney JA, Brown LR (1982) Primary mediastinal carcinoid tumors. Am J Surg Pathol 6: 195

Wilander E, Lundqvist M, El-Salhy M (1985) Serotonin in fore-gut carcinoids: a survey of 60 cases with regard to silver stains, formalin-induced fluorescence and serotonin immunocytochemistry. J Pathol 145: 251

Woeckel W, Hofmann WJ, Rolle A, Thetter O, Schmoelder A, Schopohl J, Suren H (1990) Morphologie und Klinik des Thymuskarzinoids. Dtsch Med Wochenschr 115: 412

8.4 Thymic Involvement in Malignant Lymphomas and Leukemia

E. WILLICH and E. WALTER

The mediastinum is a site of predilection for malignant lymphomas. Three types of malignant lymphoma are found in the thymus:
1. Hodgkin's disease
2. Non-Hodgkin's lymphoma of the T lymphoblastic type, including mediastinal lymphomas in the context of acute lymphatic leukemia
3. Non-Hodgkin's lymphoma of the B cell type (primary mediastinal clear cell lymphoma)

These different types can originate from the thymus, or the organ can be involved during the course of the basic disease.

8.4.1 Pathologic Features

W. J. HOFMANN and H. F. OTTO

Malignant lymphomas are the most common malignant tumors of the anterior (anterosuperior) mediastinum (LICHTENSTEIN et al. 1980). They can affect the regional (mediastinal) lymph nodes and/or the thymus.

Hodgkin's disease is predominant, since approximately 50%–60% of all mediastinal lymphomas are of the Hodgkin's type. Practically all cases of Hodgkin's disease located in the thymus region are of the nodular sclerosing type (Fig. 8.33). This

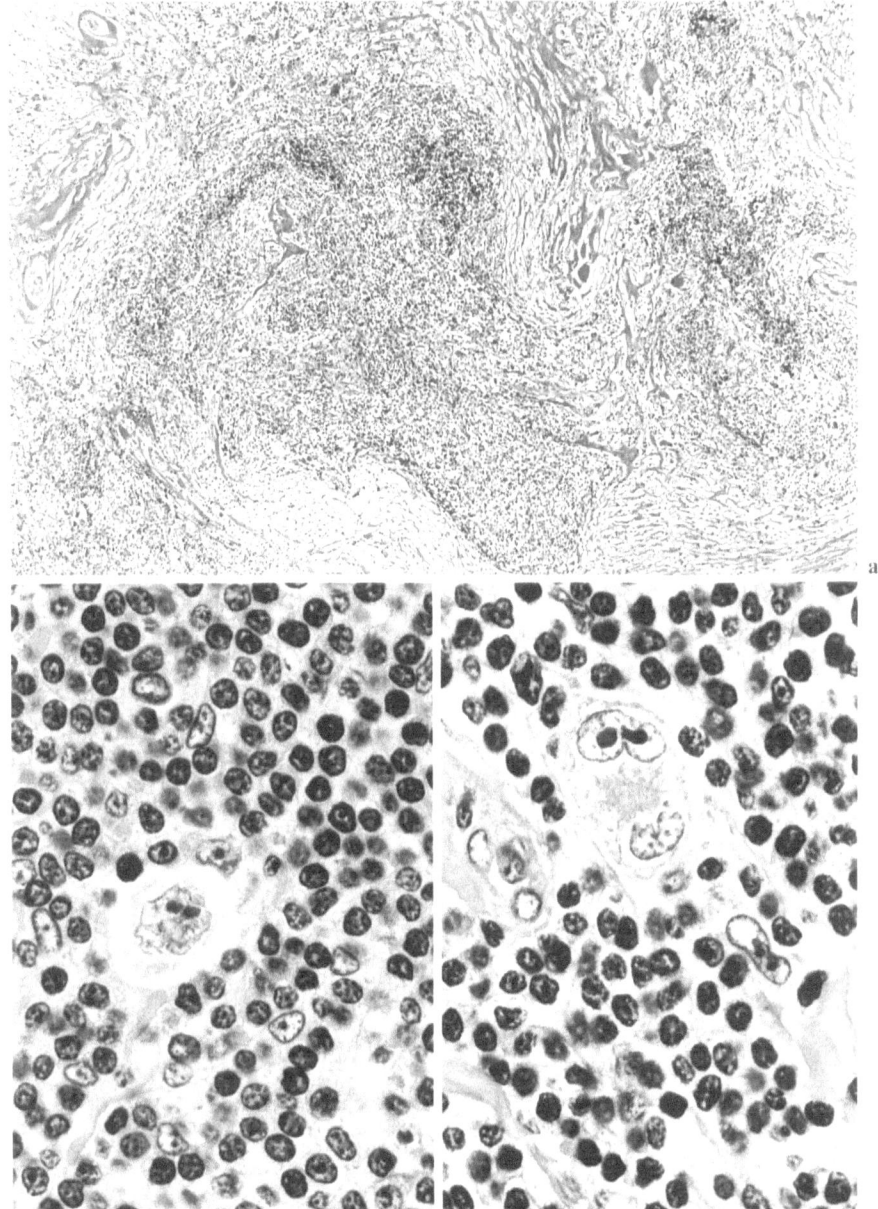

Fig. 8.33 a–c. Hodgkin's disease, nodular sclerosing type. **a** In an overview tumor nodules are visible, surrounded by dense fibrous tissue giving the typical appearance of the nodular sclerosing type. H&E, ×52. **b** Higher magnification showing a typical lacunar cell (i.e., a Hodgkin's cell with artificial shrinkage) surrounded by numerous lymphocytes and a few dendritic cells. H&E, ×637. **c** A Reed-Sternberg cell with a double nucleus and a broad cytoplasm is shown. H&E, ×637

tumor was formerly known as granulomatous thymoma ["thymoma of granulomatous type" (EWING 1916)].

The other 40%–50% cover one of the many histologic variants of non-Hodgkin's lymphomas (LENNERT 1978). In practice, two groups of mediastinal non-Hodgkin's lymphomas are very important (OTTO 1991):

1. *Malignant T lymphoblastic lymphoma of convoluted-cell type.* Most mediastinal non-Hodgkin's lymphomas in children are of this type (NATHWANI et al. 1976), which usually presents radiographically as a lobulated mediastinal mass. Frequently, patients with malignant T lymphoblastic lymphoma develop acute lymphoblastic leukemias. This syndromatic constellation was first described by STERNBERG in 1916 (*"Leukosarkomatose"* and "Myeloblastenleukämie"). This lymphoma is probably a primary thymic lymphoma ["Sternberg's lymphoma of the thymus" (LUKES and COLLINS 1974; BARCOS and LUKES 1975)].

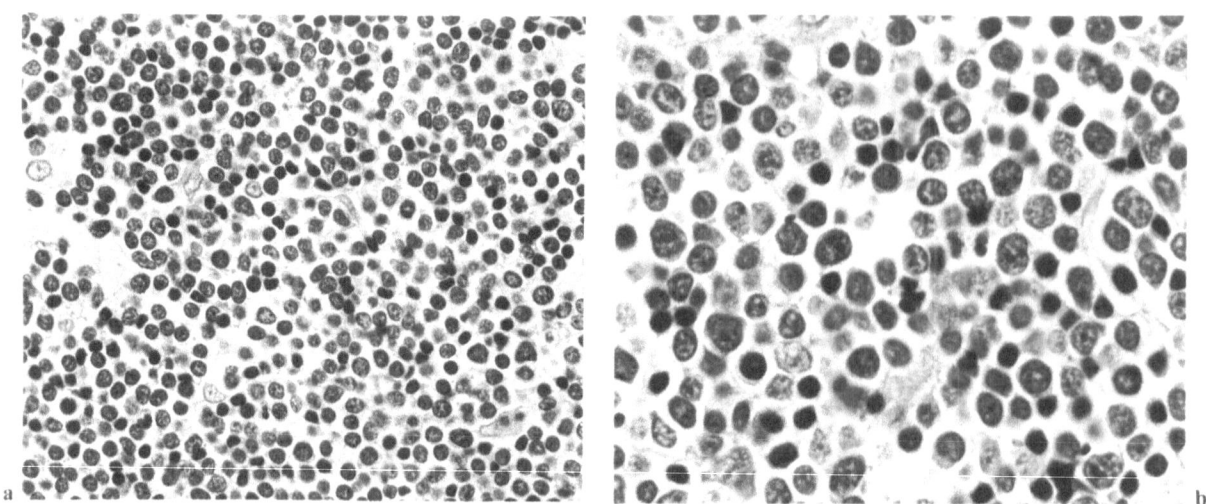

Δ

Fig. 8.34 a, b. Malignant non-Hodgkin's lymphoma, T lymphoblastic type. **a** Relatively small noncohesive tumor cells and some histiocytes. H&E, ×398. **b** Higher magnification showing pleomorphism of the tumor cells, some of which are convoluted. Mitoses and pyknotic tumor cells are visible. H&E, ×637

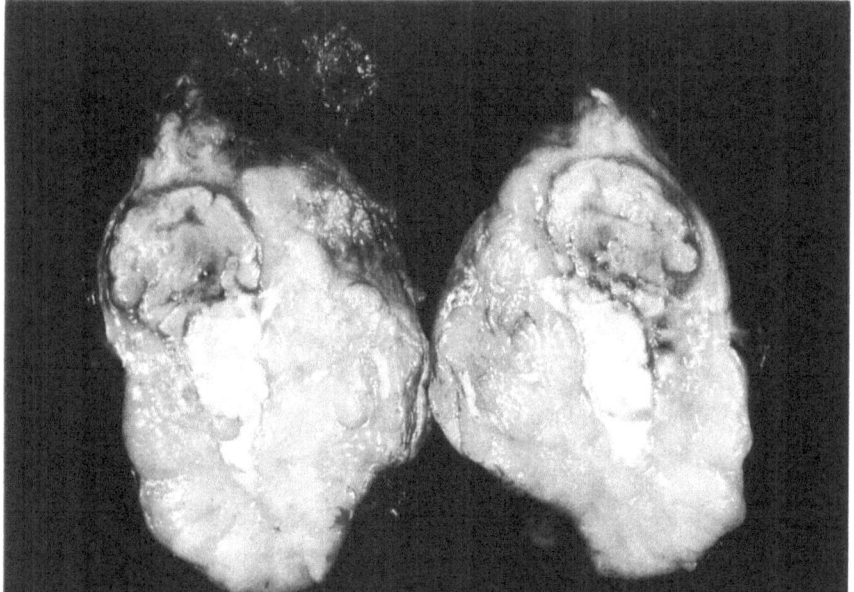

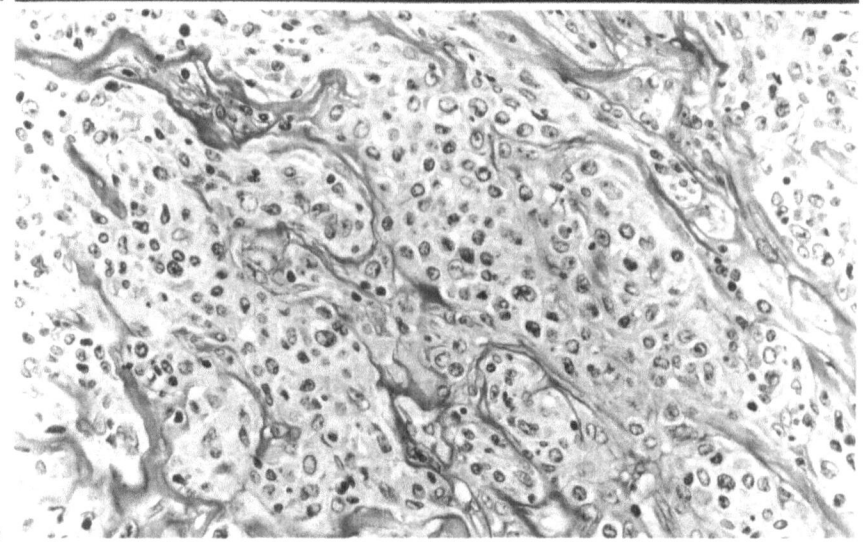

Fig. 8.35 a, b. Mediastinal clear cell lymphoma of B cell type. **a** Tumor macroscopy. The cut surface of the tumor is soft, grayish-yellow, and shows centrally located necrosis. **b** The pleomorphic tumor cells posses a broad, clear cytoplasm, show distinct cellular outlines, and are surrounded by marked fibrosis, a typical feature of some of those tumors. PAS, ×267

2. *Primary mediastinal clear cell lymphoma of B cell type.* The primary mediastinal nonlymphoblastic non-Hodgkin's lymphoma has recently been recognized as a distinct clinicopathologic entity (MENESTRINA et al. 1986; MÖLLER et al. 1986; PERRONE et al. 1986; JACOBSON et al. 1988; LAMARRE et al. 1989, DAVIS et al. 1990; ISAACSON et al. 1990). Its B cell nature was first demonstrated by MÖLLER et al. (1986). Different names have been used to describe this tumor, e.g., "mediastinal diffuse large cell lymphoma with sclerosis" (PERRONE et al. 1986) and "primary large cell lymphoma of the mediastinum" (LAMARRE et al. 1989). We, however, prefer the operational term "primary mediastinal clear cell lymphoma of B cell type" (MCCL) (MÖLLER et al. 1987; MÖLLER et al. 1989a) since it covers best the peculiar cell morphology and the immunophenotype of those tumors in which sclerosis is not an obligatory component.

The MCCLs are always situated in the thymic region of the mediastinum as a bulky mass, covered by the thymic capsule or infiltrating into the surrounding tissue and organs (Fig. 8.34). Thus, the presenting symptoms of the tumors are local ones due to the irritation of the mediastinal structures (i.e., chest pain, superior vena cava syndrome, pleural and pericardial effusions).

The tumors typically occur in young adults with a female predominance. The youngest patient we observed was a 12-year-old girl.

Histologically the tumors show a diffuse growth pattern. The cells have clear and abundant cytoplasm in common, while they vary considerably in size (Fig. 8.35) (for detailed description see MÖLLER et al. 1986a,b).

Although most of the tumors are immunoglobulin-negative, they can be classified as B cell lymphomas by the use of monoclonal antibodies against B cell differentiation antigens (MÖLLER et al. 1986; MOMBURG et al. 1987; LAMARRE et al. 1989; MÖLLER et al. 1989a,b). This can even be done on formalin-fixed and paraffin-embedded tissue using the monoclonal antibody DAKO-L26 (MÖLLER et al. 1989b).

On the basis of a small number of cases, in part initially misdiagnosed, it was thought that MCCLs carry a bad prognosis (MÖLLER et al. 1986). More recent studies, however, have revealed a 5-year survival rate of about 70% for MCCL if it is a priori diagnosed as such and if aggressive polychemotherapy protocols designed for high grade malignant, non-Burkitt non-Hodgkin's lymphoma are applied (JACOBSON et al. 1988).

There are some lines of evidence that MCCL is a tumor of thymic origin. A prerequisite for this assumption has been found in the normally occurring B cells within the thymus medulla (HOFMANN et al. 1988a,b). The location of the tumor and the involvement of the thymus also speak in favor of this assumption (MÖLLER et al. 1989b).

8.4.2 Hodgkin's Disease

E. WILLICH and E. WALTER

8.4.2.1 Occurrence

Hodgkin's disease is the most frequent malignant lymphoma in older children and adults. THOMSON (1955) was the first to suggest the Hodgkin's disease can originate from the thymus, since all the cell elements of the thymus are found to a variable extent in Hodgkin's disease. This hypothesis was confirmed subsequently by, among others, KATZ and LATTES (1969), KELLER and CASTLEMAN (1974), and KEEN and LIBSHITZ (1987); LESLIE et al. (1986) reported exclusive localization of Hodgkin's disease in the thymus. Macroscopically the tumors are usually hard and bulbous, and histologically they are almost exclusively of the nodular sclerosing type (KELLER and CASTLEMAN 1974; BERARD and DORFMAN 1974; KIM et al. 1985; and others). It is reported that primary Hodgkin's disease of the thymus is more common in young men than in women (FEDERLE and CALLEN 1979).

A more frequent occurrence than primary Hodgkin's disease of the thymus is involvement of the organ within the context of the basic illness. Involvement of the thymus is to be expected in 26%–30% of patients having Hodgkin's disease with a primary origin in a lymph node (MARSHAL and WOOD 1957; HERON et al. 1988), the figure even reaching 39% in the presence of recurrences (HERON et al. 1988).

The relative infrequency of this disease in children is documented by data from the Mayo Clinic showing that a Hodgkin's lymphoma was present in only 22 of 188 children with mediastinal tumors. In ten cases the lymphoma was restricted to the thymus alone (KING et al. 1982).

Finally it should be noted that Hodgkin's disease of the thymus can also occur in the form of a secondary tumor following treatment of a malignant testicular tumor (TARTAS et al. 1985; LESLIE et al. 1986).

8.4.2.2 Clinical Symptoms

Clinically retrosternal pain is the chief symptom, others being dyspnea, coughing, recurrent infections of the respiratory tract, weight loss, and fever (KELLER and CASTLEMAN 1974; FEDERLE and CALLEN 1979; KIM et al. 1985). A possible cause of this symptomatology is compression and/or displacement of the tracheobronchial system by the tumor; uni- or bilateral pleural effusions must also be expected.

In 75% of *children* symptoms of a different type are found, with a predominance of dyspnea, lassitude, fever, infections, etc. (CAPITANIO et al. 1984). The responsibility for the difference lies with the smaller thoracic volume in children, the higher rate of tumor malignancy, and the narrower tracheal lumen (as a consequence of which symptoms arise in children when luminal occlusion reaches 33%, whereas they do not occur in adults until occlusion of 50% is present) (MANDELL et al. 1982).

Malignant lymphoma of the thymus is rarely accompanied by other illnesses. In the case of Hodgkin's disease of the thymus only NULL et al. (1977) have described accompanying myasthenia gravis, and this disappeared completely following resection of the thymus. A coincidental concurrent appearance of the two illnesses would seem possible, but the authors believed a direct connection existed between them. In one patient with Hodgkin's disease of the thymus, WATSON et al. (1968) observed a Cushing-like symptomatology, which regressed totally after radiotherapy.

8.4.2.3 Diagnosis with Imaging Procedures

8.4.2.3.1 Conventional Radiology

In patients with malignant lymphoma of the thymus, plain chest radiographs in two planes generally reveal a usually unilateral enlargement of the mediastinal shadow on account of the position of the tumor in the anterior superior mediastinum (Fig. 8.36). However, in correspondence with the descent of the thymus, the infiltrated organ can also be situated paracardially (KAESBERG et al. 1988). Small tumors are not detected by plain chest radiography in two planes; in the cases reported by AMOUR et al. (1987) the involved organ was hidden within the mediastinal shadow.

No pathognomonic findings have been reported in the literature that permit differentiation from tumors of other histologic type (KIM et al. 1985).

Pleural effusions, be they uni- or bilateral, are a frequent occurrence and can be easily recognized on plain chest radiographs.

Conventional tomography does not permit the tumor to be distinguished from other mediastinal structures. Again, differentiation from lesions of another histologic type is not possible by means of conventional tomography, especially since calcifications are not to be expected within the tumor. Tumor-related displacement and compression of the trachea can, however, be documented by conventional tomography (LEMAITRE et al. 1987).

GÖTHLIN et al. (1977) reported on *angiographic findings*. They found vascular stenoses to be more frequent in Hodgkin's disease of the thymus than in thymomas.

8.4.2.3.2 Ultrasonography

Ultrasonographic findings in cases of malignant lymphoma and leukemia have been reported upon by LEMAITRE et al. (1987) and VON LENGERKE and SCHMIDT (1988). Employing a suprasternal approach and a 5-MHz transducer the enlarged thymus was well depicted – a finding that holds true in cases of Hodgkin's disease as well. Heterogeneous changes were observed in parts of the organ or diffusely: a mixed hyper- and hypoechoic pattern was seen relatively frequently, and a hypoechoic pattern less often. With forced respiration the contours of the enlarged thymus remain rigid; the pulmonary artery is displaced dorsally, and the ventral curved contour shows either a loss of roundness or a "truss pad" shape. This is displayed more clearly on parasternal than on transverse sections (Figs. 8.43, 8.44, p. 168).

Radiographically demonstrable displacement and compression of the trachea could also always be recognized on ultrasonograms. Tumor fixation and compression of great vessels were taken to be indicative of infiltration of neighboring organs. Additional retrosternal, para-aortic, and paratracheal lymphomas could be clearly differentiated form infiltrated thymus. The liver and spleen serve as comparative parameters when assessing the echogenicity of the thymus. Concomitant pleural or pericardial effusions can be visualized simultaneously. The reported findings cannot, however, be considered pathognomonic (LEMAITRE et al. 1987; VON LENGERKE and SCHMIDT 1988).

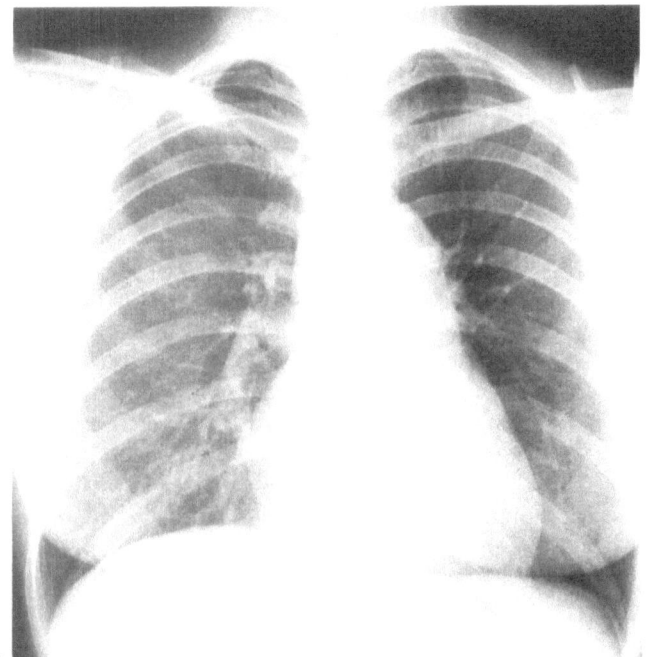

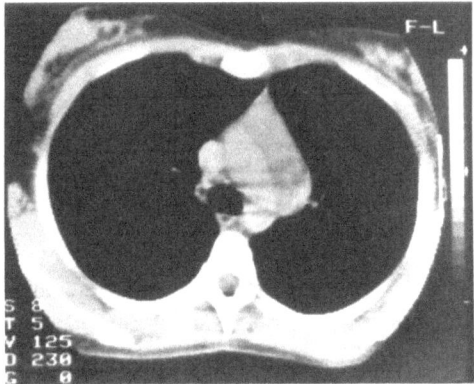

Fig. 8.36 a, b. Hodgkin's disease originating from the thymus in a 26-year-old female. Histology: nodular sclerosing type. **a** Plain posteroanterior chest radiograph: mediastinal mass, recognizable by virtue of widening and deformity of the aortopulmonary window. **b** CT scan at the aortic arch level: a dense homogeneous mass is situated para-aortally and corresponds to Hodgkin's disease originating from the thymus

8.4.2.3.3 Computed Tomography

Computed tomography of primary Hodgkin's disease of the thymus was first reported by FEDERLE and CALLEN (1979), WALTER and HÜBENER (1980), and BARON et al. (1982). According to the observations of WALTER and HÜBENER (1980) and BARON et al. (1982), so-called granulomatous thymoma (LOWENHAUPT and BROWN 1951) can be recognized as a mass of homogeneous density occupying a typical position between the sternum and the ascending thoracic aorta or the aortic arch (Fig. 8.36 b). The thymus may show diffuse enlargement with retention of its characteristic configuration (HERON et al. 1988); however, it may also appear as a tumor having a spherical shape and smooth margins (WALTER 1982; LESLIE et al. 1986) or alternatively a polycyclic border (FEDERLE and CALLEN 1979; AMOUR et al. 1987). The CT appearance then corresponds to that of a thymoma (SCHNYDER and CANDARDJIS 1987).

In our experience the attenuation values of the tumor lie between + 35 and + 55 HU, a range that is also observed in cases of Hodgkin's disease originating from lymph nodes. These values additionally correspond to those of normal thymus, of thymoma, and of chest wall musculature (WALTER and HÜBENER 1980) – although it should be pointed out that BARON et al. (1982) gave somewhat higher values for the chest wall musculature, and HERON et al. (1988) somewhat lower values. In most cases

the tumor is of homogeneous density, although inhomogeneity is also sometimes observed (AMOUR et al. 1987). After bolus injection of contrast medium, attenuation values of solid tumors increase to as high as + 108 HU, thereby somewhat exceeding those of thymoma (WEISS et al. 1987). Polycystic degeneration is a frequent occurrence in untreated lymphomas of the thymus, and has been reported whithin the radiologic literature by FEDERLE and CALLEN (1979), SCHNYDER and CANDARDJIS (1987), and NOGUES et al. (1987). Such degeneration is not, however, a regular finding (WALTER 1982), perhaps occurring in a third of cases in which cysts are present (SCHNYDER and CANDARDJIS 1987).

In general, infiltration of neighboring organs can be demonstrated reliably by means of CT. Only the region of the cranial and caudal circumference of the tumor is difficult to assess using CT, since here the tumor runs parallel to the plane of CT scan.

Of 11 patients with Hodgkin's disease reported by FRANCIS et al. (1985), eight showed a tumor in the anterior mediastinum that was larger than 12 mm, in six cases leading to a focal alteration in the mediastinal contour. In every cases CT measurement of the thickness of the thymus yielded pathologic values in comparison to a normal control group comprising 82 patients.

In *children* CT reveals inhomogeneous density, areas of reduced density, and, in more than 50 % of those with Hodgkin's disease of recent onset, tracheobronchial compression; the extent of such compression could be measured precisely (KIRKS and KOROBKIN 1980). Important diagnostic features revealed by CT are the extension of the tumor to the anterior chest wall and respiratory tract compression, which can be recognized radiographically by means of either body section radiography of the high-kV technique. The possibility of simultaneous CT of the abdomen, which permits determination of the size of the spleen and assessment of periaortic lymph nodes, is also of importance.

8.4.2.3.4 Magnetic Resonance Imaging

W. R. WEBB and G. DE GEER

Patients with Hodgkin's disease studied using MRI commonly show anterior superior mediastinal involvement, probably affecting the thymus. In 14 of 18 patients in one study employing MRI (NYMAN et al. 1989), the main part of the lymphoma was located in this region (Fig. 8.37).

In patients with lymphoma or leukemia involving the thymus MRI shows a generalized increase in the size of the thymus or, more commonly, a lo-

bulated thymic mass (Figs. 8.38, 8.39) (NYMAN et al. 1989). The overall signal intensity of the enlarged thymus is similar to that of normal thymus, but there may be a minimal relative increase in intensity on T2-weighted images. Also, a heterogeneous appearance is very common, with areas of low and high signal intensity on SE 1500/70 images. In one study (SIEGEL et al. 1989), two of seven patients with lymphoma involving the thymus had a homogeneous appearing thymus, while in the remaining five, areas of increased or decreased intensity were visible on T2-weighted images. The low intensity areas may represent fibrosis, while the high intensity areas could reflect hemorrhage or cystic degeneration. In one reported patient (SIEGEL et al. 1989), only a low intensity mass was visible. Although the MRI characteristics of lymphoma are not characteristic, the combination of a thymic mass with mass or lymph node enlargement in

Fig. 8.37a–d. Hodgkin's lymphoma. **a** T1-weighted transaxial image shows a large thymic mass, associated with right hilar and subcarinal mediastinal adenopathy. **b** With T2 weighting the masses appear inhomogeneous, a finding which is common with lymphomas. **c** T1-weighted coronal image shows the large anterior mediastinal mass, associated with a large pericardial effusion. **d** After radiation, on a T2-weighted image at the same level as **c**, the thymic mass *(arrow)* is significantly reduced in size, as are the hilar nodes

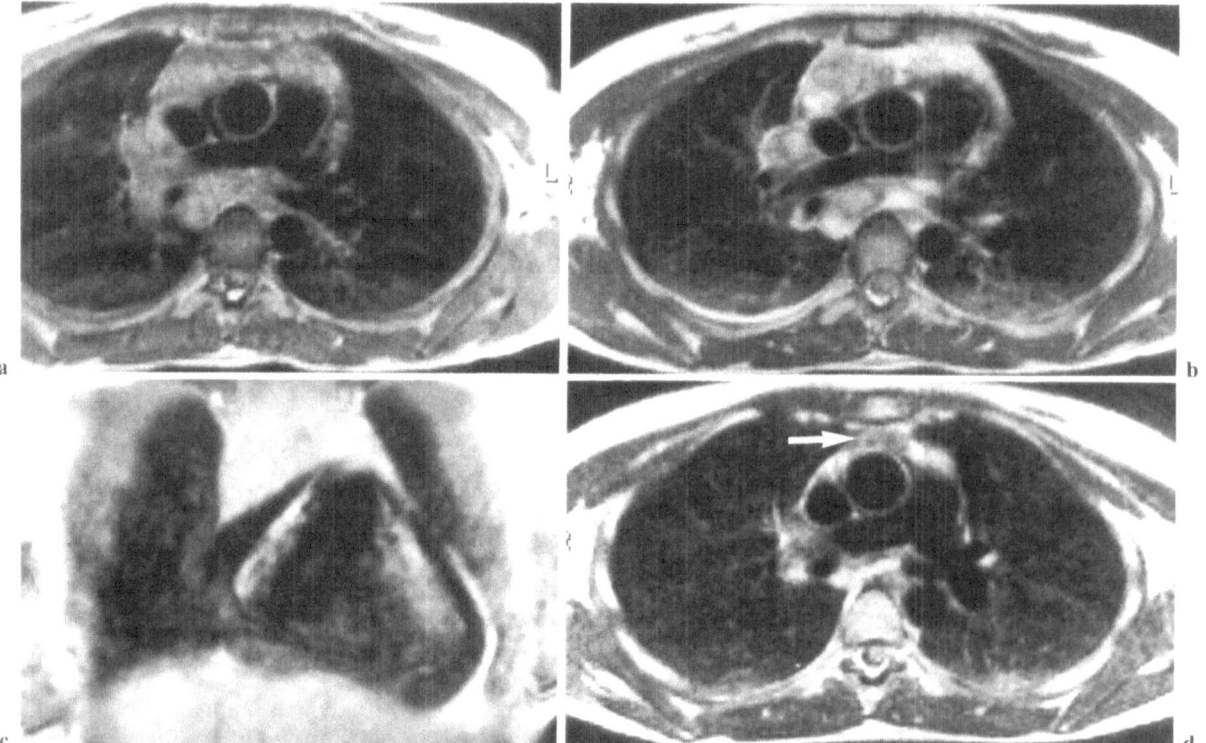

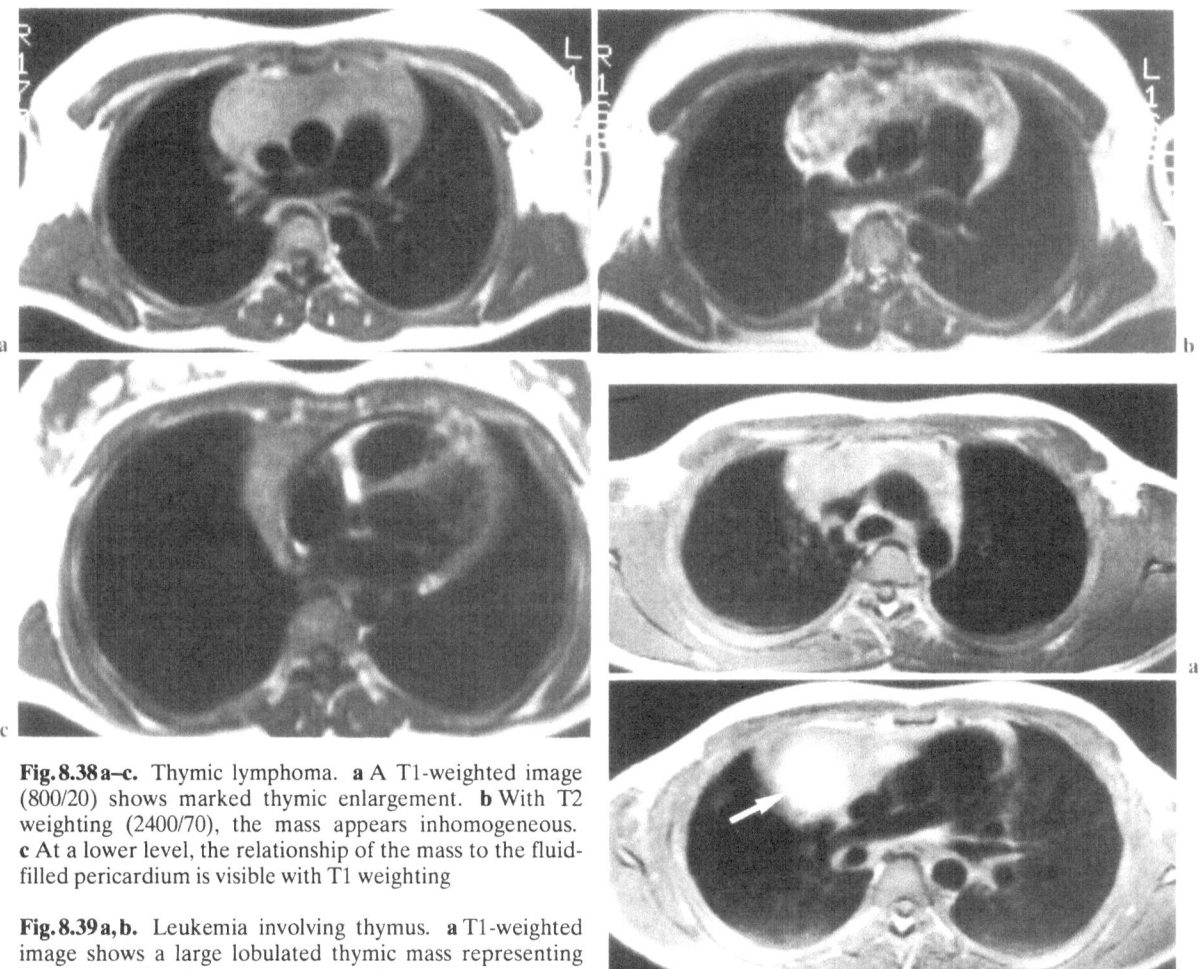

Fig. 8.38 a–c. Thymic lymphoma. **a** A T1-weighted image (800/20) shows marked thymic enlargement. **b** With T2 weighting (2400/70), the mass appears inhomogeneous. **c** At a lower level, the relationship of the mass to the fluid-filled pericardium is visible with T1 weighting

Fig. 8.39 a, b. Leukemia involving thymus. **a** T1-weighted image shows a large lobulated thymic mass representing leukemic infiltration of the thymus. **b** At a lower level, a large intense focus *(arrow)* probably represents hemorrhage

8.39

other areas of the mediastinum is very suggestive of the diagnosis.

In patients who have had radiation for lymphoma, residual mediastinal masses can make the diagnosis of residual or recurrent tumor difficult (NORTH et al. 1987; NYMAN et al. 1989). These residual masses are relatively common, and depending on the criteria used for diagnosis, are seen on chest radiographs in 12%–88% of patients following therapy (NORTH et al. 1987; WEBB 1989). Although it is generally acknowledged that most of these masses are benign and of no consequence, in one study the frequency of intrathoracic relapse was more than twice as great in patients who had residual masses after treatment (NORTH et al. 1987). Residual masses were visible in 14 of 18 patients with Hodgkin's disease studied by NYMAN et al. (1989) using MRI, and all of the masses were anterior mediastinal. The residual mass, as measured on MRI, ranged from 9% to

69% of the size (in pixels) of the pretreatment mass.

NYMAN and co-workers (1989) have shown that MRI may play a significant role in the follow-up of treated patients with mediastinal Hodgkin's disease, helping to determine that residual masses are benign. After treatment, the T2-weighted intensity of residual mediastinal masses significantly decreased in most patients (probably reflecting the residual fibrous mass). The average mass/fat intensity ratio on the T2-weighted sequence in NYMAN et al.'s study was approximately 0.8 prior to treatment, and slightly less than 0.4 after treatment. Thus, a high relative intensity with T2 weighting, although not specific for persistent or recurrent tumor, might indicate the need for biopsy or close follow-up of a residual mediastinal mass (WEBB 1989). A change in intensity from low to high during follow-up should be regarded as very significant.

8.4.2.3.5 Nuclear Medicine

E. Walter and E. Willich

No specific reports are available in respect of Hodgkin's disease of the thymus.

8.4.2.4 Hodgkin's Disease of the Thymus Before and After Radiotherapy and Chemotherapy

E. Walter and E. Willich

In rare cases, a multilobular cystic mass in the anterior mediastinum is observed within the context of Hodgkin's disease *prior to* irradiation. Such a mass is usually confused with a thymic cyst or a cystic teratoma and is first diagnosed histologically (Nogues et al. 1987; Keller et al. 1974; Eiser and Samarrai 1975).

A thymus infiltrated by Hodgkin's disease does tend toward spontaneous cystic degeneration, but this usually occurs *after* radio- or chemotherapy (Baron et al. 1981, 1982; Kim et al. 1985; among others). This means that the mediastinal mass will not regularly show a reduction in size during the course of radio- or chemotherapy; rather, its size, as observed on radiographs, tends to remain constant or even increase owing to the cystic degeneration. The development of cysts following radiotherapy can also simulate tumor recurrence. Thus Baron et al. (1981), Lindfors et al. (1985), and Heron et al. (1988) report patients with isolated Hodgkin's disease of the thymus, always of the nodular sclerosing type histologically, in whom thymogenic cysts that appeared 3–12 months after the conclusion of successful radiotherapy were at first mistakenly diagnosed as tumor recurrences on conventional radiographs. The cysts, which can be identified by CT (but also ultrasonographically), can contain up to 60 ml of fluid (Kim et al. 1985) and may be multilocular or unilocular (Murray and Parker 1984).

Like Katz et al. (1977), Lindfors et al. (1985) surmised that the cysts are a consequence of radiotherapy, possibly resulting from the degenerative changes it causes. Both Katz et al. (1977) and Lindfors et al. (1985) also point to the possibility that radiotherapy stimulates secretion by the endothelium of preexisting smaller cysts.

Cysts are easily recognized on CT sections. Their absorption behavior essentially corresponds to that of dysontogenetic thymogenic cysts, although the latter usually display a thinner cyst wall.

In addition it should be noted that enlargement of the thymus may also occur following chemotherapy as a consequence of reactive hyperplasia [in general the enlargement occurs after 4–12 months (Shin and Ho 1983; Heron et al. 1988)].

After the treatment of Hodgkin's disease enlargements of the thymus occasionally ensue that render difficult the differentiation between a recurrence of the primary disease, a mediastinal metastasis, residual mediastinal disease following irradiation, and regenerative thymic hyperplasia. Ford et al. (1987) drew attention to the occurrence of a rebound phenomenon during or after treatment. These authors recommended that a steroid test be employed first in order to avoid unnecessary invasive diagnostic measures.

8.4.3 Non-Hodgkin's Lymphoma

Non-Hodgkin's lymphoma is a highly malignant tumor that originates from lymphatic tissue, with early leukemic transformation, i.e., with involvement of the bone marrow and central nervous system. The tumor may originate from the thymus or may metastasize to or infiltrate it. Especially during childhood there are fluid transitions to acute lymphatic leukemia. Confirmation of the diagnosis is procured through lymph node biopsy.

The *clinical symptoms* resemble those of Hodgkin's disease. Dysphagia and a blockage of the upper vene cava may also be present. Testicular involvement may occur at an early stage.

In adults, *diagnostic imaging procedures* yield appearances that are scarcely distinguishable from Hodgkin's disease (Fig. 8.40). In children the mass in the anterior mediastinum is larger, the younger they are. In most cases the middle mediastinum is also involved, and lymphadenopathy is found in 37% of patients (in Hodgkin's disease the figure is 61%) (Kirks and Korobkin 1981) (Figs. 8.41, 8.42). Pleural effusion is more frequent and often contributes to the massive enlargement of the middle mediastinal shadow (Fig. 8.41 c). The radiographic appearance can be regarded as pathognomonic.

Ultrasonography (Figs. 8.43, 8.44) yields the same findings as in Hodgkin's disease (see Sect. 8.4.2.3) In children, *computed tomography* best depicts the mediastinal lymph nodes, tumors, the infiltrated thymus, and effusions; in addition, enlarged retroperitoneal lymph nodes are visualized in cases of leukemia, and abdominal metastases in non-Hodg-

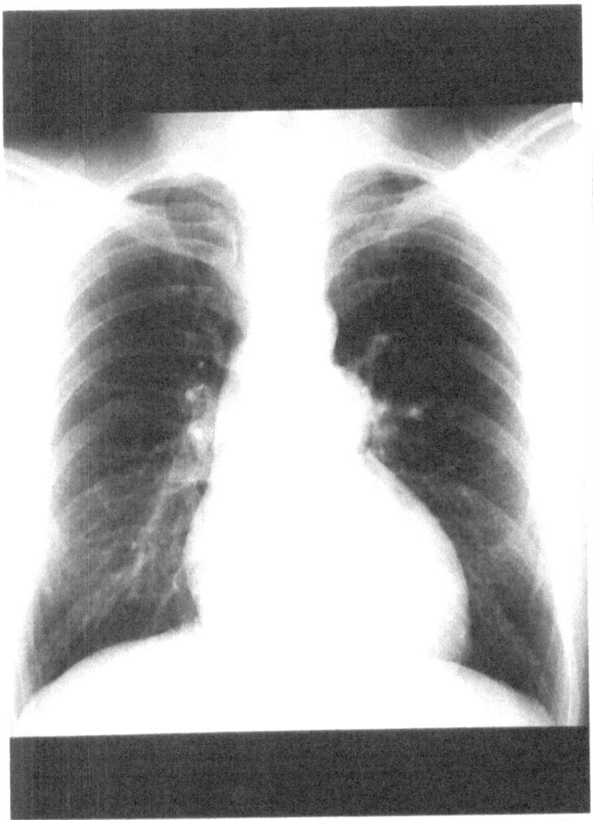

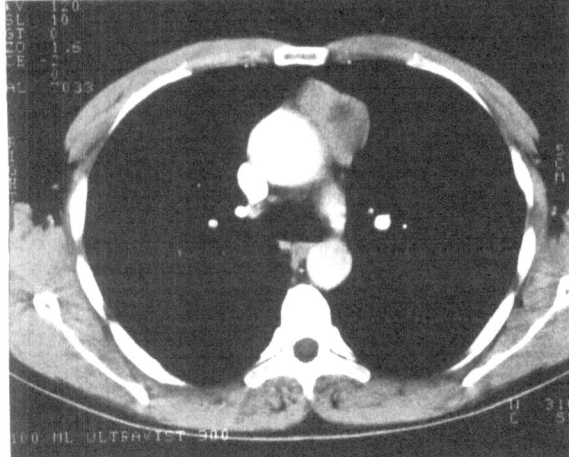

Fig. 8.40 a–c. B cell lymphoma that originated in the thymus of a 36-year-old man. **a** Plain chest radiograph: small enlargement of the mediastinum in the right hilar region; a bulging lymph node is present on the left at the same level. **b** Lateral view: the mass is localized in the anterior mediastinum above the heart. **c** CT scan: mass situated ventral to the ascending aorta, corresponding to B cell lymphoma as confirmed by operation. Central cavity: necrotic liquefaction

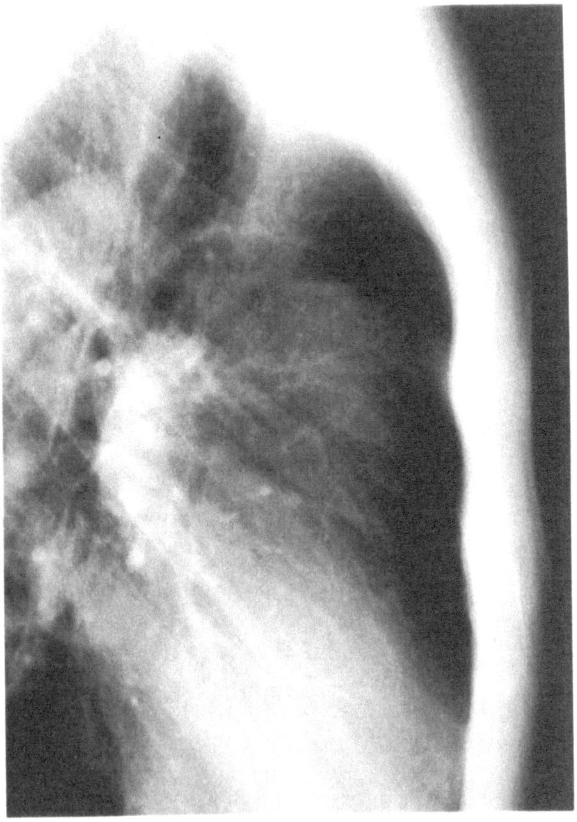

kin's lymphoma (Fig. 8.42 e). In adults, non-Hodgkin's lymphoma of the thymus resembles Hodgkin's disease (see above) in presenting as a mass that may have either clearly defined or indistinct borders depending upon its infiltration of the region. The attenuation values correspond to those of Hodgkin's disease of the thymus. Necrotic liquefaction is possible in cases of B cell lymphoma with a primary origin in the thymus (Fig. 8.40 c).

8.4.4 Leukemia

Infiltration of the thymus has to be reckoned with in cases of leukemia. In mice, involvement and infiltration of the thymus are almost always seen; indeed, frequently the thymus is the only organ to be affected (McEndy et al. 1944), and this is reflected macroscopically in corresponding thymic enlargement. However, in man leukemic infiltrates are a

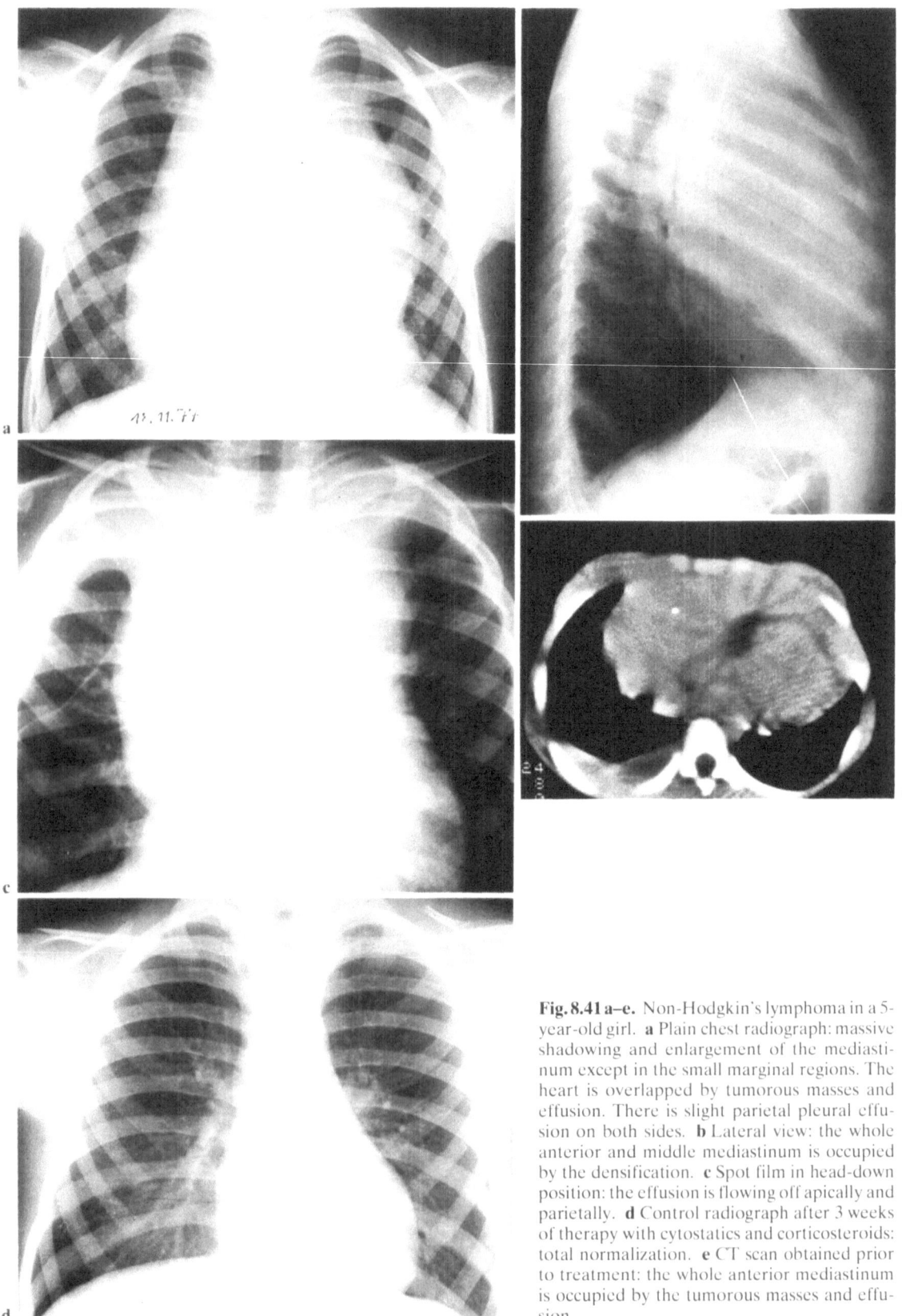

Fig. 8.41 a–e. Non-Hodgkin's lymphoma in a 5-year-old girl. **a** Plain chest radiograph: massive shadowing and enlargement of the mediastinum except in the small marginal regions. The heart is overlapped by tumorous masses and effusion. There is slight parietal pleural effusion on both sides. **b** Lateral view: the whole anterior and middle mediastinum is occupied by the densification. **c** Spot film in head-down position: the effusion is flowing off apically and parietally. **d** Control radiograph after 3 weeks of therapy with cytostatics and corticosteroids: total normalization. **e** CT scan obtained prior to treatment: the whole anterior mediastinum is occupied by the tumorous masses and effusion

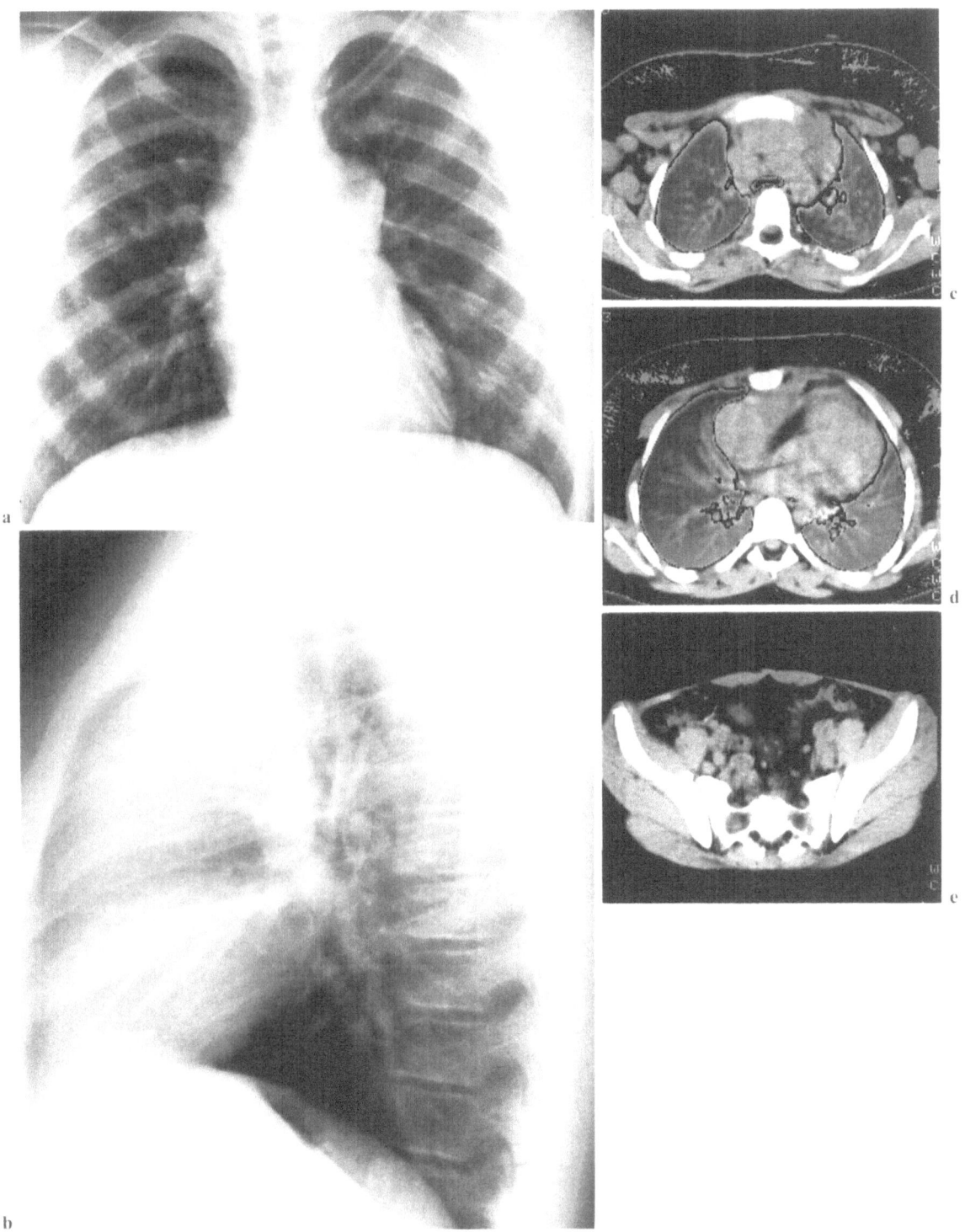

Fig. 8.42 a–e. Non-Hodgkin's lymphoma in a 13-year-old boy. **a** Plain chest radiograph: polycyclic bulging on the left, para-aortally, and in the right hilum up to 2 cm above the bifurcation. Multiple enlarged lymph nodes. **b** Lateral view: homogeneous, delimited density of the thymic region. **c,d** CT: the whole anterior mediastinum is occupied by tumorous masses. **e** Abdominal scan at the level of the pelvis: multiple lymphadenopathies (Courtesy of Prof. Dr. K. D. EBEL, Dept. of Pediatric Radiology, Children's Municipal Hospital, Cologne-Riehl, FRG)

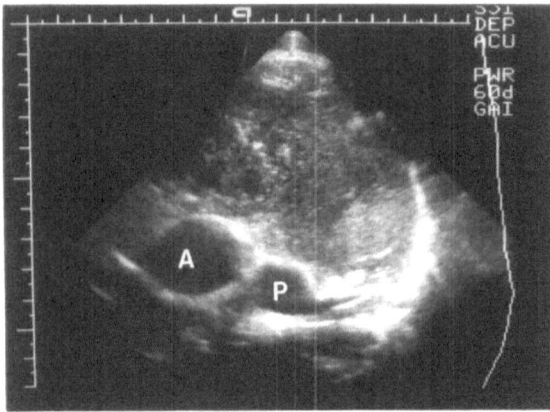

8.43

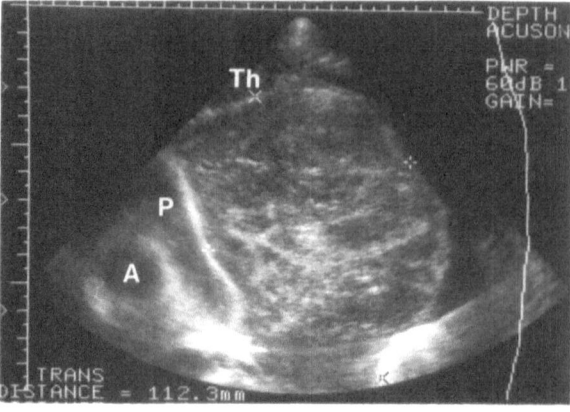

8.44

Fig. 8.43. Ultrasonogram of Non-Hodgkin's lymphoma in a 5-year-old girl. Transverse scan. Complex change of the thymic structure. The aorta *(A)* and pulmonary artery *(P)* are dislocated posteriorly. (Courtesy of Prof. Dr. H. J. von Lengerke, Münster i. W., FRG)

Fig. 8.44. Non-Hodgkin's lymphoma in a 14-year-old boy. Ultrasonogram in left parasternal transverse axis: inhomogeneous and very vascularized rigid mass with dislocation of the thymus *(Th)* and "truss pad deformation" *("Pelottierung")* of the trunk of the pulmonary artery *(P)*. Extended pleural effusion. (Courtesy of Prof. Dr. H. J. von Lengerke, Münster i. W., FRG)

relatively rare finding. According to Bichel (1947) thymic enlargement is to be found in 18% of patients with acute leukemia, while Cooke (1932) gave a figure of 24%; Gilmartin (1963) did find such enlargement in 91% (11 of 12 cases), but Klatte et al. (1963), on the other hand, observed no instances of an enlarged thymus in patients with leukemia.

While leukemia in adults is predominantly of the chronic myeloid type, in children acute lymphatic leukemia is by far the most common form, and 20%–25% of such cases are T cell leukemias. In ca. 15% of children with leukemia there is a simultaneous thymic involvement in the form of a mediastinal mass (Gilmartin 1963). Boys are affected three times more often than girls; the average age at presentation is 11 years, and most cases occur between the ages of 3 and 12 years.

While T lymphocytes are the starting matrix, not all T cell leukemias are accompanied by a mediastinal tumor.

As long ago as 1932 Cooke collected 74 cases of thymic tumors reported in the literature between 1862 and 1931. Of the 38 patients with leukemia, of whom half were less than 15 years old, one-quarter

showed thymic enlargement. Among the 22 patients reported by Bichel (1947) the proportion was one-fifth. It is noteworthy that thymic involvement in leukemia occurs more frequently *prior* to involution of the gland, i. e., it is a more common finding in children, and particularly infants (*"leucaemia thymica,"* Weicker 1962). It is still unclear whether thymic tumors in patients with leukemic alterations in the blood picture represent primary non-Hodgkin's lymphomas, as claimed by Sternberg (1915) and Webster (1961), or infiltration of the gland by leukemic cells, as assumed by Cooke (1932) and Gilmartin (1963) and as demonstrated at autopsy by Mainzer and Taybi (1971) in one case. Schey et al. (1973) believe that the actual leukemia develops indirectly, via a non-Hodgkin's lymphoma or a primary thymic sarcoma.

The *clinical symptoms* are the same as those previously mentioned in respect of non-Hodgkin's lymphomas. In T cell leukemias there is, as a rule, massive emigration of pathologic cells into the peripheral blood, so that leukocyte levels in the peripheral blood may increase to more than 100/µl (= 100000/mm³). As already mentioned, non-Hodgkin's lymphomas tend toward leukemic transformation, so that differentiation is based on the number of lymphoblasts in the bone marrow.

The findings yielded by *diagnostic imaging procedures* in children correspond to those in non-Hodgkin's lymphoma, although the enlargement of the middle mediastinal shadow tends to be less pronounced (Fig. 8.45). Pleural effusion is less common in leukemia than non-Hodgkin's lymphoma, although Mainzer and Taybi (1971) did find a pleural effusion in the early stages of acute lymphatic leukemia in four out of five children. By contrast, Gilmartin (1963) registered only one such case among 12 patients.

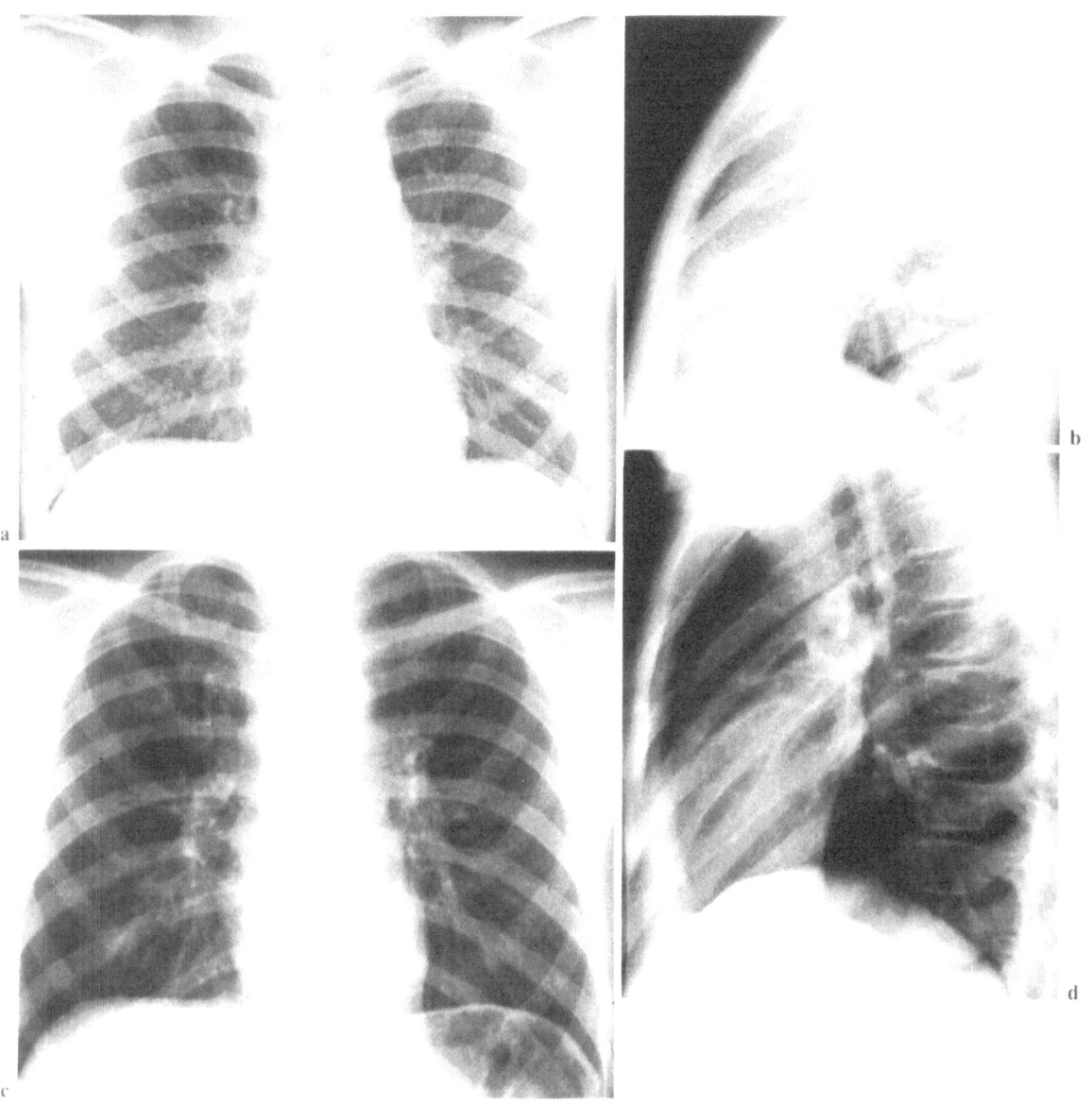

Fig. 8.45 a–c. Leukemia with thymic involvement in an 8-year-old girl. **a** Plain chest radiograph: dense and sharply delimited enlargement of the upper mediastinum. **b** Lateral view: the whole thymic space is of homogeneous density; the upper border of the heart is not visible. **c** After combined therapy over 3 months: slight diminution in the mediastinal shadow. **d** Lateral view: distinct translucence of the thymic region

Ultrasonographically the predominantly diffuse involvement of hypo- and hyperechoic structures of the enlarged thymus is conspicuous, as also is the increased vascularity (Fig. 8.46).

Computed tomography is likely to reveal diffuse enlargement of the thymus (LEMAITRE et al. 1987). The attenuation values closely resemble those of the chest wall (AMOUR et al. 1987). Pathognomonic signs are not to be expected on CT scans. No results are available in respect of MRI and angiography.

Unequivocal differentiation between non-Hodgkin's lymphoma and acute lymphatic leukemia is not possible on the basis of imaging methods alone.

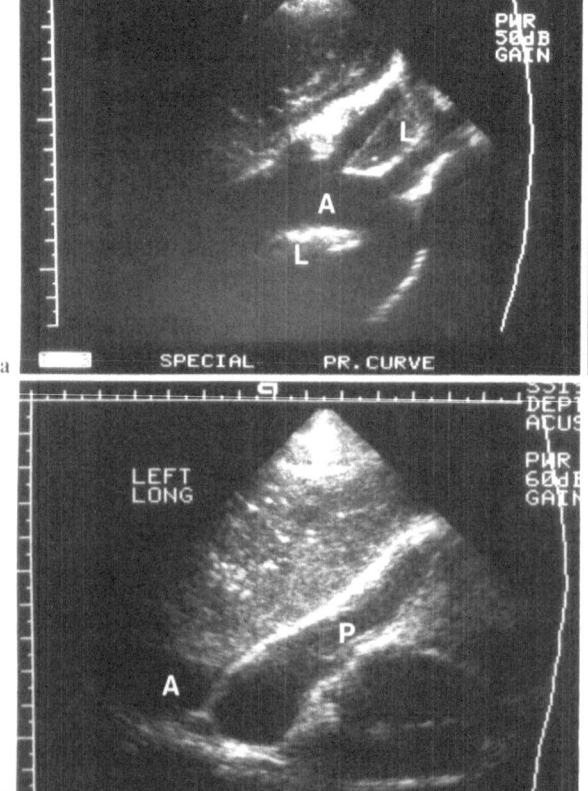

Fig. 8.46 a–c. Acute lymphatic leukemia with involvement of the thymus in a 15-year-old boy. **a** Suprasternal access: diffuse inhomogeneous infiltration of the thymus. Enlarged para-aortal lymph nodes *(L)*. *A*, aorta. **b** Right parasternal longitudinal scan: Dislocation of the great vessels posteriorly. Numerous band-shaped structures of reflexes as a sign of vascularized tumor. *SVC*, superior vena cava. **c** Left parasternal longitudinal scan: rigidity of the wall and mass of the thymus are visible at the impression of the contour of the pulmonary artery *(P)*. (Courtesy of Prof. Dr. H. J. VON LIN-GERKE, Münster i. W., FRG)

8.4.5 Non-Hodgkin's Lymphoma and Leukemia with Thymic Involvement, During and After Radiotherapy and Chemotherapy

During cytostatic or steroid therapy and after low-dose irradiation, thymic tumors, which are highly radiosensitive, tend to display complete regression within a short time, melting away like "butter in the sun" (Fig. 8.41 d). However, recurrences occur in many cases, depending upon the type of lymphoma and the mode of therapy.

In general it is non uncommon for mediastinal enlargement to develop during or after radio- or chemotherapy for malignant lymphomas, although this may also occur when such treatment forms are adopted for other malignancies in children and adults. In individual cases it is then necessary to exclude residual mediastinal tumor following irradiation, a mediastinal recurrence of the tumor, or a mediastinal metastasis (see Sect. 8.4.6). Most often, however, the cause is thymic hyperplasia due to a rebound phenomenon (FORD et al. 1987); this is best diagnosed using the steroid test, and a biopsy should be undertaken only if this fails.

The earlier assumption that thymic involvement in cases of acute lymphatic lymphoma carries a worse prognosis was disproved by CHILCOTE et al. (1984).

For further comments of relevance, the reader is referred to Sect. 8.4.2.3.

8.4.6 Differential Diagnosis

E. WALTER

On a purely morphologic basis, differentiation of lymphoma from tumors of other histology is possible only to a very limited extent using conventional radiographic procedures or CT. When there is simultaneous demonstration of mediastinal or abdominal lymph nodes and thymic enlargement, malignant lymphoma in the thymus lies at the forefront of differential diagnostic considerations. This differential diagnostic criterion naturally does not apply to a malignant lymphoma of primary origin in the thymus without manifestation in lymph nodes that are not part of the regional drainage area. Histologic differentiation of Hodgkin's disease and non-Hodgkin's lymphoma is not possible by means of CT.

If the tumorous form of malignant lymphoma occurs in the thymus, invasive or noninvasive thymoma enters the differential diagnosis. Distinction between these possibilities is very difficult radiographically. The two tumors display identical attenuation values in their solid tissue portions. After administration of a water-soluble contrast medium in bolus from there is reportedly somewhat greater contrast medium enhancement in the case of malignant lymphoma of the thymus, but the difference is insufficient to serve as a differential diagnostic criterion. Both tumors tend toward cystic degeneration and necroses. Calcifications are not found with untreated malignant lymphoma of the thymus whereas they do occur in up to 25% of cases of thymoma. If there is a clinical picture of myasthenia gravis or other accompanying disorders on an immunologic basis, thymoma is to be suspected since to date an association between malignant lymphoma and myasthenia gravis or Cushing's disease has been reported only once. If myasthenia gravis and other accompanying disorders typical for thymoma are absent, and if no calcifications are present, then thymoma can resemble a thymic lymphoma.

Differentiation between malignant lymphoma and thymic carcinoid must also be on a clinical basis, since thymic carcinoids display characteristic symptomas on account of the neuroendocrine hormone secretion. If such symptoms are lacking, differential diagnosis is not possible.

Since malignant lymphoma of the thymus can present as a diffuse enlargement of the organ without loss or alteration of its typical triangular configuration, thymic hyperplasia must be considered in the differential diagnosis. This also holds true when there is thymic enlargement in cases of leukemia. Differential diagnosis is only possible clinically when myasthenia gravis or a leukemic blood picture is present.

Unlike thymic lymphomas with cystic degeneration, dysontogenic thymic cysts typically display thin walls (1–2 mm). Persisting residual tissue is usually present in the case of thymic cysts, although in general it is localized. Bronchogenic cysts are usually located in the course of the foregut rather than in the anterior superior mediastinum.

A solitary extrathymic lymphoma is capable of resembling an intrathymic lymphoma. If isolated typical thymic remnants can be identified, this speaks against manifestation of the disease in the thymus.

Dermoid cysts and thymolipomas tend to display areas with the attenuation values of fat – a finding lacking in malignant lymphoma of the thymus.

A dystopic parathyroid adenoma is usually situated cranial to the thymus; only exceptionally is it located directly at its cranial circumference.

On fluoroscopy, vascular lesions such as aneurysms occasionally show mural calcifications and the typical arterial pulsation. Dynamic CT confirms the diagnosis of a vascular lesion by virtue of the characteristic contrast medium behavior.

The possibility of a rebound phenomenon involving thymic enlargement has already been referred to in the preceding text (cf. FORD et al. 1987).

8.4.7 Relative Value of the Imaging Procedures

Conventional chest radiography in two planes remains the basic diagnostic procedure even though it fails to reveal pathologic findings in up to 16% of patients (AMOUR et al. 1987), such cases are explained by the thymic mass not yet being sufficiently large to produce alterations in the mediastinal structures and their contours. The diagnostic methods of choice for further clarification are ultrasonography and, above all, CT, which illustrates the pathologically enlarged thymus without overlapping of structures. Tracheobronchial compression caused by the tumor is also recognizable on CT scans, so that conventional tomography is in general unnecessary.

Neither ultrasonographic nor CT findings pathognomonic for malignant lymphoma of the thymus have been described, and differential diagnosis therefore essentially relies on clinical parameters or fine needly biopsy.

Arteriography is of no differential diagnostic significance and its use consequently needs to be considered only exceptionally, for special indications.

Superior venacavography is able to demonstrate tumor-related compression or secondary thrombosis with a blockage of the upper vena cava, but CT can also fulfil this function following administration of a water-soluble contrast medium. The value of MRI cannot yet be evaluated owing to the lack of reports on the use of this technique.

References

Amour TES, Siegel MJ, Glazer HS, Nadel SN (1987) CT appearance of the normal and abnormal thymus in childhood. J Comput Assist Tomogr 11: 645

Barcos MP, Lukes RJ (1975) Malignant lymphoma of convoluted lymphocytes – a new entity of possible T cell type. In: Sinks LF, Godden JO (eds) Conflicts in childhood cancer. An evaluation of current management, vol. 4. Alan R, Liss, New York, pp 147

Baron RL, Sagel SS, Baglan RJ (1981) Thymic cysts followig radiation therapy for Hodgkin disease. Radiology 141: 593

Baron RL, Lee JKT, Sagel SS, Levitt RG (1982) Computed tomography of the abnormal thymus. Radiology 142: 127

Berard CW, Dorfman RF (1974) Histopathology of malignant lymphomas. Clin Haematol 3: 39

Bichel J (1947) Mediastinal tumors in leukosis. Acta Radiol 28: 81

Capitanio MA, Faerber EN, Gainey MA, Wolfson BJ (1984) CT of the pediatric chest. J Radiol 65: 727

Chilcote RR, Coccia P, Satzer HN, Robinson LL, Bachner RL, Nesbit ME, Hammond D (1984) Mediastinal mass in acute lymphoblastic leukemia. Med Pediatr Oncol 12: 9

Cooke JV (1932) Mediastinal tumor in acute leukemia. A clinical and roentgenologic study. Am J Dis Child 44: 1153

Davis RE, Dorfman RF, Warnke RA (1990) Primary large-cell lymphoma of the thymus: A diffuse B-cell neoplasm presenting as primary mediastinal lymphoma. Hum Pathol 21: 1262

Eiser NM; Samarrai AA (1975) Thymic lymphoma. An unusual presentation. Thorax 30: 588

Ewing J (1916) The thymus and its tumors. Report of three cases of thymoma. Surg Gynecol Obstet 22: 461

Federle MP, Callen PW (1979) Cystic Hodgkin's lymphoma of the thymus: computed tomography appearance. J Comput Assist Tomogr 3: 542

Francis JR, Glazer GM, Bookstein FL, Gross BH (1985) The thymus: reexamination of age-related changes in size and shape. AJR 145: 249

Ford EG, Lockhart SK, Sullivan MP, Andrassy RJ (1987) Mediastinal mass following chemotherapeutic treatment of Hodgkin's disease: recurrent tumor or thymic hyperplasia? J Pediatr Surg 22: 1155

Gilmartin D (1963) Leukaemic involvement of the thymus in children. Br J Radiol 36: 211

Göthlin J, Jonsson K, Lunderquist A, Rausing A, Albuquerque LM (1977) The angiographic appearance of thymic tumors. Radiology 124: 47

Heron CW, Husband JE, Williams MP (1988) Hodgkin disease: CT of the thymus. Radiology 167: 647

Hofmann WJ, Momburg F, Möller P (1988a) Thymic medullary cells expressing B lymphocyte antigens. Hum Pathol 19: 1280

Hofmann WJ, Momburg F, Möller P, Otto HF (1988b) Intra- and extrathymic B cells in physiological and pathological conditions. Immunohistochemical study on normal thymus and lymphofollicular hyperplasia of the thymus. Virchows Arch [A] 412: 431

Isaacson PG, Chan JKC, Tang C, Addis BJ (1990) Low-grade B-cell lymphoma of mucosa-associated lymphoid tissue arising in the thymus. A thymic lymphoma mimicking myoepithelial sialadenitis. Am J Surg Pathol 14: 342

Jacobson JO, Aisenberg AC, Lamarre L, Willet CG, Linggood RM, Miketic LM, Harris NL (1988) Mediastinal large cell lymphoma. An uncommon subset of adult lymphomas curable with combined modality therapy. Cancer 62: 1893

Kaesberg PR, Foley DB, Pellett J, Hafez GR, Ershler WB (1988) Concurrent development of a thymic cyst and mediastinal Hodgkin's disease. Med Pediatr Oncol 16: 293

Katz A, Lattes R (1969) Granulomatous thymoma or Hodgkin's disease of thymus? A clinical and histologic study and a re-evaluation. Cancer 23: 1

Katz M, Piekarski JD, Bayle-Weisgerber C, Laval-Jeantet M, Teillet F (1977) Masses médiastinales résiduelles post-radiothérapiques au cours de la maladie de Hodgkin. Ann Radiol 20: 667

Keen SJ, Libshitz H (1987) Thymic lesions. Experience with computer tomography in 24 patients. Cancer 59: 1520

Keller AR, Castleman B (1974) Hodgkin's disease of the thymus gland. Cancer 33: 1615

Kim HC, Nosher J, Haas A, Sweeney W, Lewis R (1985) Cystic degeneration of thymic Hodgkin's disease following radiation therapy. Cancer 55: 354

King RM, Telander RL, Smithson WA, Banks PM, Mao-Tang Han (1982) Primary mediastinal tumors in children. J Pediatr Surg 17: 512

Kirks DR, Korobkin M (1980) Chest computed tomography in infants and children. An analysis of 50 patients. Pediatr Radiol 10: 75

Kirks DR, Korobkin M (1981) Computed tomography of the chest in infants and children: techniques and mediastinal evaluation. Radiol Clin North Am 19: 409

Klatte EC, Yardley J, Smith EB, Rohn R, Campbell JA (1963) The pulmonary manifestations and complications of leukemia. AJR 89: 598

Lamarre L, Jacobson JO, Aisenberg AC, Harris NL (1989) Primary large cell lymphoma of the mediastinum. A histologic and immunophenotypic study of 29 cases. Am J Surg Pathol 13: 730

Lemaitre L, Leclerc F, Marconi V, Taboureau O, Avni FE, Remy J (1987) Ultrasonographic findings in thymic lymphoma in children. Eur J Radiol 7: 125

Lennert K (1978) Malignant lymphomas other than Hodgkin's disease. Springer, Berlin Heidelberg New York

Leslie MD, Brada M, Peckham MJ (1986) Hodgkin's disease during surveillance of stage I testicular teratoma. Br J Radiol 59: 1230

Lichtenstein AK, Levine A, Taylor OR, Boswell W, Rossman S, Feinstein DI, Lukes RJ (1980) Primary mediastinal lymphoma in adults. Am J Med 68: 509

Lindfors KK, Meyer JE, Dedrich CG, Hassell LA, Harris NL (1985) Thymic cysts in mediastinal Hodgkin disease. Radiology 156: 37

Lowenhaupt E, Brown R (1951) Carcinoma of the thymus of granulomatous type. A clinical and pathological study. Cancer 4: 1193

Lukes RJ, Collins RD (1974) Immunologic characterization of human malignant lymphomas. Cancer 34: 1488

Mainzer F, Taybi H (1971) Thymic enlargement and pleural effusion: an unusual roentgenographic complex in childhood leukemia. AJR 112: 35

Mandell GA, Lautieri R, Goodman LR (1982) Tracheobronchial compression in Hodgkins lymphoma in children. AJR 139: 1167

Marshal AHE, Wood C (1957) The involvement of the thymus in Hodgkin's disease. J Pathol Bacteriol 73: 163

McEndy DP, Boon MC, Furth J (1944) On the role of thymus, spleen, and gonads in the development of leukemia
in a high-leukemia stock of mice. Cancer Res 4: 377

Menestrina F, Chilosi M, Bonetti F et al. (1986) Mediastinal
large cell lymphoma of B-type, with sclerosis: histopathological and immunohistochemical study of eight cases.
Histopathology 10: 589

Möller P, Lämmler B, Eberlein-Gonska M, Feichter GE,
Hofmann WJ, Schmitteckert H, Otto HF (1986) Primary
mediastinal clear cell lymphoma of B-cell type. Virchows
Arch [A] 409: 79

Möller P, Lämmler B, Herrmann B, Otto HF, Moldenhauer G, Momburg F (1986) The primary mediastinal
clear cell lymphoma of B-cell type has variable defects in
MHC antigen expression. Immunology 59: 411

Möller P, Matthaei-Maurer DU, Hofmann WJ, Dörken B,
Moldenhauer G (1989a) Immunophenotypic similarities
of mediastinal clear-cell lymphoma and sinusoidal
(monocytoid) B cells. Int J Cancer 43: 10

Möller P, Hofmann WJ, Mielke B, Otto HF (1989b) Das
primär mediastinale, hellzellige B-Zell-Lymphom ist ein
epithelassoziiertes Thymuslymphom. Pathologe 10: 234

Möller P, Moldenhauer G, Momburg F, Lämmler B, Eberlein-Gonska M, Kiesel S, Dörken B (1987) Blood 69:
1087

Momburg F, Herrmann B, Moldenhauer G, Möller P
(1987) B-cell lymphomas of high-grade malignancy frequently lack HLA-DR, -DP and -DQ antigens and associated in variant chain. Int J Cancer 40: 598

Murray JA, Parker AC (1984) Mediastinal Hodgkin's disease and thymic cysts. Acta Haematol 71: 282

Nathwani BN, Kim H, Rappaport H (1976) Malignant lymphoma, lymphoblastic. Cancer 38: 964–983

Nogués A, Tovar JA, Sunol M, Palacio M, Albisu J (1987)
Hodgkin's disease of the thymus: a rare mediastinal cystic
mass. J Pediatr Surg 22: 996

North LB, Fuller LM, Sullivan-Halley JA, Hagemeister FB
(1987) Regression of mediastinal Hodgkin disease after
therapy: evaluation of time internal. Radiology 164: 599

Null JA, LiVolsi VA, Glenn WWL (1977) Hodgkin's disease of the thymus (granulomatous thymoma) and myasthenia gravis. Clin Pathol 67: 521

Nyman RS, Rehn SM, Glimelius BLG, Hagberg HE,
Hemmingsson AL, Sundström CJ (1989) Residual mediastinal masses in Hodgkin disease: prediction of size
with MR imaging. Radiology 170: 435

Otto F (1984) Pathologie des Thymus. In: Doerr W, Seifert G (eds) Spezielle pathologische Anatomie, vol.17.
Springer, Berlin Heidelberg New York

Otto HF (1991) Tumors of the thymus and their nomencla-
ture. Virchows Arch A (in press)

Perrone T, Frizzera G, Rosai J (1986) Mediastinal diffuse
large cell lymphoma with sclerosis: a clinicopathologic
study of 60 cases. Am J Surg Pathol 10: 176

Schey WL, White H, Conway JJ, Kidd JM (1973) Lymphosarcoma in children. A roentgenologic and clinical evaluation of 60 children. AJR 117: 59

Schnyder P, Candardjis G (1987) Computed tomography of
thymic abnormalities. Eur J Radiol 7: 107

Shin MS, Ho K-J (1983) Diffuse thymic hyperplasia following chemotherapy for nodular sclerosing Hodgkin's disease. Cancer 51: 30

Siegel MJ, Glazer HS, Wiener JI, Molina PL (1989) Normal
and abnormal thymus in childhood: MR imaging. Radiology 172: 367

Sternberg C (1915) Leukosarkomatose and Myeloblastenleukämie. Beitr Path Anat 61: 75

Tartas NE, Korin J, Dengra CS, Barazzutti LM, Blasetti A,
Sanchez Avalos JC (1985) Diffuse thymic enlargement in
Hodgkin's disease. JAMA 254: 406

Thomson AD (1955) The thymic origin of Hodgkin's disease. Br J Cancer 9: 37

Von Lengerke H-J, Schmidt H (1988) Mediastinalsonographie im Kindesalter. Ergebnisse bei 310 Untersuchungen.
Radiologe 28: 460

Walter E (1982) Computertomographische Diagnostik des
Thymus. In: Lissner J, Doppman JL (eds) CT 82, Internationales Computertomographie Symposium, Seefeld/Ti-
rol. Schnetztor, Konstanz

Walter E, Hübner K-M (1980) Computertomographische
Charakteristika raumfordernder Prozesse im vorderen
Mediastinum und ihre Differentialdiagnose. ROFO 133:
391

Watson RR, Weissel W, O'Connor TM (1968) Thymic neoplasms. Arch Surg 97: 230

Webb WR (1989) MR imaging of treated mediastinal
Hodgkin disease. Radiology 170: 315

Webster R (1961) Lymphosarcoma of thymus: its relation
to acute lymphatic leukaemia. Med J Aust 48: 542

Weicker H (1962) Tumoren im Kindesalter. In: Bartelhei-
mer H, Maurer HJ (eds) Diagnostik der Geschwulst-
krankheiten. Thieme, Stuttgart

Weiss C, Dinkel E, Wimmer B, Schildge J, Grosser G
(1987) Der Thymus im Computertomogramm. Normalbefunde und Pathologie. Radiologe 27: 414

8.5 Mesenchymal Tumors (Thymolipoma)

E. WALTER

According to a classification proposed by OTTO (1984), mesenchymal tumors include "myoid cell" sarcoma (myosarcoma), presumably originating from myoid cells of the thymus, and histiocytic tumors. Both types of tumor are rare.

Only thymolipoma is of greater clinical significance, it being by far the most common tumor of this group (BOETSCH et al. 1966; RINGE et al. 1979). To date radiographic findings are available solely in respect of thymolipomas; consequently the discussion here will be restricted to this tumor type.

8.5.1 Pathologic Features

W. J. HOFMANN and H. F. OTTO

Thymolipoma was first described by LANGE in 1916 ("lipoma of the thymus"). In 1949, HALL introduced the term *thymolipoma* for the diagnosis of these unusual tumors. He suggested that the tumor is a true mixed tumor of adipose and thymic tissue.

Grossly, thymolipomas are always yellowish, soft, and pliable and are often lobate with thin edges (Fig. 8.47). The majority (68%) of the reported thymolipomas have weighed over 500 g, and 23% have weighed over 2000 g (BIGELOW and EHLER 1952; DUNN and FRKOVICH 1956; KORHONEN and LAUSTELA 1968). The largest tumor weighed over 12 kg (MOIGNETEAU et al. 1967).

Thymolipomas are well encapsulated (Fig. 8.47). They may adhere to the pleura or pericardium and may displace adjacent mediastinal organs, but invasion has never been documented (OTTO et al. 1982; OTTO 1984; HOFMANN and OTTO 1989). Histologically, they are composed of large lobules of mature adipose tissue with interspersed islands of normally structured thymic tissue with Hassall's corpuscles (Thymolipoma with striated myoid cells: ISEKI et al. 1990).

The nature of thymolipoma is still unknown. Various theories have been proposed for the pathogenesis of this lesion of the thymus, but all of them are unsatisfactory explanations of this tumor and its development (ALMOG et al. 1977; OTTO et al. 1982; OTTO 1984).

Only a few patients with thymolipoma have associated systemic disease, including Graves' disease (BENTON and GERARD 1966), aplastic anemia (BARNES and O'GORMAN 1962), hypogammaglobulinemia (cf. Table 8.9), and myasthenia gravis (REINTGEN et al. 1978; OTTO et al. 1982). TRITES (1966) described an unusual case in which lipomas were present in the thyroid gland, thymus, and aryepiglottic fold of the same patient. With regard to thymoliposarcoma, see HAVLICEK and ROSAI (1984) and OKUMORI et al. (1983).

8.5.2 Occurrence and Clinical Symptoms

E. WALTER

8.5.2.1 Occurrence

The thymolipoma described by LANGE in 1916 weighed 1600 g and consisted of fat, residual thymic tissue, and Hassall's corpuscles. HEUER and ANDRUS (1940) named this type of tumor a benign

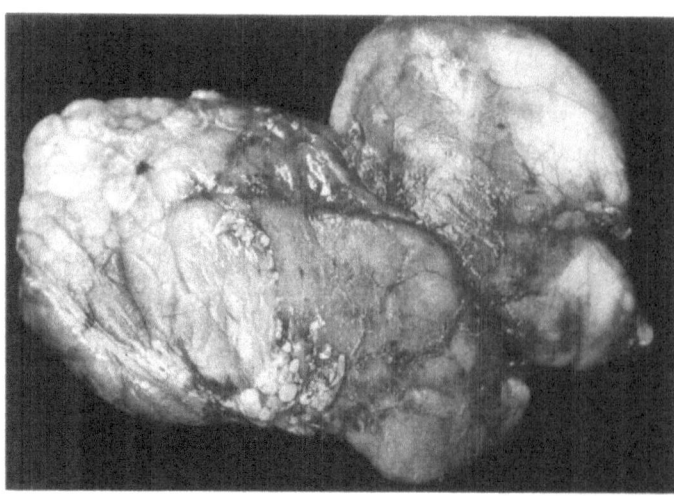

Fig. 8.47. Thymolipoma with well-formed capsule and soft yellow uniform surface (93 g, 56-year-old man with symptoms of myasthenia gravis)

Table 8.9. Thymolipoma: summary of clinical features, Institute of Pathology, University of Hamburg

Case	Age (yrs)	Sex	Symptoms	Duration of symptoms	Clinical diagnosis	Findings on chest radiograph	Weight and size (cm) of tumor	Follow-up
1	5	M	Anemia, intercurrent infections	9 mo	Erythrocyte hypoplasia, hypogammaglobulinemia	Widened anterior mediastinum	320 g $17 \times 9 \times 7$	9 yr, alive and well
2	32	M	Asymptomatic	–	Abnormal chest radiograph, possible tumor	Widened anterior mediastinum	270 g $12 \times 9 \times 5$	7 mo, alive and well
3	57	F	Asymptomatic	–	Abnormal chest radiograph, possible tumor	Widened anterior mediastinum	420 g $19 \times 11 \times 8$	6 yr, alive and well
4	64	M	Asymptomatic	–	Abnormal chest radiograph, possible tumor	Widened anterior mediastinum	120 g $7 \times 6 \times 6$	4 yr, alive and well
5	56	M	Ptosis	4 yr	Myasthenia gravis; thymoma?	Normal CT scan: mediastinal lipomatosis (cf. Fig. 8.47)	93 g $13 \times 7 \times 5$ $7 \times 5 \times 4$	Transient remission following thymectomy; after few months, myasthenic reaction

thymoma (LANGE's report had simply been entitled "On a lipoma of the thymus" – *"Über ein Lipom des Thymus"*), while SCHANHER and HODGE (1949) used the term "lipoma with the inclusion of thymic remnants"; as already mentioned, the term "thymolipoma" was first proposed by HALL (1949). In the English-language literature the tumor is also referred to a "lipothymoma" (BIGELOW and EHLER 1952). TEPLICK et al. (1973) reviewed ca. 50 cases reported in the English-language literature to that date.

Thymolipoma is a rare benign tumor of the mediastinum that accounts for 2%–9% of all thymic tumors (MATHEY et al. 1962; MOIGNETEAU et al. 1967; OTTO and HÜSSELMANN 1978; OTTO et al. 1982; OTTO 1984). Mediastinal lipomas/lipomatosis of nonthymic origin are more common (RUBIN and MISHKIN 1954). Thymolipomas can occur at any age; thus a review of the literature by HEIMANN et al. (1987) revealed an age range of 3–60 years. Adolescents and young adults are, however, most frequently affected, clinical manifestation of the tumor predominantly occurring in the second to third decades. OTTO (1984) reported the average age at presentation to be 22 years. LEVINE et al. (1986) stated that men are twice as often affected as women, whereas TEPLICK et al. (1973) and HEIMANN et al. (1987) did not find any sex-related difference in occurrence.

8.5.2.2 Clinical Symptoms

Between 40% and 50% of patients fail to display clinical symptoms. In such cases the thymolipoma is identified on routine control chest radiographs or at autopsy (LEVINE et al. 1968; PEAKE and ZEIGLER 1977). Even lipomas weighing as much as 2000 g and occupying the caudal two-thirds of a hemithorax can remain clinically silent (FEDRIGA et al. 1989).

In general thymolipomas have a slow rate of growth. Thus YEH et al. (1983) reported one case in which a thymolipoma ultimately coming to weigh 940 g developed over a time span of 12 years. Because of the slow growth rate, clinical manifestation of the tumor occurs at a late stage; this in turn explains their high weight. The clinical symptoms observed with the larger tumors are neither uniform nor specific, and arise as a result of space occupation, compression, and pressure effects. Bronchial compression can be observed endoscopically even though the thymolipoma usually follows the contours of preexistent anatomic structures (WINARSO et al. 1982). Dyspnea, coughing, and nonspecific thoracic pain are especially frequent symptoms, and less often there is sanguineous sputum or, in the case of poststenotic bronchial infection, purulent sputum (BOETSCH et al. 1966; CSAPO and SZENOHRADSZKY 1970; PAN et al. 1988; FAERBER et al. 1990; and others). In isolated cases there is weight loss, fatigue (SHUB et al.

1979), cyanosis, and compression of the vene cava causing raised JVP with edema of the cranial region (WEINGARTEN and GORDON 1955).

Thymolipomas tend to grow caudally, originating from the anterior superior and middle mediastinum. They are then situated paracardially, either uni- or bilaterally. As a consequence the appearance on routine chest radiographs simulates that of cardiomegaly in 40% of cases (ROSEFF et al. 1958; SUNDSTRÖM 1976; FAERBER et al. 1990), and may also resemble that of a cardiac defect such as a combined mitral valve defect (WINARSO et al. 1982). The specific cardiologic diagnostic procedures that are then employed, such as echocardiography, electrocardiography, and cardiac function tests, reveal no pathologic findings in respect of the heart itself (MATSUYAMA et al. 1986; ALMOG et al. 1977; YEH et al. 1983).

Thymolipoma is seldom accompanied by other illnesses. In general myasthenia gravis is not observed in conjunction with thymolipoma (TEPLICK et al. 1973; ROSENBERG 1985), only seven such cases having been described in the literature (REINTGEN et al. 1978; OTTO et al. 1982; OLANOW et al. 1982; MIKKELSEN 1984; ALFARO et al. 1982; PAN et al. 1988). PAN et al. (1988) reported that myasthenia gravis and thymolipoma occurred in conjunction in 2.8% of their own patients, although their review of the literature expect a figure of ca. 10%. Such cases are more frequent among the elderly. Due to the fact that their clinical symptomatology causes them to be discovered at an earlier stage, the size of the thymolipoma is lower than that in patients without accompanying myasthenia gravis (PAN et al. 1988). In addition there have been single case reports of associations between thymolipoma and hyperthyroidism (BENTON and GERARD 1966; ALFARO et al. 1982), aplastic anemia (BARNES and O'GORMAN 1962; OTTO et al. 1982), and endocarditis (TEPLICK et al. 1973). A curious case was described by TRITES (1966), in which a 2350-g thymolipoma occurred in combination with a lipoma of the thyroid and pharynx.

8.5.3 Diagnosis with Imaging Procedures

8.5.3.1 Conventional Radiology

As already mentioned, thymolipomas generally present as relatively large tumors owing to their slow growth and the late appearance of symptoms. Thus conventional chest radiography in two planes shows irregular contours and enlargement of,

usually, the anterior superior mediastinum (Fig. 8.48), whereby the mediastinum and heart may be displaced. In the case of large unilateral tumors, caudal displacement of the diaphragm and thus – when there is a left-sided location – of the gastric air bubble and the air-containing colon has been observed (HEIMANN et al. 1987). Thymolipomas with the clinical symptomatology of myasthenia gravis or hyperthyroidism are discovered at an earlier stage owing to the basic disease and are generally correspondingly small. The lipoma described by OTTO et al. (1982) in conjunction with myasthenia gravis weighed 93 g and could not be recognized on the plain chest radiograph and conventional tomography.

Since the tumor frequently rests on the heart base and in addition tends to follow the contours of the heart in growing caudally, the appearance on chest radiographs in two planes may mimic cardiomegaly. On fluoroscopy one can then observe strikingly slight (GUNNELLS et al. 1963) or absent (SHUB et al. 1979) pulsation of the heart contour. When the tumor occupies a paracardiac position, it may simulate a pericardial cyst (HUI and GUO 1987).

The fat content of thymolipomas led TEPLICK et al. (1973) to recommend a Bucky film, since in such cases it should be possible to distinguish the tumor from the heart on account of the former's lower radiation absorption. According to ALMOG et al. (1977) it should be possible to distinguish the heart within the tumor when the plain chest radiograph is inspected more carefully, since thymolipomas display a mature fatty tissue content of up to 90% (OTTO et al. 1982). For this reason MOK et al. (1980) recommend a hard chest radiograph in two planes, and in particular a hard lateral film. It should also be noted that the high-fat thymolipoma displays more radiolucent margins.

Conventional tomography is not of differential diagnostic significance; calcifications are not to be expected (TEPLICK et al. 1973; PEAKE and ZEIGLER 1977).

In the past arteriographic investigations were more frequently performed for the differential diagnosis of cardiomegaly (PEAKE and ZEIGLER 1977). Angiocardiography yielded normal findings (LEVINE et al. 1968). As regards thymolipoma itself, GUNNELLS et al. (1963) described multiple, smooth, and harmoniously coursing vessels in a case of paracardially situated thymolipoma. PEAKE and ZEIGLER (1977), too, failed to find neovascularization in the sense of pathologic vessels.

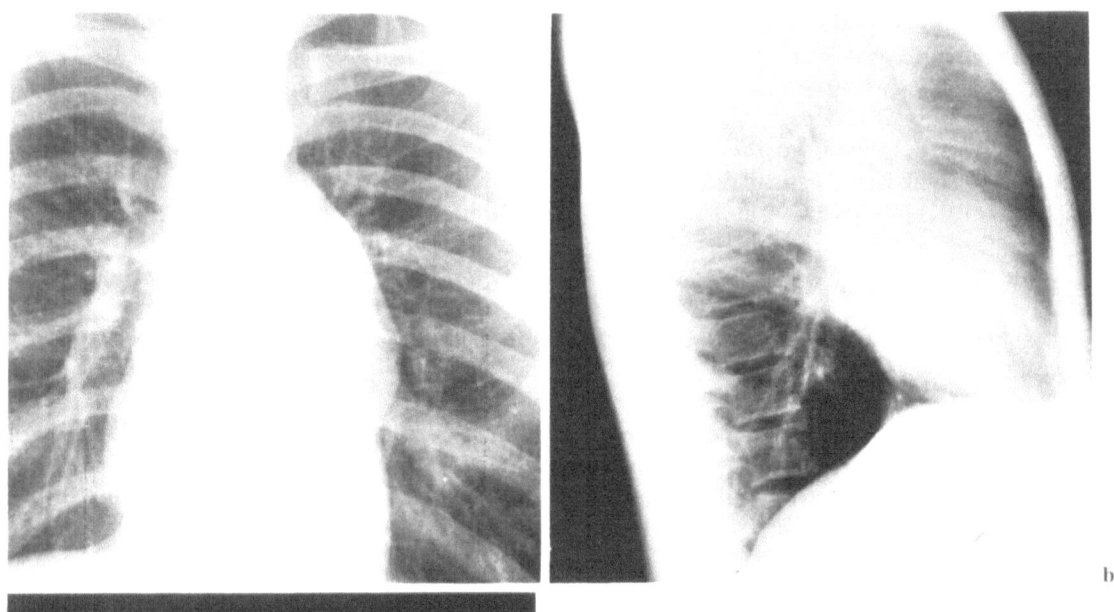

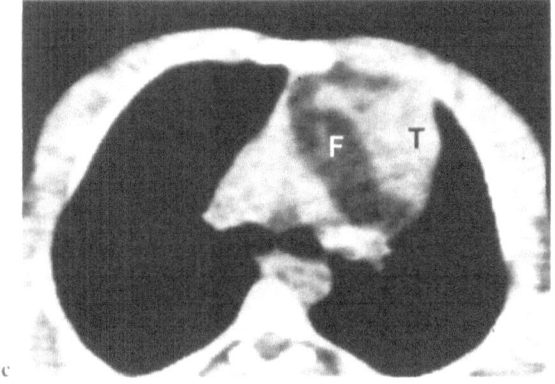

Fig. 8.48 a–c. Thymolipoma in a 26-year-old patient. a,b Chest radiography in two planes, standing position. On the posteroanterior view there is mediastinal enlargement to the left, at the level of the heart base. In the lateral projection there is indistinct densification of the retrosternal space, caused by the mediastinal mass. c CT with visualization of the characteristic components of thymolipoma: areas of fatty tissue (F) and solid thymic tissue (T)

Since thymolipomas generally follow the contours of anatomic structures, esophageal displacement (MOK et al. 1982) is not to be expected.

8.5.3.2 Ultrasonography

Several authors have reported ultrasonographic findings obtained in patients with thymolipoma. Both HEIMANN et al. (1987) and FEDRIGA et al. (1989) describe thymolipoma as a hyperechoic tumor, while YEH et al. (1983) report a homogeneous echo pattern, with the tumor being more highly echogenic than normal liver parenchyma.

8.5.3.3 Computed Tomography

This benign tumor is well differentiated from neighboring structures on CT scans on account of its fibrous capsule (Fig. 8.48 c), and this especially holds true for paracardially situated thymolipomas. The capsule itself, however, is not visualized. The tumor displays highly variable attenuation values in accordance with its heterogeneous anatomic structure. Thus while areas of mature fatty tissue yield attenuation values of between -80 and -120 HU, areas corresponding to solid thymic tissue display values of between $+30$ and $+60$ HU (WALTER 1982). In addition to the easily distinguishable areas of uniform tissue comprising fat or thymus (Fig. 8.48 c), the tumor also contains extensive mixtures of the histologic components (FEDRIGA et al. 1989; FAERBER et al. 1990). Significant enhancement is not to be expected after administration of a water-soluble contrast medium (FAERBER et al. 1990). In correspondence with its pathoanatomic extension, the tumor in the anterior superior mediastinum frequently also displays a paracardiac location (YEH et al. 1983), and exceptionally is to be found in the right cardiophrenic angle (GUILFOIL and MURRAY 1955).

As with other imaging procedures, calcifications are not usually to be observed on CT scans. It is true that CSAPO and SZENOHRADSZKY (1970) found calcifications of Hassall's corpuscles, but these escape detection by CT owing to their small size. Only WINARSO et al. (1982) have described CT demonstration of calcareous foci in a thymolipoma.

8.5.3.4 Magnetic Resonance Imaging

To date only SHIRKHODA et al. (1987) and FEDRIGA et al. (1989) have reported MRI findings in respect of thymolipoma, the tumors in question weighing 2140 and 2000 g respectively. On T1-weighted spin-echo images the predominant fatty nature of the neoplasm results in strong signal intensity because of its short T1 (SHIRKHODA et al. 1987). MRI is of value in demonstrating the size, extension, and borders of the tumor, as well as its mediastinal origin.

8.5.4 Differential Diagnosis

As neoplasms with heterogeneous density, other fatty tumors are of prime differential diagnostic significance.

Liposarcomas are typically located in the posterior mediastinum (MENDEZ et al. 1979) but they are occasionally observed in the anterior mediastinum (CICCIARELLI et al. 1964). In contrast to thymolipomas, liposarcomas can be polycentric and usually invade neighboring organs as an expression of their malignancy.

Mediastinal lipomatosis extends diffusely within the anterior mediastinum; solid tissue portions are lacking. This also applies to localized pure lipomas, which additionally tend to be located in the paracardiac region rather than in the region of the thymus (CICCIARELLI et al. 1964). As masses of heterogeneous density, teratogenic cysts, and in particular dermoid cysts, must also receive consideration in the differential diagnosis. In this case, however, the fatty portions, corresponding to sebaceous matter, are centrally situated and are surrounded by solid tissue (WALTER and HÜBENER 1980).

The good delineation of a thymolipoma from the heart achieved with CT (especially after administration of a water-soluble contrast medium to improve visualization of the pericardial cavity and great vessels) permits differential diagnosis against cardiomegaly, pericardial effusion, pericardial tumors, pericardial cysts (FREDELL and PERLMUTTER 1961), or aneurysms of the ascending thoracic aorta when these are suspected on the basis of plain chest radiography. Ultrasonography can also aid in differential diagnosis. Cardiography and pneumomediastinography (GUILFOIL and MURRAY 1955) are superfluous nowadays.

If imaging procedures are inconclusive, histologic confirmation can be achieved by means of fine needle biopsy. HEIMANN et al. (1987) report that a 20-gauge Chiba needle is adequate for the purpose. In the cytologic aspirate from a thymolipoma they found mature fatty tissue, large epithelial cells, and cells representing the remnants of Hassall's corpuscles. By contrast aspiration at multiple sites in lipomas yields only fat cells. Aspirates from liposarcomas – the symptomatology of which is in general pronounced – show lymphoblasts.

8.5.5 Relative Value of the Imaging Procedures

Chest radiography in two planes remains the basic investigative procedure. Whether the tumor occupies the typical position or there is an appearance of cardiomegaly, CT and to a lesser extent ultrasonography will be necessary for differential diagnosis against other types of tumor or a paracardiac mass such as pericardial effusion, pericardial tumor, pericardial cyst, or cardiomegaly.

Today CT occupies the central position in differential diagnosis. Evaluation of the role of MRI is not possible, given the paucity of reports on this method. According to HEIMANN and co-workers (1987), in cases of doubt fine needle biopsy with a 20-gauge Chiba needle is suitable for establishing the diagnosis and histologic classification of the tumor.

8.5.6 Therapy and Prognosis

Thymolipomas are usually resected surgically. This is in general easily achieved given the benign character of the tumor and its fibrous capsule. Recurrences are not to be expected.

References

Alfaro A, Gilsanz A, Cervelló MA, Antolin MA, Albero-la C, Villoslada C (1982) Oftalmoplejia crónica en un caso de miastenia grave, hipertiroidismo y timolipoma. Med Clin (Barcelona) 79: 236

Almog CH, Weissberg D, Herczeg E, Pajewski M (1977) Thymolipoma simulating cardiomegaly: a clinicopathological rarity. Thorax 32: 116

Barnes RDS, O'Gorman P (1962) Two cases of aplastic anaemia associated with tumors of the thymus. J Clin Pathol 15: 264

Benton C, Gerard P (1966) Thymolipoma in a patient with Graves' disease. J Thoracic Cardiovasc Surg 51: 428

Bigelow NH, Ehler AA (1952) Lipotomoma: an unusual benign tumor of the thymus gland. J Thorac Surg 23: 528

Boetsch CH, Swoyer GB, Adams A, Walker JH (1966) Lipothymoma. Report of two cases. Dis Chest 50: 539

Cicciarelli FE, Soule EH, McGoon DC (1964) Lipoma and liposarcoma of the mediastinum: A report of 14 tumors including one lipoma of the thymus. J Thoracic Cardiovasc Surg 47: 411

Csapó Z, Szenohradszky J (1970) Thymolipom. Zbl allg Path 113: 401

Dunn BH, Frkovich G (1956) Lipomas of the thymus gland. With an illustrative case report. Am J of Path 32: 41

Faerber EN, Balsara RK, Schidlow DV, Marmon LM, Zaeri N (1990) Thymolipoma: Computed tomographic appearances. Pediatr Radiol 20: 196

Fedriga E, Chiesa G, Ravini M (1989) Apporto della tomografia computerizzata e della risonanza magnetica alla caratterizzazione del timolipoma. Radiol Med 78: 395

Fredell CH, Perlmutter AD (1961) Thymolipoma. Report of a Case. Arch Surg 83: 898

Guilfoil PH, Murray H (1955) Thymolipoma. Report of a Case. Surgery 38: 406

Gunnells JC, Miller DE, Jacoby WJ, May RL (1963) Thymolipoma simulating cardiomegaly: Opacification of the tumor by cineangiocardiography. Am Heart J 66: 670

Hall GFM (1949) A case of thymolipoma with observations on a possible relationship to intrathoracic lipomata. Br J Surg 36: 321

Havlicek F, Rosai J (1984) A sarcoma of thymic stroma with features of liposarcomas. Am J Clin Pathol 83: 217

Heimann A, Sneige N, Shirkhoda A, DeCaro LF (1987) Fine needle aspiration cytology of Thymolipoma. A case report. Acta Cytologica 31: 335

Heuer GJ, Andrus WD (1940) The surgery of Mediastinal tumors. Am J Surg 5: 146

Hui YZ, Guo QX (1987) Thymolipoma simulating pericardial cyst. A clinicopathologic rarity. Chin Med J 100: 809

Hofmann WJ, Otto HF (1989) Pathology of tumors of the thymic region. In: Thoracic Surgery: Frontiers and uncommon neoplasms (Martini N, Vogt-Moykopf I, eds) pp 157–175. The CV Mosby Company, St. Louis Baltimore Toronto

Iseki M, Tsuda N, Kishikawa M, Shimada O, Hayashi T, Kawahara K, Tomita M (1990) Thymolipoma with striated myoid cells. Histological, immunohistochemical, and ultrastructural study. Am J Surg Pathol 14: 395–398

Korhonen LK, Laustela E (1968) Thymolipoma. Scand J Thorac Cardiovasc Surg 2: 147

Lange I (1916) Über ein Lipom des Thymus. Centralbl allg Path pathol Anat 27: 97

Levine S, Labiche H, Chandor S (1968) Thymolipoma. Am Rev Resp Dis 98: 875

Mathey J, Renauld P, De Saint-Florent G, Galey J-J, Binet J-P (1962) A propos des 61 interventions sur le thymus. Nouv Press med 70: 2191

Matsuyama K, Nakagawa T, Horio Y, Hongo H, Miyauchi Y, Yasue H (1986) Thymolipoma Simulating Cardiomegaly: Diagnostic usefulness of computed tomography. Jap Circ J 50: 839

Mendez G, Isikoff MB, Isikoff SK, Sinner WN (1979) Fatty tumors of the thorax demonstrated by CT. AJR 133: 207

Mikkelsen B (1984) Thymolipoma in association with lateonset myasthenia gravis. J Neurol NeuroSurg Psychiatr 47: 216

Mok CK, Ho FCS, Nandi P, Ong GB (1980) Lipothymoma. Med J Aust 1: 272

Moigneteau C, Cornet E, Gordeef A, Dubigeon P, Delajartre A, Guillement JM (1967) Le thymo-lipome. J Chir (Paris) 94: 509

Nuruddin R, Daud A (1988) CT and sonographic diagnosis of thymolipoma. Case report. Australas Radiol 32: 497

Olanow CW, Lane RJM, Roses AD (1982) Thymectomy in late-onset myasthenia gravis. Arch Neurol 39: 82

Okumori M, Mabuchi M, Nakagawa M (1983) Malignant thymoma associated with liposarcoma of the mediastinum: a case report. Jpn J Surg 13: 512

Otto HF (1984) Pathologie des Thymus. In: Doerr W, Seifert G, Uehlinger E (eds) Spezielle pathologische Anatomie. Bd 17. Springer, Berlin Heidelberg New York

Otto HF, Hüsselmann H (1978) Klinisch-pathologische Studie zur Klassifikation und Prognose von Thymustumoren. Teil I. Histologische und Ultrastrukturpathologische Untersuchungen. Z Krebsforsch 91: 81

Otto HF, Löning T, Lachenmayer L, Janzen RWC, Gürtler KF, Fischer K (1982) Thymolipoma in association with myasthenia gravis. Cancer 50: 1623

Pan CH, Chiang CY, Chen SS (1988) Thymolipoma in patients with myasthenia gravis: report of two cases and Review Acta Neurol Scand 78 (1988) 16

Peake JB, Zeigler MG (1977) Thymolipoma: Report of three cases. Am Surg 43: 477

Reintgen D, Fetter BF, Roses A, McCarty KS (1978) Thymolipoma in association with myasthenia gravis. Arch Pathol Lab Med 102: 463

Ringe B, Dragojevic D, Frank G, Borst HG (1979) Thymolipoma – A rare, benign tumor of the thymus gland. Two case reports and review of the literature. Thorac cardiovasc Surgeon 27: 369

Rosai J, Levine CD (1976) Tumor of the thymus. In: Atlas of tumor pathology, 2 d series, Fascicle 13, Washington, DC, Armed Forces Institute of Pathology, p 162

Roseff I, Levine B, Gilbert L (1958) Lipothymoma simulating cardiomegaly: Case Report. Am Heart J 56: 119

Rosenberg JC (1985) Neoplasms of the mediastinum. In: DeVita VT, Hellman S, Rosenberg SA (eds). Cancer Principles and practice of oncology. 2nd. edn. Lippincott, Philadelphia

Rubin M, Mishkin S (1954) The relationship between mediastinal lipomas and the thymus. J Thorac Surg 27: 494

Schanher PW, Hodge GB (1949) Mediastinal Lipoma with inclusion of remnants of thymus gland. Am J Surg 77: 376

Shirkhoda A, Chasen MH, Eftekhari F, Goldman AM, DeCaro LF (1987) MR Imaging of mediastinal thymolipoma. J Comput Assist Tomogr 11: 364

Shub C, Parkin TW, Lie JT (1979) An unusal mediastinal lipoma simulating cardiomegaly. Mayo Clin Proc 54: 60

Sundström C (1976) Thymolipoma simulating cardiomegaly. Upsala J Med Sci 81: 135

Teplick JG, Nedwich A, Haskin ME (1973) Roentgenographic features of thymolipoma. Am J Roentgenol 117: 873

Trites AEW (1966) Thyrolipoma, thymolipoma and pharyngeal lipoma: A syndrome. Canad Med Ass J 95: 1254

Walter E (1982) Computertomographische Diagnostik des Thymus. In: Lissner J, Doppman JL (Hrsg) CT 82, Internationales Computertomographie Symposium, Seefeld/Tirol. Schnetztor, Konstanz

Walter E, Hübener KH (1980) Computertomographische Charakteristika raumfordernder Prozesse im vorderen Mediastinum und ihre Differentialdiagnose. ROFO 133: 391

Weingarten W, Gordon G (1955) Thymoma: diagnosis and treatment. Ann Int Med 42: 283

Winarso P, Isherwood I, Photiou S, Donnelly RJ (1982) Short reports. Thymolipoma simulating cardiomegaly: use of computed tomography in diagnosis. Thorax 37: 941

Yeh H-C, Gordon A, Kirschner PA, Cohen BA (1983) Computed tomography and sonography of thymolipoma. AJR 140: 1131

8.6 Germ Cell Tumors and Teratomas

E. WALTER

Primary extragonadal germ cell tumors occur along the midline of the body. It is claimed that they can originate from the thymus, although the histogenesis has not yet been completely clarified. The following mechanism is suspected: During the course of embryogenesis the urogenital ridge extends from C6 to L4. This ridge lies very close to the thymus so that germ cells can migrate to the organ (COHEN et al. 1988). While OTTO and HÜSSELMANN (1978) and ROSENBERG (1985) recognize the thymus as a source of germ cell tumors, OTTO (1984) classifies the latter within the group of tumors that are of differential diagnostic importance. Leaving aside the question of their primary origin, the fact that germ cell tumors do occur within the thymus makes it appropriate that they be discussed here.

Various histologic appearances of germ cell tumors have been described (see Sect. 8.6.1). Since, moreover, mediastinal seminomas are mentioned much more frequently in the literature than nonseminomatous, pure or mixed germ cell tumors, pure primary mediastinal seminomas and nonseminomatous germ cell tumors should be distinguished and considered separately, as suggested by MARTINI et al. (1974).

8.6.1 Pathologic Anatomy

W. J. HOFMANN and H. F. OTTO

Germ cell tumors (and teratomas) are a group of neoplasms that characteristically arise from the testes and ovaries. They are though to arise from primitive cells that differentiate into embryonic and extraembryonic structures, resulting in a spectrum of benign and malignant neoplasms that are listed in Table 8.10.

Teratomas (GONZALEZ-CRUSSI 1982) are neoplasms composed of several tissue components that recapitulate abnormally the development of all embryonic layers (ectoderm, endoderm, and mesoderm).

It is well known that tumors of germ cell origin and teratomas can appear in extragonadal location. As mentioned above, they are usually situated along the body midline, in the mediastinum, retroperitoneum, sacrococcygeal area, or pineal body.

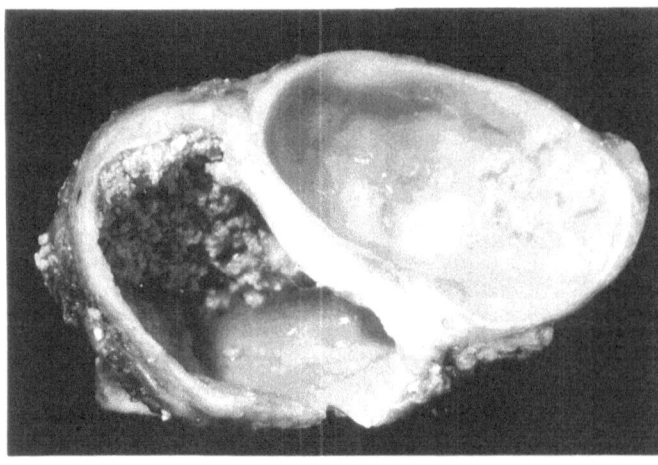

Fig. 8.49. Mature teratoma of the anterior mediastinum ($8 \times 7 \times 5$ cm). The double-spaced tumor contained a yellowish fluid, sebaceous material, and hairs

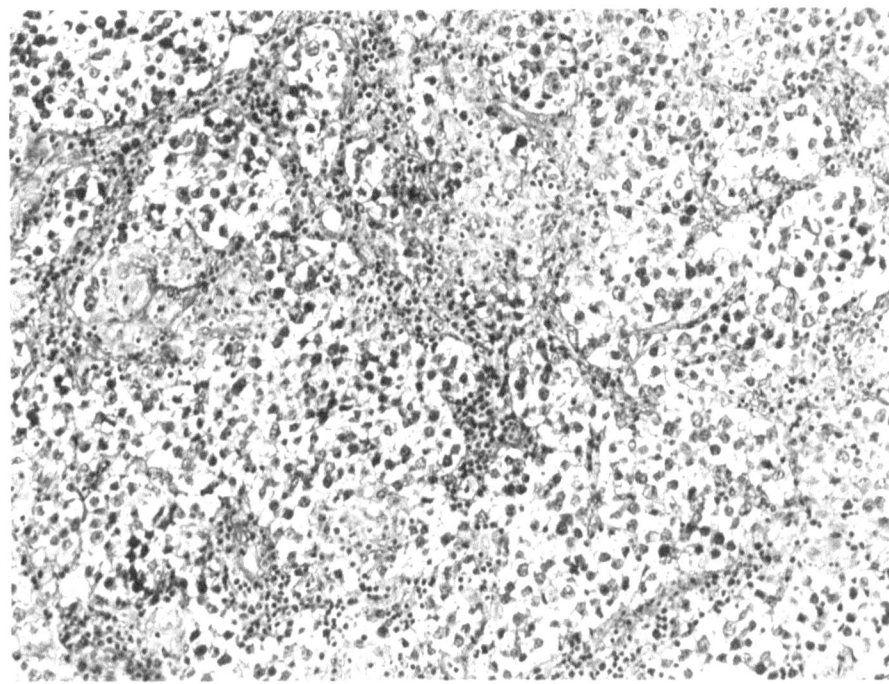

△

Fig. 8.50. Seminomatous tumor of the mediastinum. Sheets of loosely cohesive tumor cells are surrounded by lymphocytes. Note the granulomatous reaction. H&E, ×200

Fig. 8.51. Yolk sac carcinoma (endodermal sinus tumor) of the mediastinum. PAS, ×270. *Inset:* Schiller-Duval body. PAS ×320
▽

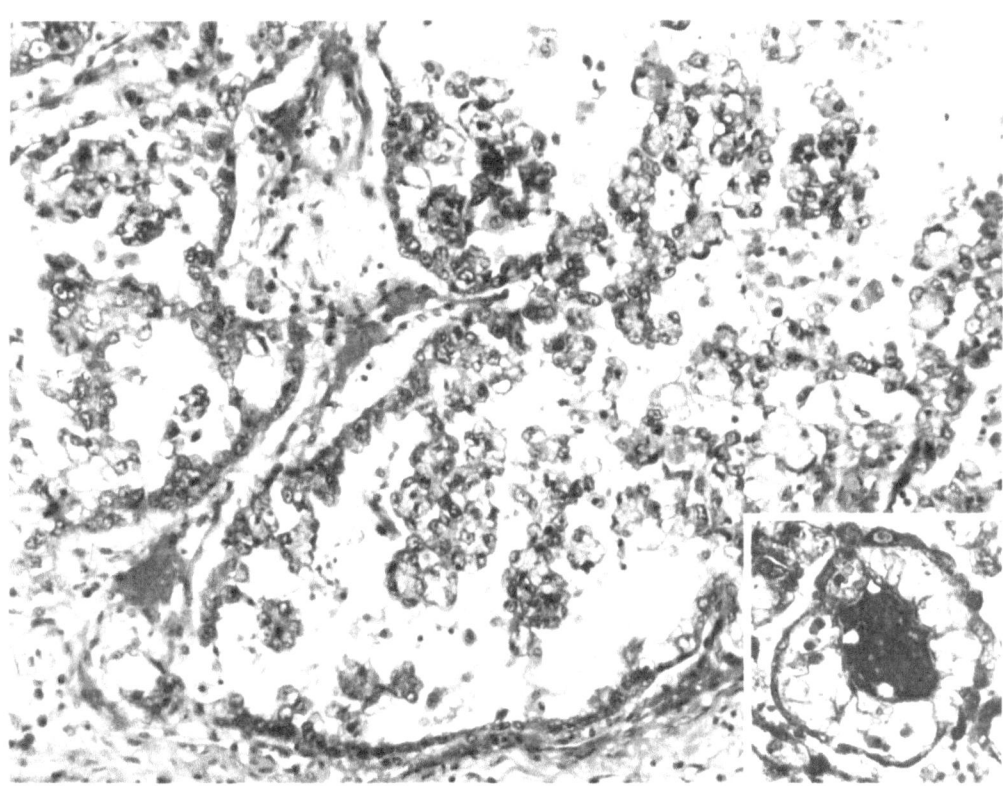

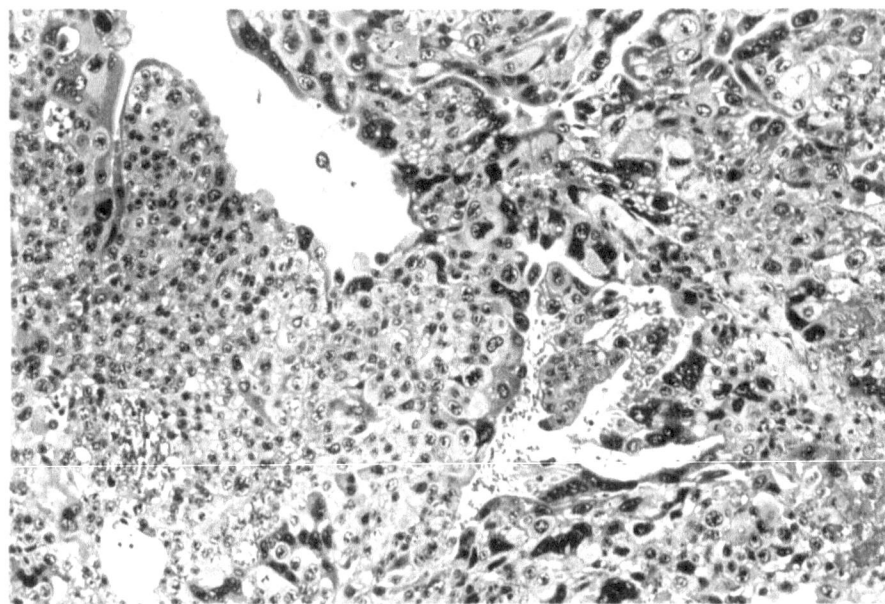

Fig. 8.52. Mediastinal choriocarcinoma. Large clusters of cytotrophoblastic cells alternate with elongated syncytiotrophoblastic component. H&E, ×180

The mediastinum is one of the most frequent sites of origin of extragonadal germ cell tumors and teratomas. Approximately 20% of all anterior superior mediastinal tumors and cysts are germ cell tumors. All microscopic variants of germ cell tumors have been found in the mediastinum, including mature (Fig. 8.49) and malignant teratoma (teratocarcinoma), seminoma (Fig. 8.50) (dysgerminoma), embryonal carcinoma, endodermal sinus tumor (yolk sac tumor) (Fig. 8.51), choriocarcinoma (Fig. 8.52), and mixed germ cell tumors. These mediastinal germ cell tumors have the same pathologic features as their gonadal counterparts.

Seminoma (Fig. 8.50) is the most common tumor type. It represents 25%–30% of all malignant mediastinal germ cell tumors. It has often been described as seminomatous thymoma, pseudoseminomatous thymoma, primary thymic seminoma, or seminoma-like tumor of the thymus.

Germ cell tumors of the mediastinum are often misinterpreted as metastatic, poorly differentiated carcinomas. In questionable cases, the tumor material should be examined by immunhistologic techniques to detect specific tumor markers [e.g., α-fetoprotein (AFP) and/or human chorionic gonadotropin (hCG)].

8.6.2 Seminoma

E. WALTER

8.6.2.1 Occurrence and Clinical Symptoms

Seminomas, also referred to as "seminomatous thymomas" (OTTO and HÜSSELMANN 1978), are the most common mediastinal germ cell tumor (HURT et al. 1982; OTTO 1984). Approximately 40% of germ cell tumors of the thymus are pure seminomas. BESZNYAK et al. (1973) listed all cases published to that date (74 cases, cited according to author); up to 1979, 103 cases had been reported in the English-language literature (compilation by POLANSKY et al. 1979). In the review of thymic tumors by OTTO and HÜSSELMANN (1978), 1.8% were reported to be primary mediastinal seminomas.

A review of our own cases and of the literature (POLANSKY et al. 1979), as well as of those cases re-

Table 8.10. Histopathologic variants of germ cell tumors/teratomas

Teratoma
  Mature, solid
  Cystic (dermoid cyst)
  Immature
  Malignant (teratocarcinoma)
  Mixed

Seminoma (dysgerminoma)

Embryonal carcinoma

Endodermal sinus tumor (yolk sac tumor)

Choriocarcinoma

Mixed germ cell tumor

ported by WALTER (1982), LIVESAY et al. (1979), and others, revealed all primary mediastinal seminomas to be located within the anterior superior mediastinum. To date there have been no reports of "seminomatous thymoma" in a dystopic thymus.

Men between the age of 20 and 40 years are most frequently affected (SCHANTZ et al. 1972; COX 1975; STERCHI and CORDELL 1975); up to 5% of cases occur in women (POLANSKY et al. 1979). Among 107 patients with primary mediastinal seminomas, six were women.

According to POLANSKY et al. (1979) and HURT et al. (1982), between 15% and 30% of primary mediastinal seminomas are asymptomatic; such cases are discovered accidentally on chest radiographs in two planes. In addition to general symptoms such as tiredness and weight loss there are also specific symptoms caused by compression and infiltration of mediastinal organs, i.e., thoracic pressure symptoms (retrosternally and radiating into the arm), thoracic pain, cough, dyspnea, hoarseness, and dysphagia (COX 1975; HURT et al. 1982; SLAWSON et al. 1983; and others).

Obstruction of the superior vena cava with venous congestion, which is often the first clinical symptom, is observed in 10% of patients (POLANSKY et al. 1979). Unlike patients with thymomas, those with primary mediastinal seminoma do not suffer from myasthenia gravis of systemic thymic-related disease (SHIELDS et al. 1966; POLANSKY et al. 1979).

In the case of "impure" seminomas, i.e., when there is admixture with germ cell tumors of other histology, hormones originating from within the tumor can give rise to clinical signs or symptoms such as gynecomastia.

Unlike thymomas, mediastinal seminomas often metastasize. Metastasis most frequently occurs to the regional and supraclavicular lymph nodes, the lungs, and the skeleton (BESNYAK et al. 1973; COX 1975; POLANSKY et al. 1979; HURT et al. 1982), but may also occur to the liver (HURT et al. 1982), the spleen (STEINMETZ and HAYS 1961), the tonsils (STEINMETZ and HAYS 1961), the thyroid (KOUNTZ et al. 1963), the adrenal gland (STEINMETZ and HAYS 1961), skin (WOOLNER et al. 1955), spinal cord (EL-DOMEIRI et al. 1968; BESZNYAK et al. 1973), and brain (HURT et al. 1982). Diffuse abdominal carcinomatosis has also been reported (HURT et al. 1982).

8.6.2.2 Diagnosis with Imaging Procedures

8.6.2.2.1 Conventional Radiologic Procedures

On conventional radiographs the appearance of primary mediastinal seminoma closely resembles that of a thymoma or lymph node tumor (Figs. 8.53 a–c, 8.54 a). Thus WALTER and HÜBENER (1980) and WALTER (1982) described mediastinal enlargement at a typical location.

Additional information is not to be expected from the use of conventional tomography (WALTER 1982), particularly since calcification within the tumor cannot always be recognized on conventional tomograms (POLANSKY et al. 1979). The informational content delivered by modern computed tomography (CT) far exceeds that provided by conventional tomography (GRAEBER et al. 1984). Displacement of the trachea dorsally (O'GARA et al. 1958; OBERMAN and LIBCKE 1964; KLEITSCH et al. 1967) or of the bronchi (KLEITSCH et al. 1967; NICKELS and FRANSSILA 1972; LARMI and KÄRKÖLÄ 1974) has been reported as a tumor-related finding. Such displacement can be visualized by means of conventional tomography but this can equally be achieved with CT.

Since obstruction of the superior vena cava with venous congestion is the first clinical symptom in 10% of patients (POLANSKY et al. 1979), superior venacavography is a conventional procedure that retains some significance even today. Angiographic findings have been reported by DÜX (1977) (Fig. 8.54).

8.6.2.2.2 Ultrasonography

No findings have been reported in the literature.

8.6.2.2.3 Computed Tomography

Computed tomographic findings in respect of primary mediastinal seminomas were first reported by LIVESAY et al. (1979), WALTER and HÜBENER (1980), WALTER (1982), and HURT et al. (1982).

Pathoanatomically, such tumors are solid and appear relatively homogeneous; owing to their infiltrative growth they display a poorly defined border. Cystic regression seldom occurs, but necroses and hemorrhages are common.

In accordance with the brief preceding description of its pathoanatomic characteristics, primary mediastinal seminoma usually presents as an ir-

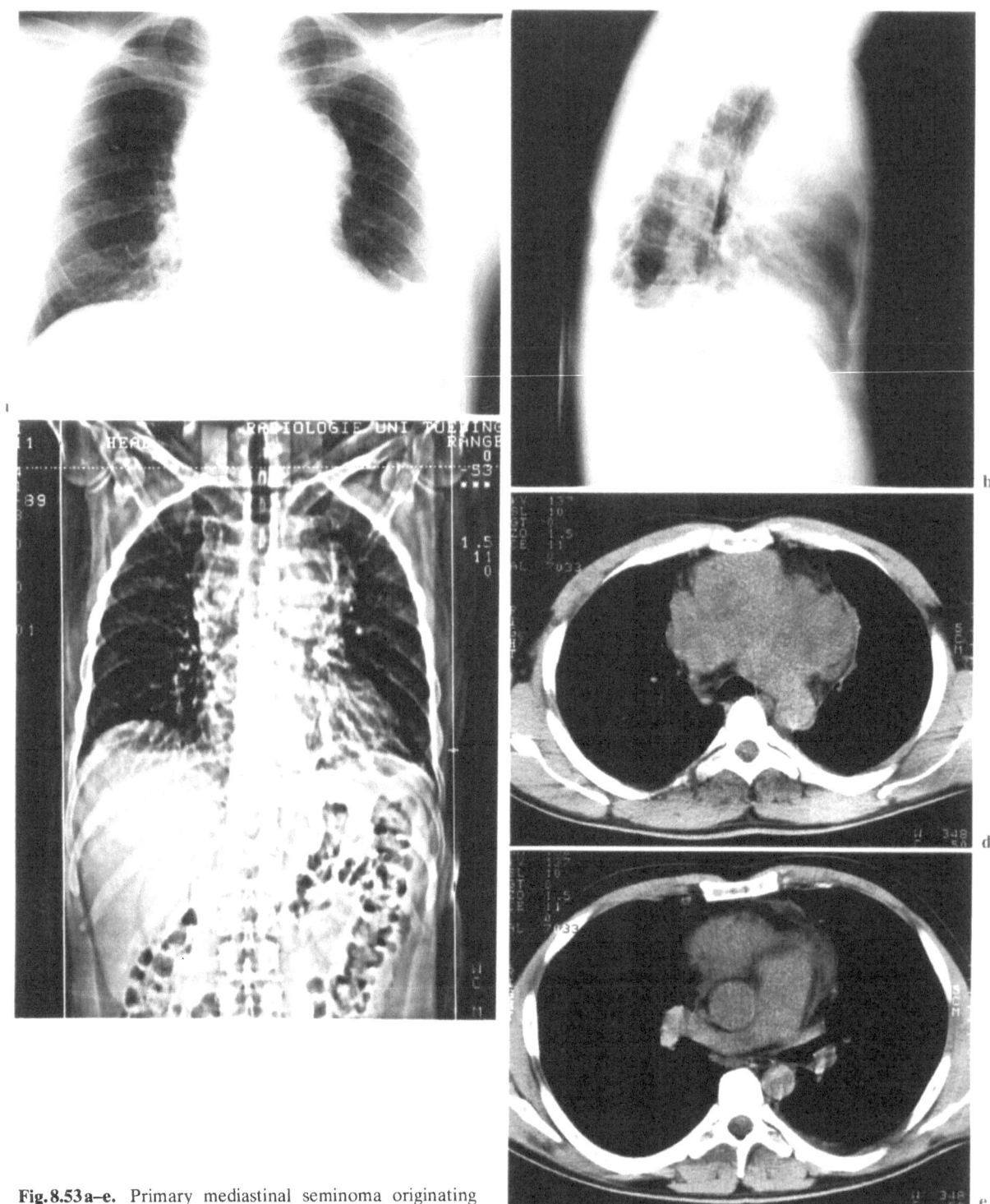

Fig. 8.53 a–e. Primary mediastinal seminoma originating from the thymus in a 39-year-old man. **a,b** Chest radiograph in two planes in the standing position. Pronounced mediastinal enlargement is evident; according to the lateral film this enlargement concerns the anterior superior mediastinum. Accompanying effusion is present on the left. **c** Digital radiography. Again, it is not possible to distinguish the tumor from the remaining mediastinal structures. No additional information that might be of use in differential diagnosis is provided. **d,e** Computed tomography of the chest. **d** An irregularly bordered mass is situated anterior to the trachea. A few small hypodense areas are present as an expression of necrotic tissue. There is extensive contact between the mass and the arch of the aorta, so that infiltration of its wall must be assumed. **e** Plane of section through the pulmonary trunk. There are signs of percardial infiltration

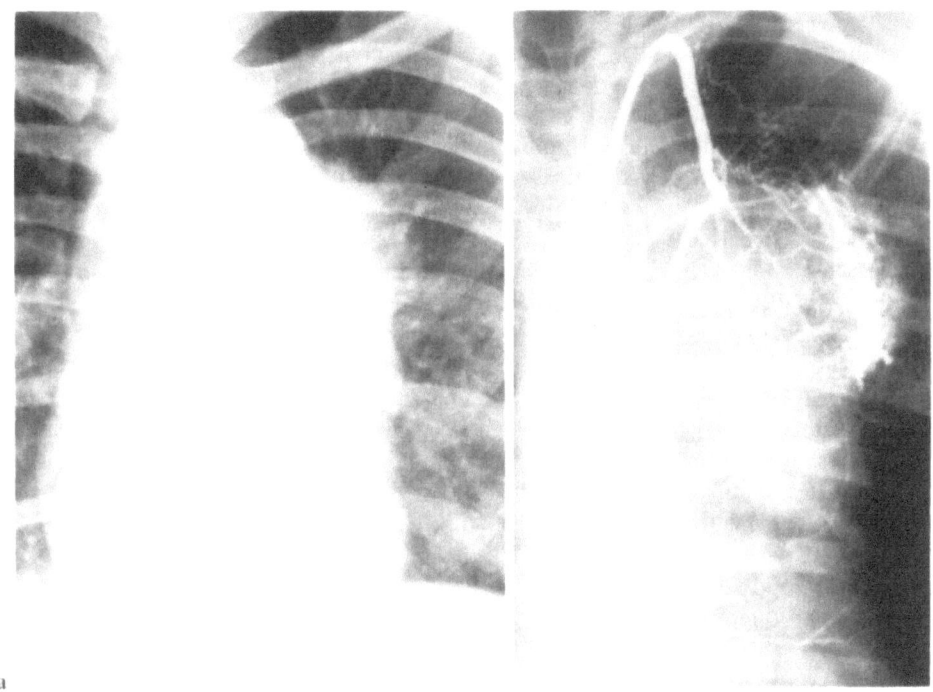

a   b

regularly bordered mass in the anterior superior mediastinum, at the typical position of the thymus between the sternum and the ascending thoracic aorta or the arch of the aorta (Fig. 8.53 d). It displaces mediastinal structures and its margins may be unclear as an expression of its infiltrative growth. Infiltration of adjacent structures such as blood vessels and the pericardium has been described (LIVESAY et al. 1979; WALTER 1982) (Fig. 8.53 e).

The attenuation values, at ca. 40 HU, correspond not only to those of the surrounding musculature but also to those of thymomas and lymph node conglomerate tumors. The standard deviation of ± 10 HU (cf. LIVESAY et al. 1979) is relatively high, this being attributable to the abovementioned necroses and hemorrhages that are frequently observed. After bolus administration of a water-soluble contrast medium, diffuse enhancement with values of ca. 20–30 HU occurs in areas of vital tumor tissue (SCHNYDER and CANDARDJIS 1987). The administration of a water-soluble contrast medium does not, however, help further in differential diagnosis against other tumors.

LEVINE and ROSAI (1978) report that seminomas originating from the thymus occasionally display polycystic, i.e., clearly marginated malacia, although according to the pathologist OTTO (1984) such a feature is rare. GRAEBER et al. (1984) de-

Fig. 8.54 a, b. Mediastinal seminoma in a 16-year-old male. **a** Posteroanterior chest radiograph showing a mediastinal mass. **b** Selective angiography of the left internal thoracic artery reveals a heterogeneously vascularized tumor and neovascularization. Again there are no pathognomonic findings that would permit the diagnosis of a primary mediastinal seminoma origination from the thymus. (Case by courtesy of Prof. A. DÜX, Mönchengladbach, FRG)

scribed clinical examples of cysts within seminomas of the thymus. SCHNYDER and CANDARDJIS (1987) have reported that calcifications are frequently found within the tumor, but in the three cases that we ourselves have observed to date, we have not once seen cysts, necrotic malacia, or calcifications.

8.6.2.2.4 Magnetic Resonance Imaging

No reports are as yet available on the use of this technique.

8.6.2.2.5 Nuclear Medicine

In rare cases, marked uptake of gallium 67 within the tumor has been reported (POLANSKY et al. 1979).

8.6.2.3 Differential Diagnosis and Relative Value of the Imaging Procedures

Conventional radiography does not permit distinction between mediastinal seminoma and masses of other origin, with the exception of arterial aneurysms.

In the absence of pseudocystic changes, cysts, or calcifications, CT, too, does not permit differential diagnosis between mediastinal seminoma and a conglomerate tumor of lymph nodes (malignant lymphoma, lymph node metastases) (WALTER and HÜBENER 1980). The CT findings are consequently unspecific (SCHNYDER and CANDARDJIS 1987), and distinction from a thymoma can be difficult with both CT and conventional procedures (SCHNYDER and CANDARDJIS 1987). The advantage of CT lies in its ability ot determine the precise size of the mass and its relation to neighboring organs, including, in particular, their infiltration.

8.6.2.4 Therapy and Prognosis

At the time of discovery of the tumor, advanced disease is usually present, with infiltration in the tumor's vicinity. Complete resection of the tumor is consequently possible in only 20% of patients (MARTINI et al. 1974; HURT et al. 1982).

Seminomas are regarded as radiosensitive (BAGSHAW et al. 1969; COX 1975); according to BUSH et al. (1981) 45–60 Gy should be administered within 6 weeks. In such cases a 10-year survival rate of 69% and a recurrence-free survival rate of 54% can be expected. In addition to radiation therapy as the sole method of treatment, primary surgery and surgery combined with subsequent irradiation also come into consideration. Corresponding therapeutic suggestions have been described in detail by BUSH et al. (1981), CLAMON (1983), and SLAWSON et al. (1983).

8.6.3 Nonseminomatous, Pure or Mixed Germ Cell Tumors

Histologically, nonseminomatous germ cell tumors include the following: adult teratomas (including dermoid cysts), embryonal carcinomas (teratocarcinomas), choriocarcinomas (for a review of cases see YURICK and OTTOMAN 1960), and mixed germ cell tumors (see Sect. 8.6.1). Detailed studies have been reported by HUNTINGTON and BULLOCK (1970), SCHANTZ et al. (1972), UTZ and BUSCEMI

(1971), MARTINI et al. (1974), COX (1975), FRIEDMAN et al. (1982), LEVITT et al. (1984), and ROSENBERG (1985).

8.6.3.1 Occurrence and Clinical Symptoms

Nonseminomatous germ cell tumors occur primarily in men. MARTINI et al. (1974) identified 20 not purely seminomatous germ cell tumors between 1949 and 1971, of which 14 were in men. The survey by COX (1975) revealed only 10% of germ cell tumors to occur in women. Clinical manifestation is usually between 20 and 40 years of age (MARTINI et al. 1974; COX 1975; LEVITT et al. 1984), though SAURE and FREYSCHMIDT (1976) reported on a cystic teratoma in a 6-year-old.

Patients with Klinefelter's syndrome are reputed to be particularly prone to suffer from germ cell tumors (RECONDO and LIBSHITZ 1978; CURRY et al. 1981).

As with seminomas, the clinical manifestations of these tumors comprise unspecific symptoms and signs such as pleuralgia or substernal pain, dyspnea, hemoptysis, and tussis, which are caused by tumor-related tracheal constriction. In the case of choriocarcinoma, gynecomastia is present in more than 50% of patients (SICKLES et al. 1974). Approximately 70% of patients with nonseminomatous germ cell tumors are reported to have raised fetoprotein levels (ECONOMOU et al. 1982), and choriocarcinoma is reported to be associated with elevated levels of hCG (JERNSTROM and McLAUGHLIN 1962).

Infiltrations per continuitatem may involve the ribs, pleura, and lungs, but also the regional lymph nodes. In addition metastases to the regional and supraclavicular lymph nodes are observed (COX 1975). According to MARTINI et al. (1974), hematogenous metastases of embryonal carcinoma may occur to the following organs (frequency in percent): lungs (85%), pleura (70%), pericardium (50%), thorax (20%), axillary and cervical lymph nodes (25%), liver (20%), and heart (15%); less frequently, and in descending order of frequency, they occur to the brain, kidneys, bones, and pancreas (cf. also RECONDO and LIBSHITZ 1978). Finally, metastasis to the intestine war reported in one case by SICKLES et al. (1974).

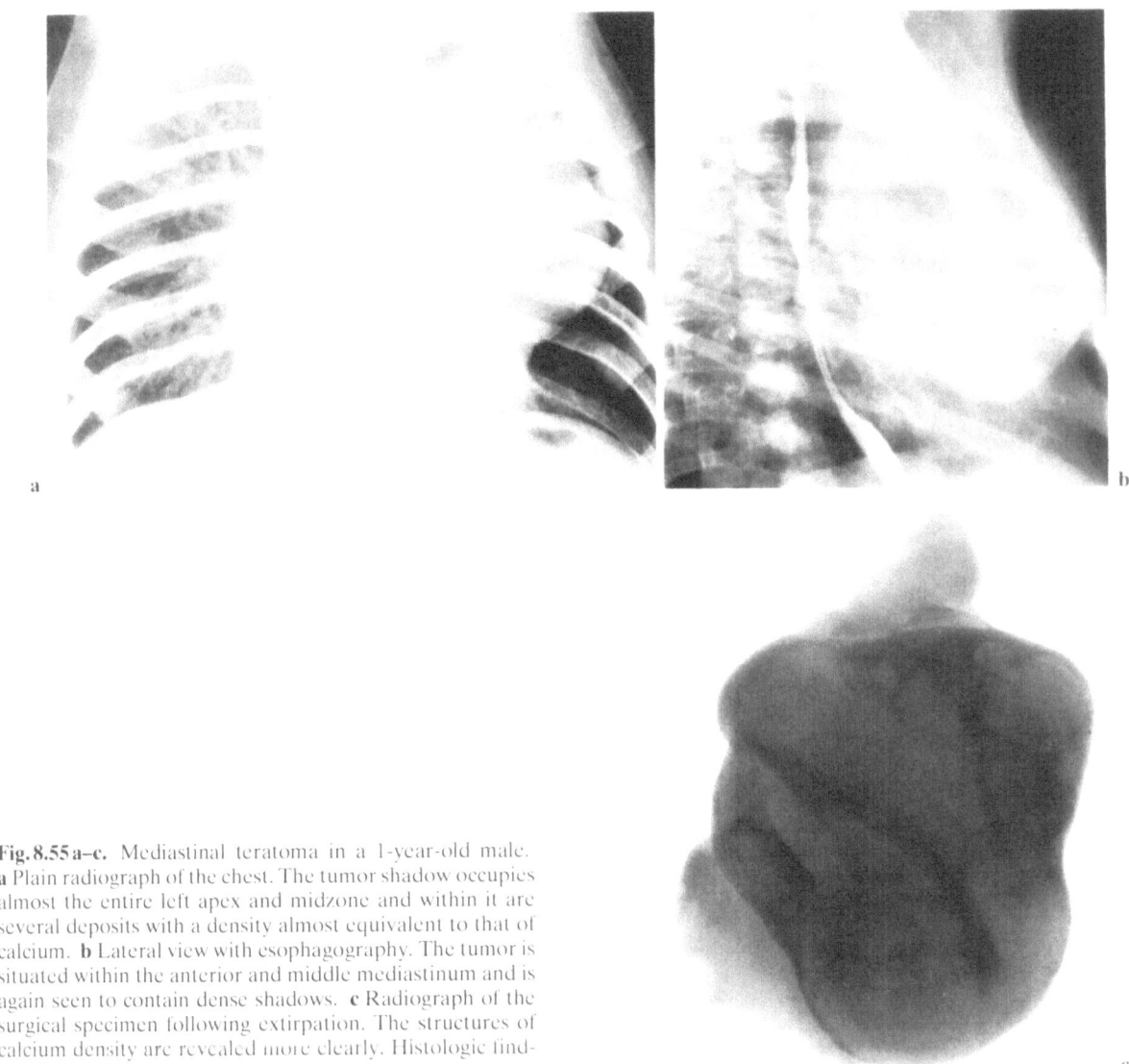

Fig. 8.55 a–c. Mediastinal teratoma in a 1-year-old male. **a** Plain radiograph of the chest. The tumor shadow occupies almost the entire left apex and midzone and within it are several deposits with a density almost equivalent to that of calcium. **b** Lateral view with esophagography. The tumor is situated within the anterior and middle mediastinum and is again seen to contain dense shadows. **c** Radiograph of the surgical specimen following extirpation. The structures of calcium density are revealed more clearly. Histologic finding: benign teratoma

8.6.3.2 Diagnosis with Imaging Procedures

8.6.3.2.1 Conventional Radiologic Procedures

Using chest radiography in two planes one is generally able to recognize large, typically lobulated masses that are clearly differentiated from the lung (Fig. 8.55) and can enlarge both the right and the left mediastinum. As a consequence, tracheal and bronchial displacement is a frequent occurrence (RECONDO and LIBSHITZ 1978). The tumors display a tendency to grow around blood vessels; this can cause constriction, particularly of the venous vessels, which can be demonstrated by means of superior venacavography.

Plain radiographs do not permit differential diagnosis against masses of other origin. Conventional tomography does demonstrate bronchial and tracheal displacement and stenosis, and also occasionally teeth or bones in cases of teratoma or teratocarcinoma.

Osteolytic metastases (TEMPLETON 1961) can usually be easily recognized using conventional radiology.

8.6.3.2.2 Ultrasonography

As yet experience with this technique is lacking.

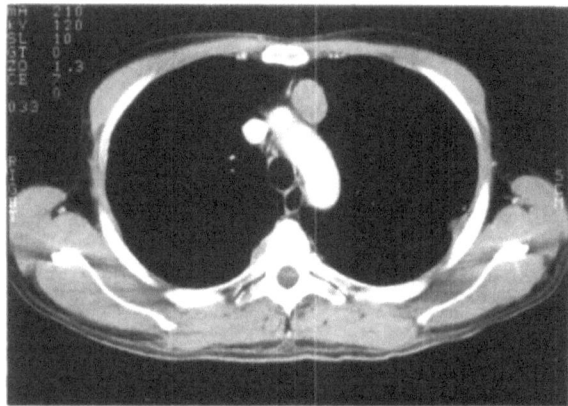

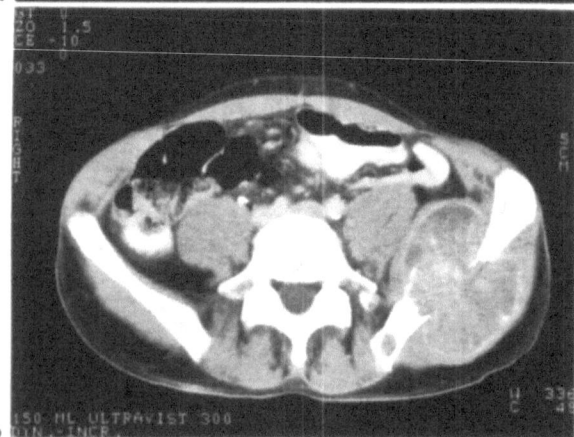

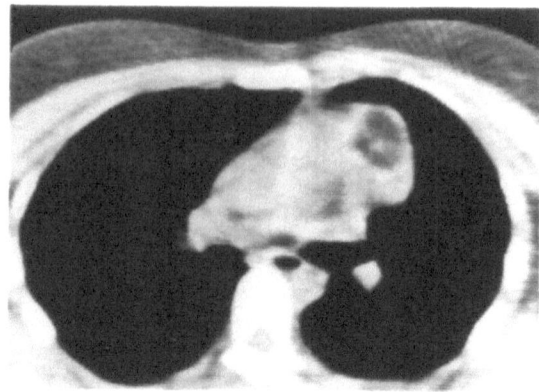

Fig. 8.57. CT appearance of a dermoid cyst containing seba-ceous matter (attenuation values equivalent to those of fat) in a 33-year-old woman. The fatty areas are located in the central portions of the tumor and are surrounded by solid tissue structures. This can be regarded as a differential diag-nostic criterion vis-à-vis thymolipoma (cf. Fig. 8.48)

Fig. 8.56 a, b. Extragonadal germ cell tumor of the mixed type (nonseminomatous) situated primarily in the thymus in a 43-year-old man. **a** CT of the anterior superior mediasti-num: histologically confiremd metastasis in the region of the thymus. **b** Large pelvic metastasis with osseous destruction, compression and infiltration of the gluteal musculature, in-filitration of the iliac muscle, and compression of the psoas muscle anteriorly and medially

8.6.3.2.3 Computed Tomography

The most important report on CT findings in pa-tients with germ cell tumors is that by MORI et al. (1987), but such findings have also been described by BARON et al. (1982), LEVITT et al. (1984), AMOUR et al. (1987), and SCHNYDER and CANDARDJIS (1987). Like all thymogenic tumors, germ cell tu-mors are typically situated in the anterior middle and superior mediastinum (Fig. 8.56 a). At the time of diagnosis the tumor is usually already relatively large and in some cases is also irregularly bor-dered (BARON et al. 1982).

Dermoid cysts (Fig. 8.57), which comprise two germ layers, are usually benign and consequently are clearly defined on CT scans. The cyst wall, which is thick in comparision to that of thymogenic cysts, surrounds an area of fatty tissue correspond-ing to sebaceous matter, the attenuation values of which are similar to those of adult fatty tissue (WALTER and HÜBENER 1980). Calcifications of the cyst wall are possible (PANTOJA et al. 1975).

Benign, noninvasive germ cell tumors of the thy-mus are well defined and almost invariably display a central cystic area with attenuation values of 7–17 HU. The wall of such a tumor is relatively thick (MORI et al. 1987). Malignant, i. e., invasive germ cell tumors are, by contrast, poorly demarcated on CT scans.

The great advantage of CT over conventional procedures lies in its ability to demonstrate tumor infiltration of adjacent mediastinal structures, e. g., the anterior chest wall (LEVITT et al. 1984). Malig-nant germ cell tumors also display inhomogeneous attenuation values owing to the dual presence of solid and cystic structures (MORI et al. 1987). In contrast to conventional procedures, CT reveals all tissues typical for teratomas, i. e., fatty structures, teeth, and bones whereas glands, cartilage, muscle and nerves – in CT isodense – cannot be differen-tiated (TEMPLETON 1961; FRIEDMAN et al. 1982); conventional procedures only permit the recogni-tion of calcified structures. In addition to cystic de-generation and necroses, calcifications are also ob-served in cases of teratoma. According to MORI et al. (1987) such calcifications are to be expected in 70% of patients regardless of whether the tumor is benign or malignant; these calcifications may be plaque-like or shell-like.

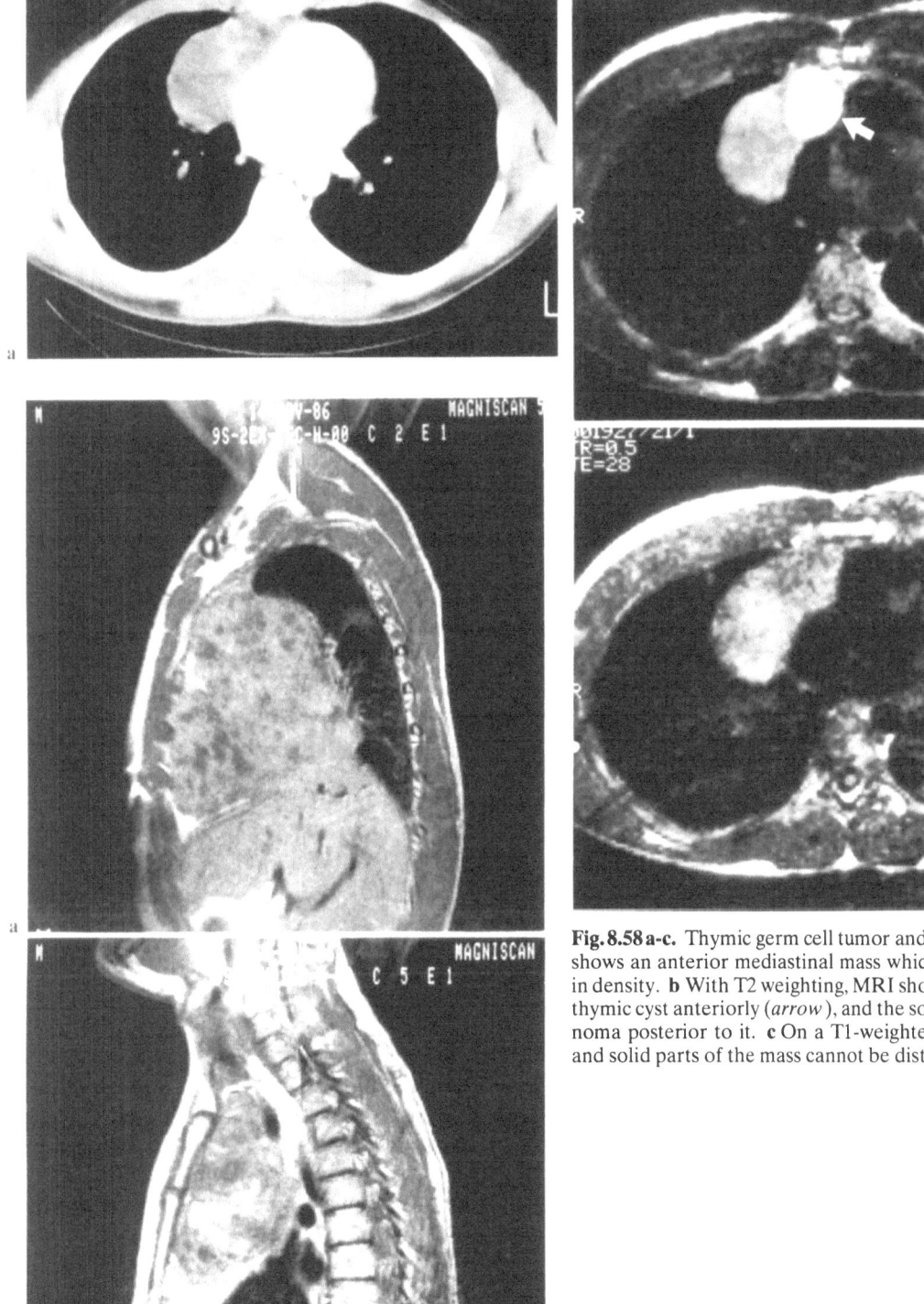

Fig. 8.58 a-c. Thymic germ cell tumor and thymic cyst. **a** CT shows an anterior mediastinal mass which is homogeneous in density. **b** With T2 weighting, MRI shows a high intensity thymic cyst anteriorly (*arrow*), and the solid germ cell carcinoma posterior to it. **c** On a T1-weighted image the cystic and solid parts of the mass cannot be distinguished

Fig. 8.59 a, b. Embryonal carcinoma. **a** T1-weighted sagittal image shows a large inhomogeneous mass. **b** Near the midline, the mass can be seen to be arising in the anterior mediastinum. Pericardial invasion has resulted in hemopericardium (*arrow*)

Osseous metastases from teratomas are osteolytic (TEMPLETON 1961). Depending on the region under investigation they can be discovered simultaneously using CT (in the bone window) (Fig. 8.56 b). Sometimes further clarification by means of ^{99m}Tc-MDP bone survey or conventional radiography is appropriate.

8.6.3.2.4 Magnetic Resonance Imaging

W. R. WEBB and G. DE GEER

In one patient with a thymic germ cell tumor we have studied, a homogeneous appearing mass was visible (Fig. 8.58); it was similar in intensity to other thymic tumors which we have seen, and which have been reported. As with other thymic tumors, germ cell tumors can appear inhomogeneous or cystic (Fig. 8.59).

In one patient with a cystic teratoma who has been reported (SIEGEL et al. 1989), the mass appeared inhomogeneous on both T1- and T2-weighted images. The cystic components of the mass were visible as areas of high intensity on T2-weighted images. Areas of low intensity probably reflected fibrous stroma and areas of calcification.

8.6.3.2.5 Nuclear Medicine

E. WALTER

There is no experience with nuclear medical techniques for diagnosis of the primary tumor. Osteolytic metastases are recognizable on bone scintiscans.

8.6.3.3 Differential Diagnosis and Relative Value of the Imaging Procedures

The following CT signs are suggestive of a germ cell tumor: a relatively large mass in the presence of comparatively low-grade clinical symptomatology, and a tendency towards hemorrhage and necroses. The diagnosis of teratoma is established if teeth and bones can be detected.

Given the heterogeneity of the anatomic structures, retrosternal goiter enters the differential diagnosis. The heterogeneous attenuation values are the result of colloid cysts, solid tissue portions, and areas of calcification. In the presence of retroster-

nal goiter, the organ can be continuously traced on CT scans from its orthotopically positioned portion at the neck into the superior mediastinum (WALTER and HÜBENER 1980). True dystopia is extremely rare, having an incidence of 0.1%–0.3% (JACKSON 1953; STREICHER 1957). Thyroidal scintigraphy is also capable of yielding findings of use in differential diagnosis. Owing to the cystic changes that are particularly evident with benign germ cell tumors, consideration must be given to a dysontogenetic thymic cyst. The wall of such a cyst is typically uniformly 1–2 mm thick, and only localized thymic remnants can be demonstrated.

Areas of calcification, cystic degeneration, and necroses are also to be found with thymomas, particularly invasive forms. Differential diagnosis can be impossible on the basis of the radiographic appearance, and the clinical syndromes that accompany thymomas, such as myasthenia gravis, must be taken into consideration. Elevated fetoprotein levels or gynecomastia as a sign of hormone release from a choriocarcinoma are unknown in patients with thymoma.

Carcinoids tend still to be small at the time of clinical diagnosis, which typically is made at an early stage owing to their characteristic hormone release (LEVITT et al. 1984). Malignant lymphomas customarily display neither hemorrhage nor necrosis.

Chest radiography in two planes is the basis for diagnosis. It should be followed immediately by CT; administration of a water-soluble contrast medium, however, provides no further information of relevance for differential diagnosis. The value of CT resides in its demonstration of the germ cell tumor itself and of its topographic relationship to adjacent organs, in the proof it offers of malignancy, recognizable by virtue of the infiltrative growth, and in its demonstration on metastases to the lungs, liver, and lymph nodes. In addition, CT has acquired a central role in the planning of radiation therapy. Unequivocal histologic classification of a tumor in the anterior mediastinum is not possible with the diagnostic imaging procedures currently available, instead requiring either fine needle biopsy or exploratory thoracotomy.

8.6.3.4 Therapy and Prognosis

Nonseminomatous germ cell tumors are not quite as radiosensitive as purely seminomatous tumors. Permanent cure cannot be achieved despite the relatively good radiosensitivity, and the average length of survival is only 7 months (MARTINI et al. 1974) owing to early metastasis (SICKLES et al. 1974). Survival is also very limited when chemotherapy is employed (COX 1975).

References

Amour TES, Siegel MJ, Glazer HS, Nadel SN (1981) CT appearance of the normal and abnormal thymus in childhood. J Comput Assist Tomogr 11: 645

Bagshaw MA, McLaughlin WT, Earle JD (1969) Definitive radiotherapy of primary mediastinal seminoma. AJR 105: 86

Baron RL, Lee JKT, Sagel SS, Levitt RG (1982) Computed tomography of the abnormal thymus. Radiology 142: 127

Besznyák I, Sebestény M, Kuchár F (1973) Primary mediastinal seminoma. A case report and review of literature. J Thorac Cardiovasc Surg 65: 930

Bush SE, Martinez A, Bagshaw MA (1981) Primary mediastinal seminoma. Cancer 48: 1877

Clamon GH (1983) Management of primary mediastinal seminoma. Chest 83: 263

Cohen II, Templeton A, Philips AK (1988) Tumors of the thymus. Med Pediatr Oncol 16: 135

Cox JD (1975) Primary malignant germinal tumors of the mediastinum. A study of 24 cases. Cancer 36: 1162

Curry WA, McKay CE, Richardson RL, Greco FA (1981) Klinefelter's syndrome and mediastinal germ cell neoplasms. J Urol 125: 127

Düx A (1977) Mediastinum. In: Teschendorf W, Anakker H, Thurn P (eds) Röntgenologische Differentialdiagnostik, vol I, part 2. Thieme, Stuttgart

Economou JS, Trump DL, Holmes EC, Eggleston JE (1982) Management of primary germ cell tumors of the mediastinum. J Thorac Cardiovasc Surg 83: 643

El-Domeiri AA, Hutter RVP, Pool JL, Foote FW Jr (1968) Primary seminoma of anterior mediastinum. Ann Thorac Surg 6: 513

Friedman AC, Pyatt RS, Hartman DS, Downey EF Jr, Olson WB (1982) CT of benign cystic teratomas. AJR 138: 659

Gonzalez-Crussi F (1982) Extragonadal teratomas. Atlas of tumor pathology, second series, fascicle 18. Armed Forces Institute of Pathology, Washington DC

Graeber GM, Thompson LD, Cohen DJ, Ronnigen LD, Jaffin J, Zajtchuk R (1984) Cystic lesion of the thymus. J Thorac Cardiovasc Surg 87: 295

Huntington RW, Bullock WK (1970) Yolk sac tumors of extragonadal origin. Cancer 25: 1368

Hurt RD, Bruckman JE, Farrow GM, Bernatz PE, Hahn RG, Earle JD (1982) Primary anterior mediastinal seminoma. Cancer 49: 1658

Jackson AS (1953) Intrathoracic goiter. J Int Coll Surg 20: 485

Jernstrom P, McLaughlin H (1962) Choriocarcinoma of the thymus. JAMA 182: 147

Kleitsch WP, Taricco A, Haslam GJ (1967) Primary seminoma (germinoma) of the mediastinum. Ann Thorac Surg 4: 249

Kountz SL, Connolly JE, Cohn R (1963) Seminoma-like (or seminomatous) tumors of the anterior mediastinum. J Thorac Cardiovasc Surg 45: 289

Larmi TKI, Kärkölä P (1974) Mediastinal seminoma. Ann Chir Gynaecol Fenniae 63: 351

Levine GD, Rosai J (1978) Thymic hyperplasia and neoplasia: a review of current concepts. Hum Pathol 9: 495

Levitt RG, Husband JE, Glazer HS (1984) CT of primary germ-cell tumors of the mediastinum. AJR 142: 73

Livesay JJ, Mink JH, Fee HJ, Bein ME, Sample WF, Mulder DG (1979) The use of computed tomography to evaluate suspected mediastinal tumors. Ann Thorac Surg 27: 305

Martini N, Golbey RB, Hajdu SI, Whitmore WF, Beattie EJ (1974) Primary mediastinal germ cell tumors. Cancer 33: 763

Mori K, Eguchi K, Moriyama H, Miyazawa N, Kodama T (1987) Computed tomography of anterior mediastinal tumors. Differentiation between thymoma and germ cell tumor. Acta Radiol 28: 395

Nickels J, Franssila K (1972) Primary seminoma of the anterior mediastinum. Acta Pathol Microbiol Scand [A] 80: 260

Oberman HA, Libcke JH (1964) Malignant germinal neoplasms of the mediastinum. Cancer 17: 498

O'Gara RW, Horn RC, Enterline HT (1958) Tumors of the anterior mediastinum. Cancer 11: 562

Otto HF (1984) Pathologie des Thymus. In: Doerr W, Seifert G (eds) Spezielle pathologische Anatomie, vol 17. Springer, Berlin Heidelberg New York

Otto HF, Hüsselmann H (1978) Klinisch-pathologische Studie zur Klassifikation und Prognose von Thymustumoren. Teil I. Histologische und ultrastrukturpathologische Untersuchungen. Z Krebsforsch 91: 81

Pantoja E, Wendth AJ, Cross VF (1975) Radiographic manifestations of teratoma. NY State J Med 75: 2353

Polansky SM, Barwick KW, Ravin CE (1979) Primary mediastinal seminoma. AJR 132: 17

Recondo J, Libshitz HI (1978) Mediastinal extragonadal germ cell tumors. Urology 11: 369

Rosai JG, Levine ED (1976) Tumors of the thymus. Atlas of tumor pathology, second series, fascicle 13. Armed Forces Institute of Pathology, Washington DC, p 1

Rosenberg JC (1985) Neoplasms of the mediastinum. In: De Vita VT, Hellman S, Rosenberg SA (eds) Cancer. Principles and practice of oncology, 2nd edn. Lippincott, Philadelphia

Saure D, Freyschmidt J (1976) Verbreiterung des Herzschattens durch ein Teratom im Thymus. Z Kinderchir 19: 197

Schantz A, Sewall W, Castleman B (1972) Mediastinal germinoma. A study of 21 cases with an excellent prognosis. Cancer 30: 1189

Schnyder P, Candardjis G (1987) Computed tomography of thymic abnormalities. Eur J Radiol 7: 107

Shields TW, Fox RT, Lees WM (1966) Thymic tumors. Classification and treatment. Arch Surg 92: 617

Sickles EA, Belliveau RE, Wiernik PH (1974) Primary mediastinal choriocarcinoma in the male. Cancer 33: 1196

Siegel MJ, Glazer HS, Wiener JI, Molina PL (1989) Normal and abnormal thymus in childhood: MR imaging. Radiology 172: 367

Slawson R, Aygun C, Carbone D, Hafiz M, Attar S, Whitley N (1983) Primary mediastinal seminoma. RadioGraphics 3: 100

Steinmetz WH, Hays RA (1961) Primary seminoma of the mediastinum. Report of case with an unusual site of metastasis and review of the literature. AJR 86: 669

Sterchi M, Cordell AR (1975) Seminoma of the anterior mediastinum. Ann Thorac Surg 19: 371

Streicher A (1957) Substernale Strumen. Langenbecks Arch Klin Chir 287: 201

Templeton AW (1961) Malignant mediastinal teratoma with bone metastases. Radiology 76: 245

Utz DC, Buscemi MF (1971) Extragonadal testicular tumors. J Urol 105: 271

Walter E (1982) Computertomographische Diagnostik des Thymus. In: Lissner J, Doppman JL (eds) CT 82, Internationales Comutertomographie Symposium, Seefeld/Tirol. Schnetztor, Konstanz

Walter E, Hübener K-H (1980) Computertomographische Charakteristika raumfordernder Prozesse im vorderen Mediastinum und ihre Differentialdiagnose. ROFO 133: 391

Woolner LB, Jamplis RW, Kirklin JW (1955) Seminoma (germinoma) apparently primary in the anterior mediastinum. N Engl J Med 252: 653

Yurick BS, Ottoman RE (1960) Primary mediastinal chorioncarcinoma. Radiology 75: 901

8.7 Rare Tumors of the Thymus

According to a survey by TESSERAUX (1953), benign tumors such as fibroma, lipoma, myxoma, xanthoma, myxolipoma, lymphangioma, lymphoendothelioma, reticuloma, and epithelioma are all rare. No results in respect of these tumors have been recorded in radiologic papers in recent years; thus no experience of modern examination techniques is available. However, hemangioma of the thymus does constitute a sole exception to the foregoing.

8.7.1 Hemangioma of the Thymus

According to a literature survey by COHEN et al. (1987), to that date 103 hemangiomas had been well documented within the mediastinum. They account for only 1.08% of mediastinal tumors and are usually to be found in the anterior mediastinum (WASSNER et al. 1970).

BRICCOLI et al. (1974) reported 58 hemangiomas from the literature. The topographic anatomy was only given in 29 cases; 25 of these tumors were located in the anterior mediastinum. No connection to the thymus was reported. LYONS et al. (1959) found only one hemangioma (of the myocardium) among 782 mediastinal tumors.

Hemangioma of the thymus is thus rarely observed. BROWN et al. (1983), LUNGENSCHMID et al. (1990), and NIEDZWIECKI and WOOD (1990) all report only one case. The principal clinical symp-

toms in the $2^1/_2$-year-old child reported by NIEDZWIECKI and WOOD (1990) were recurrent bronchitis and pneumonia. The case reported by LUNGENSCHMID et al. (1990) was accidentally discovered on a routine chest radiograph of a patient suffering from an extended influenzal infection. BROWN et al. (1983) examined by means of CT 11 cases with tumors interpreted as thymoma in patients suffering from myasthenia, and found only one cavernous hemangioma of the thymus.

Chest radiography in two planes shows a nonspecific tumors within the mediastinum. In the patient reported by LUNGENSCHMID et al. (1990) extensive calcifications up to 0.5 cm in diameter could be seen; morphologically these could be described as phleboliths. The tumor described by NIEDZWIECKI and WOOD (1990) was misinterpreted as a large thymus in the still small child.

On CT scans hemangiomas of the thymus are typically seen to lie in the anterior mediastinum between the ascending thoracic aorta and the sternum.

The hemangioma described by BROWN et al. (1983) showed a CT appearance similar to that of a thymoma so that the tumor was diagnosed as such. Thus a bolus of contrast medium was not administered. The cavernous hemangioma of the thymus described by LUNGENSCHMID et al. (1990) was seen on CT to be a tumor of inhomogeneous density. The calcifications (phleboliths) already seen on the plain film could be recognized on the CT scan. As would be expected on the basis of experience with CT to date, the administration of contrast medium produced clear enhancement. Only SIEGEL et al. (1989) and NIEDZWIECKI and WOOD (1990) report experience with magnetic resonance imaging. SIEGEL et al. (1989) reported one patient with a thymic hemangioma in whom both high and low intensity areas were evident within the tumor on T2-weighted images; the former probably reflected cystic areas within the tumor, and the latter possibly fibrous stroma or septa. NIEDZWIECKI and WOOD (1990) found a tumor well demarcated from the neighboring mediastinal structures. The tumor was of an inhomogeneous structure with isointense and hyperintense regions representing vessels with slow (hyperintense) flow and solid tissue. There was no invasion of neighboring structures. No results of angiographic methods are available.

8.7.2 Choristoma of the Thymus

Choristoma also ranks among the rare tumors of the thymus (BRECKLER and JOHNSTON 1956; ROSAI and LEVINE 1976). It is a tumor that not only shows cystically altered thymic tissue but also contains salivary and parathyroid tissue.

On conventional chest radiography in two planes the patient described by BRECKLER and JOHNSTON (1956) showed an ipsilateral effusion. On drainage a tumor could be seen that had a smooth surface and filled almost the whole of the right hemithorax. The tumor was of a homogeneous density. Differentiating procedures such as tomography, pneumomediastography, and angiography were not performed.

Ultrasonographic, CT, and MRI results are not yet available in respect of choristoma of the thymus.

References

Breckler IA, Johnston DG (1956) Choristoma of the thymus. AMA J Dis Child 92: 175

Briccoli A, Guernelli N, Mastrorilli R, Vecchi R (1974) Gli Emolinfoangiomi Mediastinici. Arch Chir Torac Cardiovasc 31: 175

Brown LR, Muhm JR, Sheedy PF, Unni KK, Bernatz PE, Hermann RC (1983) The value of computed tomography in myasthenia gravis. AJR 140: 31

Cohen AJ, Sbaschnig RJ, Hochholzer L, Lough FC, Albus RA (1987) Mediastinal hemangiomas. Ann Thorac Surg 43: 656

Lungenschmid D, Schöpf R, Dietze O, Furtschegger A (1990) Computertomographische Diagnose eines kavernösen Thymushämangioms und seine Abgrenzbarkeit gegen andere mediastinale Hämangiome. Röntgenblätter 43: 301

Lyons HA, Calvy GL, Sammons BP (1959) The diagnoses and classification of mediastinal masses. Ann Intern Med 51: 897–932

Niedzwiecki G, Wood BP (1990) Thymic hemangioma. Am J Dis Child 144: 1149

Rosai JG, Levine D (1976) Tumors of the thymus. Atlas of tumor pathology, second series, fascicle 13. Armed Forces Institute of Pathology, Washington DC, p 1

Siegel MJ, Glazer HS, Wiener JI, Molina PL (1989) Normal and abnormal thymus in childhood: MR imaging. Radiology 172: 367

Tesseraux H (1953) Physiologie und Pathologie des Thymus unter besonderer Berücksichtigung der pathologischen Morphologie. Barth, Leipzig

Wassner UJ, Alai H, Helmstadt ER (1970) Geschwülste im Mediastinum. Chirurg 41: 12

8.8 Metastases to the Thymus

Little is known regarding metastatic deposits in the thymus. MIDDLETON (1966) found thymic metastases in ca. 7% of 102 carcinoma patients on whom autopsies were conducted. The primary tumors were reported to be carcinomas of the breast, lung, stomach, and larynx.

A regular feature of these cases was already advanced general tumor dissemination, which was especially evident in the mediastinum.

Reference

Middleton G (1966) Involvement of the thymus by metastatic neoplasms. Br J Cancer 20: 41

9 Tumor-like (Nonneoplastic) Conditions of the Thymus and/or Mediastinum

E. WALTER, E. WILLICH, W. J. HOFMANN, H. F. OTTO, W. R. WEBB, and G. DE GEER

The pathology of nonneoplastic conditions of the thymus and/or mediastinum includes thymic and mediastinal or cervical cysts as well as the various forms of thymic hyperplasia (see Sect. 7.4), giant lymph node hyperplasia [angiofollicular lymph node hyperplasia or Castleman's disease (CASTLE-MAN et al. 1956; ROSAI and LEVINE 1976; OTTO 1984)], inflammatory tumor-like conditions [granulomatous or sclerosing mediastinitis (MARCHEVSKY 1990)], endocrine lesions, and neurogenic and mesenchymal tumors and tumor-like conditions.

9.1 Thymogenic Cysts

9.1.1 Pathologic Anatomy

W. J. HOFMANN and H. F. OTTO

The majority of thymic cysts (for review see LEONG 1990) are probably congenital in origin and derive from persistence of the thymopharyngeal duct. KRECH and co-workers (1954) divided thymic cysts into three groups: inflammatory, congenital, and neoplastic (Table 9.1). Inflammatory cysts of the thymus are very rare (Dubois' abscesses, Bednar's cysts, hydatid disease).

In the mediastinum, thymic cysts are round, whereas in the neck they are elongated and tubular. They are often multiloculated, have a thin fi-

Table 9.1. Thymic cysts (KRECH et al. 1954)

1	Congenital
2	Inflammatory
2.1	Syphilis (Dubois' abscess)
2.2	Tuberculosis
2.3	Hydatid disease
3	Neoplastic
3.1	Cystic thymoma
3.2	Cystic teratoma
3.3	Lymphangioma
3.4	Hemangioma

Table 9.2. Mediastinal cysts

1	*Congenital*
	Bronchogenic (tracheobronchogenic)
	Esophageal
	Tracheoesophagaeal
	Gastroenteric
	Pericardial
	Mesothelial
	Thymic (cf. Table 9.1)
	Meningocele
2	*Acquired*
2.1	Thoracic duct
2.2	Neoplastic
	Thymoma
	Teratoma
	Lymphangioma
	Hemangioma
2.3	Inflammatory (cf. Table 9.1)
	Dubois' abscesses
	Tuberculosis
	Hydatid disease
	Pancreatic pseudocysts
2.4	Cystic hematoma

brous wall, and contain a straw-colored fluid (ROSAI and LEVINE 1976; OTTO 1984).

The differential diagnosis of thymic cysts includes neoplastic cysts of the thymus (cystic thymomas and teratomas, lymphangiomatous and hemangiomatous lesions) and all forms of mediastinal cysts (Table 9.2).

9.1.2 Occurrence and Clinical Symptoms

E. WALTER and E. WILLICH

According to PODOLSKY et al. (1962), SOUPAULT (1897) was the first to describe a thymogenic cyst, observed during the postmortem examination of an 18-year-old girl.

The majority of authors report that 1% of all mediastinal tumors are thymogenic cysts (RASTE-GAR et al. 1980; CEUPPENS 1984; etc.). The largest survey of mediastinal tumors is that by WYCHULIS et al. (1971), who found 19 thymogenic cysts (1.7%) among 1064 mediastinal tumors over a period of 40 years. Combining the results of ZANCA et al. (1965), SELTZER et al. (1968), and WHITTAKER and LYNN (1973), among 438 mediastinal tumors there were 16 thymogenic cysts (3.7%). PODOLSKY et al. (1962) and MIKAL (1974) cite a larger number of thymogenic cysts from the literature, i.e., 39 and 34 respectively. WAGNER et al. (1988) collected from the literature 75 cases of cervical thymic cysts in patients under 20 years of age. Among 188 pediatric tumors KING et al. (1982) found only two thymic cysts.

Whereas according to FAHMY (1974) thymogenic cysts are twice as frequent in boys as in girls, DAY and GEDGAUDAS (1984) and GRAEBER et al. (1984) could not find any difference in incidence between the sexes.

In principle thymogenic cysts can occur at all ages (ALLEE et al. 1973); they have even been reported in neonates (RAINES and ROWE 1981; ROSEVEAR and SINGER 1981). Most authors, however, have observed cysts in the young. FAHMY (1974) found two-thirds of the cysts during the first decade, 13% during the second decade, and only occasional tumors at later ages. According to WELCH et al. (1979), 50% of thymic cysts are found in children, and the cases described by GRAEBER et al. (1984) were all in patients under 40. Only ALLEE et al. (1973) show a predilection for clinical manifestation between the third and sixth decades.

In accordance with the migration of the thymus, thymogenic cysts are found throughout the thymolymphatic duct, i.e., from the mandible to the paracardial region. In most cases they are found in the mediastinum (KRECH et al. 1954; SCHILLHAMMER and TYSON 1962). A literature survey (PODOLSKY et al. 1962; SHIN and LEVOWITZ 1973; GRAEBER et al. 1984) covering a total of 136 patients revealed 65.4% of the thymogenic cysts to have a mediastinal location, 22.1% a cervical location, and 12.5% both a mediastinal and a cervical location. The left side is favored (FAHMY 1974).

A connection between thymic cysts in the neck and an orthotopically positioned thymus is frequently found, consisting of either strips of solid thymus tissue or fibrous material.

Clinical symptoms. The location and size of the cysts determines the clinical symptoms. Thymogenic cysts located cervically usually show clinical symptoms during childhood and can be recognized as painless tumors. They are usually positioned in the anterior cervical triangle, ante-

rior to the sternocleidomastoid muscle. They sometimes extend under the sternocleidomastoid muscle or into the region between the lateral angle of the mandible and the manubrium sterni (RÖSSLEIN et al. 1988).

Sometimes cysts are found lying against the rear wall of the pharynx (BIEGER and MCADAMS 1966) or extending into the base of the skull (RATNESAR 1971). Where clinical symptoms appear they are usually dysphagia (present in 7% of patients with cervically positioned cysts), dyspnea, pain, and affections of the vocal cords causing hoarseness.

Palpation shows an engorged, elastic, nonpulsating tumor (HURLEY 1977; JOHNSEN and BRETLAU 1976).

Valsalva's maneuver, coughing, or shouting are reported to produce a change in the size of the cyst (STROME and ERAKLIS 1977; WELCH et al. 1979).

Incomplete descent in the mid neck region can produce thymogenic cysts which often occupy a parathyroid location (RADHNAKRISHNA et al. 1989) and therefore can be confused scintigraphically with a cold thyroid tumor (BENVENISTE et al. 1980).

Thymogenic cysts in the mediastinum usually produce no symptoms and are discovered on a routine chest radiograph or during fluoroscopy of the thoracic organs, usually in childhood. Symptomatic cysts produce disturbances to the breathing of differing intensity, even in newborns (RAINES and ROWE 1981). These disturbances vary from respiratory distress to recurrent infections of the upper respiratory tract, coughing, dyspnea, tachypnea, and hoarseness. Large cysts can produce the usual symptoms of a tumor of the mediastinum, namely dysphagia, dyspnea, and pressure in the chest. Sudden thoracic pain is due to acute bleeding within the cyst with secondary enlargement of the cystic tumor (YOUNG et al. 1973).

Accompanying thymus-specific syndromes must be expected since typical thymic tissue with Hassall's bodies is almost always found in the wall of the cyst (FAHMY 1974; OTTO and HÜSSELMANN 1978; REINER et al. 1980). A thymogenic cyst in combination with myasthenia gravis has only been described by FUNGI et al. (1957), ALLEE et al. (1973) and BROWN et al. (1983).

KUHLMAN et al. (1988) also described a cystic tumor in the mediastinum accompanying myasthenia gravis; however, no thymogenic antecedents could be proved. Two cases of thymogenic cyst occurring with aplastic anemia have been reported (DEHNER et al. 1977; MOSKOWITZ et al. 1980). The observation that thymogenic cysts occur more often following radiation treatment (e.g., for

Hodgkin's disease; BARON et al. 1982) is referred to in the section on malignant lymphoma (see Sect. 8.4).

Malignant degeneration of a thymogenic cyst has not yet been reported.

9.1.3 Diagnosis with Imaging Procedures

9.1.3.1 Conventional Techniques

The results of conventional radiography vary according to the topographic position of the cyst. When the cyst is positioned within the neck, compression of the trachea or esophagus (OTTO 1984; WAGNER et al. 1988) can be demonstrated by esophagography or tomography of the trachea.

Thymogenic cysts in the region of the parathyroids, discovered through visible or palpable swelling, are often thought to be connected with the thyroid. Such cases show up on the scintiscan of the thyroid as a "cold" node lateral to the thyroid. They can be confused sonographically with a thyroid cyst adjacent to or within the thyroid (BENVENISTE et al. 1980).

On conventional chest radiographs a cyst in the mediastinum is seen as a widening and deformation of the mediastinal border, which varies according to the size of the cyst and its position within the mediastinum (Figs. 9.1 a, b, 9.2 a). The picture is similar to that of a solid tumor of the thymus. Depending on the internal pressure, the cyst is either round or oval (DÜX 1977); the contour is usually smooth but can also be lobulated (YOUNG et al. 1973). At already mentioned, the paracardiac position of the cyst can cause it to be confused with cardiomegaly (SCHLUGER et al. 1968; YOUNG et al. 1973; and others). Thymogenic cysts can become so large that they block out the whole of a hemithorax (DANYLEWICZ-WYTRYCHOWSKA 1981). A rapid increase in size indicates bleeding within the cyst. Calcification of the wall is only rarely seen (YOUNG et al. 1973; GUASAY 1977; RASTEGAR et al. 1980; Fig. 9.3).

Fluoroscopy shows an accompanying pulsation, and kymography yields a similar result. Conventional tomography produces no further information and does not permit histologic differentiation; now that computed tomography (CT) is available, it can be dispensed with. Before CT was in general use, selective angiography was recommended to distinguish a cyst from a solid tumor (DÜX 1977). Moreover angiography could exclude the differential diagnosis of vascular swelling (YOUNG et al.

1973). On angiography (Fig. 9.2 b, c) a thymogenic cyst appears as an avascular tumor (ZANCA et al. 1965). Like pneumomediastinography, angiography is no longer necessary.

In conclusion it should also be mentioned that the extent of a cyst can be demonstrated by aspiration and injection of a soluble contrast medium (YOUNG et al. 1973; HURLEY 1977).

9.1.3.2 Ultrasonography

YOUNG et al. (1973) were the first to examine the thymus ultrasonographically. Ultrasonography of the thymus in the young has since developed into one of the prime methods of examination, irrespective of the position of the thymus in the mediastinum or neck, and, unlike in adult patients, precedes CT in the examination order.

Due to their fluid content, thymogenic cysts of the neck or mediastinum are typically transonic (RAINES and ROWE 1981; RÖSSLEIN et al. 1988; and others). Internal bleeding can be seen as hyperechoic areas. The capsule can be differentiated on the ultrasonogram (CLAUS and COPPENS 1984; GRAEBER et al. 1984; NGOVAN et al. 1985; WAGNER et al. 1988; LYONS et al. 1989). Where there is a parathyroidal position the cystic lesion can be so close to the thyroid that it is confused with a thyroid cyst (BENVENISTE et al. 1980). Ultrasonography can usually differentiate between a cyst and a solid lesion in the neck.

9.1.3.3 Computed Tomography

When a thymogenic cyst is situated in the anterior mediastinum, CT displays the tumor and allows determination of its size and relationship to neighboring organs (Fig. 9.1 c). With large cysts, displacement of the great vessels (usually after injection of a contrast medium) and mediastinal organs can be seen. In conformity with the pathologic anatomy, the cyst is sharply contoured and the attenuation values of the contents are between +5 and +15 HU. The wall of the cyst is regular and thin (1–2 mm). Usually persistent thymic tissue can be recognized histologically (OTTO and HÜSSELMANN 1978; WELCH et al. 1979; CEUPPENS 1984), although not always with CT (LIVESAY et al. 1979; SCHNYDER and CANDARDJIS 1987). The attenuation values of the cyst wall and persistent thymic tissue typically lie between +30 and +50 HU, i.e., they are similar to those of the muscles of the chest wall.

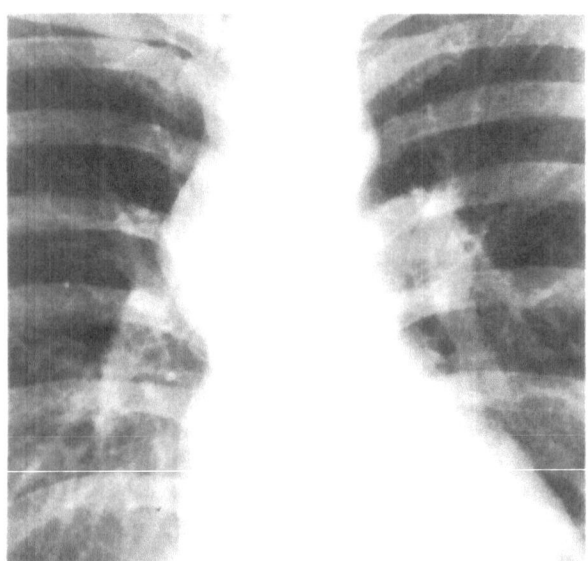
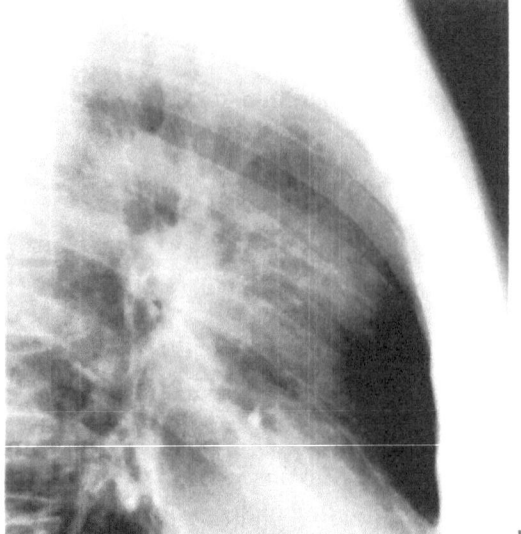

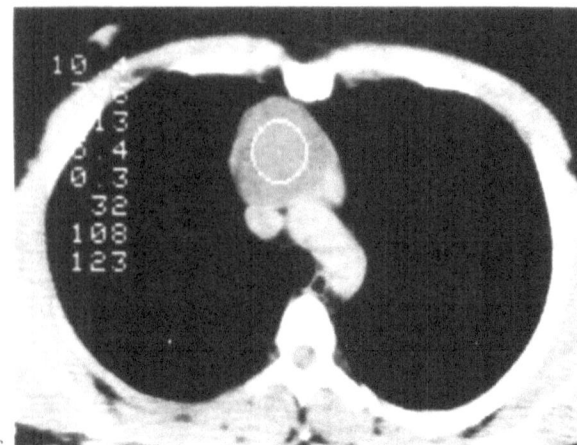

Fig. 9.1 a–c. Thymogenic cyst in an asymptomatic 30-year-old patient. **a,b** Chest radiography in two planes in the standing position. A smooth mediastinal mass is present that is well differentiated from the lung. In the lateral view it appears as a poorly defined mass located retrosternally in the anterior mediastinum. **c** CT of the retrosternally situated thymic cyst reveals attenuation values of ca. + 10 HU, which are characteristic for cystic content

Fig. 9.2 a–c. Thymogenic cyst. **a** Posteroanterior chest radiograph showing a mass in the mediastinum with mediastinal enlargement towards the left. **b,c** Selective arteriography of the internal thoracic artery, revealing an avascular mass with stretched vascular courses. There is no pathologic vascularization. (By courtesy of Prof. A. DÜX, Mönchengladbach, FRG)

▽

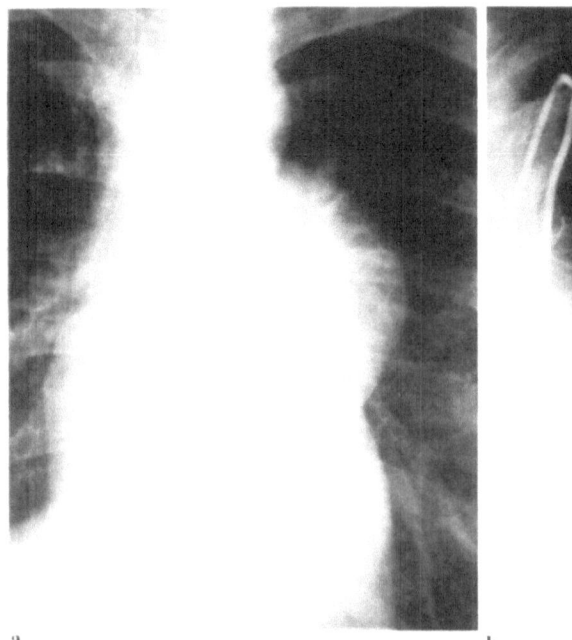
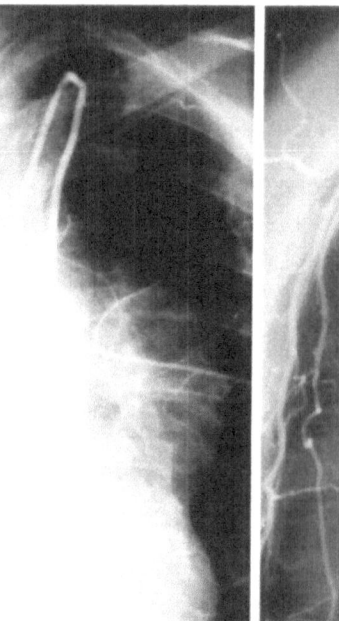
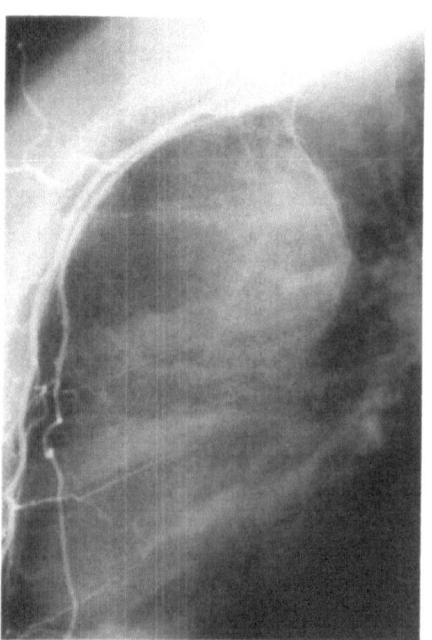

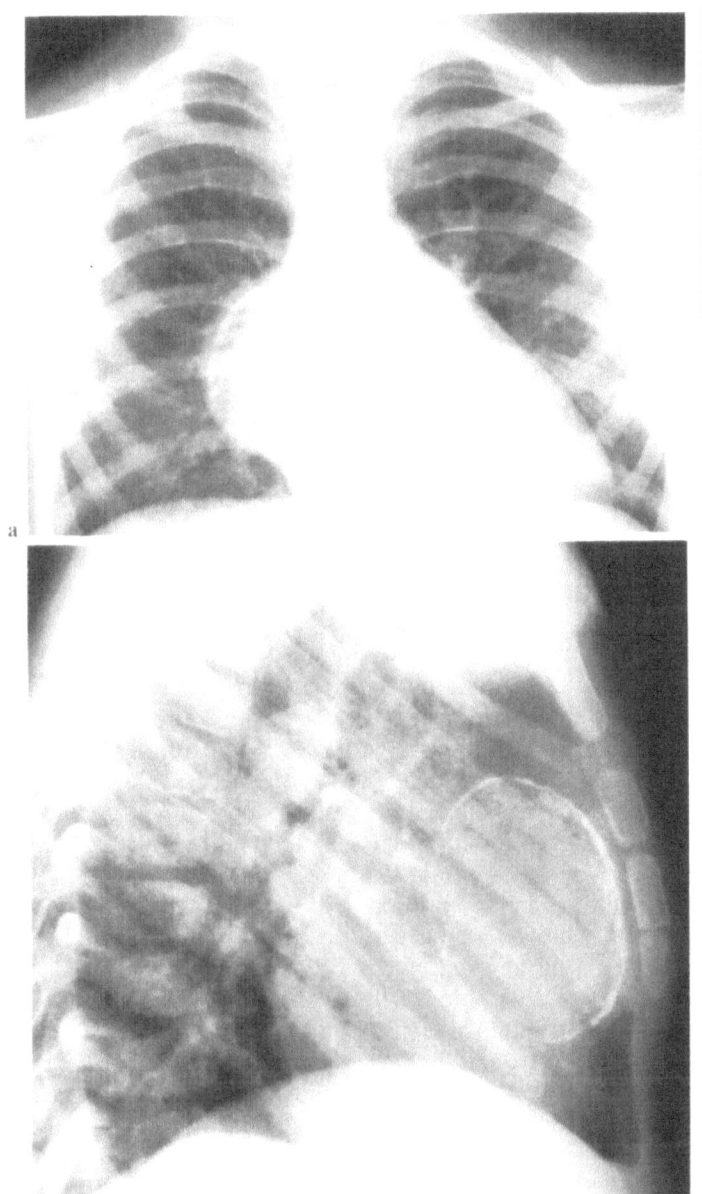

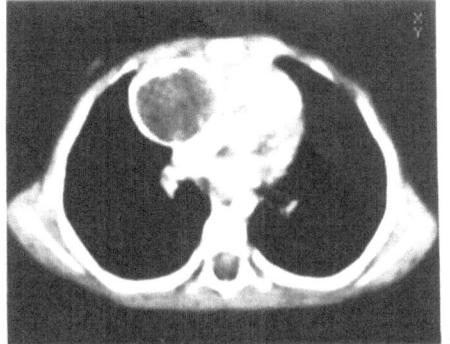

Fig. 9.3 a–c. Thymic cyst with calcified cyst wall in a $3^1/_2$-year-old child without clinical symptoms. **a** The chest radiograph shows bulging of the right cardiac contour with shell-like linear calcification. **b** Frontal view: the linear calcification surrounds the whole mass in the anterior mediastinum. **c** CT: On the right there is a retrosternally situated cyst with a homogeneous structure; it is clearly delimited and is surrounded by a calcified rim. Total extirpation was performed. Histology: benign thymic cyst

Upon administration of a contrast medium, slight enhancement can be seen in the cyst wall or persistent thymic tissue; however, detailed results are not available (SCHNYDER and CANDARDJIS 1987). Cell detritus within the cyst and hemorrhages (YOUNG et al. 1973; DEHNER et al. 1977) produce higher radiation absorption by the cystic content. Values of up to +50 HU are reported (SCHNYDER and CANDARDJIS 1987). Thus the CT appearance can resemble that of a solid tumor (GRAEBER et al. 1984). BROWN et al. (1983) did indeed mistake a thymogenic cyst for a solid tumor. Attenuation values as low as −30 HU have, however, been seen, owing to cholesterol deposits (SIEGELMANN et al. 1984).

The rare calcifications of the cystic border (RASTEGAR et al. 1980) are easily recognized on CT scans (Fig. 9.3). This is especially true of the 12.5% of thymogenic cysts with cervicomediastinal spread (GOSKE RUDICK and WOOD 1980; BARAT et al. 1985; LEVINE 1988; LYONS et al. 1989).

The CT appearance of thymogenic cysts in the neck is similar to that of those in the mediastinum. This also holds true for the paracardiac area, where the thymic cyst is sharply defined against the heart (CEUPPENS 1984). Thymic cysts can consist of one chamber but can also be bilobate (YOUNG et al. 1973). They are usually unilocular; however, in up to 35% of cases a multilocular appearance must be expected (WYCHULIS et al. 1971). Thus the CT examination should cover the entire course of the thymolymphatic duct, from the lateral cervical triangle right into the paracardiac region, in the search for further cysts (WALTER and HÜBENER 1980; WALTER 1982). The cordlike connections usually found between the individual thymic cysts or, when there is an eccentric position, with the thymus itself, elude detection by CT.

9.1.3.4 Magnetic Resonance Imaging

W. R. WEBB and G. DE GEER

As stated above, fluid-filled (cystic) or necrotic masses can be detected using magnetic resonance imaging (MRI) because of long T1 and T2 values. In patients with fluid-containing lesions, scans performed with long TR and TE values (T2-weighted images) show a significant increase in signal from the fluid within the cyst and can demonstrate inhomogeneity invisible with short TR and TE values. In some patients, cystic or fluid-filled masses can be diagnosed on MRI when they cannot on CT; in one patient with a thymic cyst we studied (Fig. 8.58) using both CT and MRI, MRI clearly showed the cyst, when this was not possible on CT. In addition to thymic cysts, thymic lymphoma, thymoma, teratoma, and other thymic neoplasms can have cystic or necrotic components (DE GEER et al. 1986; SIEGEL et al. 1989).

To some extent, the nature of the fluid contents of a thymic cyst can be predicted using MRI. Low protein or serous fluids are very low in intensity on T1-weighted images, which allows them to be distinguished from solid masses, and increase significantly with T2 weighting (WEBB et al. 1984). Cysts containing a large amount of protein mimic solid masses with T1 weighting but markedly increase in intensity with T2 weighting, often becoming more intense than fat. Blood has varying appearances on MRI, depending on its age and the state of the hemoglobin-derived iron within it. The presence of blood within a cyst can sometimes be suggested because of high intensity on both T1- (Figs. 8.39 b and 8.59) and T2-weighted images.

9.1.3.5 Nuclear Medicine

E. WALTER and E. WILLICH

Results of nuclear medical examinations giving positive proof of thymogenic cysts are not available; thus nuclear medical examinations are only of use in the differential diagnosis.

It should be noted that unlike thymogenic cysts, protogaster cysts can show ^{99m}Tc uptake, if they contain gastric mucosa; this can be of value in differential diagnosis. Where there is a question of cysts in the parathyroid region a scintiscan of the thyroid with ^{99m}Tc or ^{131}I can occasionally help in distinguishing between cysts arising from the thyroid and cysts arising from the thymus (BENVENISTE et al. 1980; GRAEBER et al. 1984).

9.1.4 Differential Diagnosis

On chest radiography in two planes, thymogenic cysts with a paracardiac location can be confused with cardiomegaly or a cardiac anomaly (SCHLUGER et al. 1968; YOUNG et al. 1973; ALLEE et al. 1973; GRAEBER et al. 1984; and others). This has occasionally led to lengthy treatment with digitalis (ALLEE et al. 1973). LE ROUX et al. (1984) described compression of the right atrium by a thymogenic cyst, with obstruction of the ventricular outflow.

All cystic structures of the mediastinum must be included in the differential diagnosis.

Bronchogenic cysts, which arise through embryonal malformation during the development of the foregut, are topographically usually found closely related to the bronchial system, often near the tracheal bifurcation. Thymogenic cysts, however, are usually (in 65% of cases according to statistical data) located in the anterior mediastinum. No differential diagnosis can be made on the basis of the attenuation values. On the other hand, a cyst dystopic to the thymus speaks against a thymogenic origin (although it is not proof thereof). CT cannot show connections of tissue between a dystopic thymic cyst and the thymic remnant.

When the thymic cyst occupies a paracardiac position, a pericardial cyst must receive consideration in the differential diagnosis. Neither conventional radiology (SCHLUGER et al. 1968; CEUPPENS 1984) nor ultrasonography and CT allow the differential diagnosis because pathognomonic results are lacking, particularly since thymic tissue remaining next to a thymogenic cyst can rarely be seen on CT scans.

This almost certainly also holds true for MRI. Thus the differential diagnosis is based on the topographic position of the cystic process. Up to 60% of pericardial cysts are to be found in the right cardiodiaphragmatic angle, up to 30% in the left cardiodiaphragmatic angle, and only 10% in other parts of the pericardium. Thymogenic cysts are extremely rarely found in a paracardiac location, in the cardiodiaphragmatic angle, so a cyst in this position is statistically more likely to be a pericardial cyst.

In this region lymphogenic cysts must also be considered. Again, certain differential diagnosis is impossible in spite of modern methods.

Cysts within the thymus can also be the result of radiation treatment of a malignant lymphoma (BARON et al. 1982); the case history is of help here.

Thymic cysts can sometimes be confused with cystic degeneration of a thymoma (LACKNER 1960), and occasionally differentiation can be difficult even for the pathologist. The cyst wall is rarely homogeneous in a thymoma with cystic degeneration; it is usually thicker than 1–2 mm and solid structures can be recognized on the cyst wall. The invasively growing thymoma also shows infiltration of the neighboring organs.

Before CT came into general use the differential diagnosis had to include solid tumors. Only very rarely does interior bleeding and/or cell detritus produce attenuation values similar to a solid tumor. BROWN et al. (1983) report a thymogenic cyst that was misinterpreted as a thymoma. Because today every thymogenic tumor should, if possible, be removed surgically, differential diagnosis with arteriography no longer seems necessary.

It remains to be seen whether MRI can help with the differential diagnosis.

The possibility of a branchial cyst must receive consideration when there is a dystopic position within the neck. However, such cysts usually do not show clinical manifestations until the third decade, only 2% doing so within the first decade (BHASKAR and BERNIER 1959).

Last but not least, a close topographic relationship to the thyroid can cause difficulties that cannot be resolved even by nuclear medical procedures. Aspiration of colloid–serous fluid from the cyst can help with the differential diagnosis.

9.1.5 Relative Value of the Imaging Procedures

The value of the various diagnostic methods depends on the age of the patient and the localization of the thymic cyst. When the cyst is within the mediastinum, conventional chest radiography in two planes forms the basis for diagnosis, especially because the majority of cases are discovered accidentally. Conventional tomography, pneumomediastinography, and kymography are no longer necessary. In children ultrasonography ranks second behind chest radiography in two planes (because of the absence of calcification of the sternum), whereas in adults CT is in second position. Ultrasonography and even more so CT can show the cyst's size, position, consistency, and relationship to neighboring organs. Arteriography need be considered only occasionally. Venography is practically no longer indicated unless venous congestion must be clarified.

Ultrasonography is the prime method in both children and adults when there is a thymogenic cyst in the neck, followed by CT in adults. Both methods display fluid-filled tumors and can distinguish them from solid lesions such as lymphoma or nodes of the thyroid gland. Conventional radiologic methods are only of supplementary diagnostic value.

It remains to be seen what use can be made of MRI as enough results have not yet been published.

9.1.6 Therapy and Prognosis

The prognosis of thymogenic cysts is considered to be good. The cyst should, especially in children, be removed surgically because of its tendency to grow and because histologic confirmation is then possible (ROSSLEIN et al. 1988; LYONS et al. 1989). There were no deaths among 39 patients with thymogenic cysts of the neck or mediastinum operated on between 1965 and 1982 (GRAEBER et al. 1984). KUHLMAN et al. (1988) recommend as an alternative aspiration of the cyst when it occupies a suitable anatomic position. RASTEGAR et al. (1980) recommend regular checkup of thoracic thymic cysts that produce no clinical symptoms. Surgical removal is not considered necessary.

Further information is given in the book by GIVEL et al. (1990).

9.2 Hydatidosis of the Thymus

Hydatid cysts of the thymus were first reported by UGON et al. (1952), and a second observations followed from GIRAUD et al. (1963). No further observations have been reported in recent years. The posteroanterior chest radiograph showed a dense tumor sharply demarcated against the lung, while the lateral projection revealed an oval, sharply demarcated tumor in the typical position of the thymus. Tomography showed no calcification (GIRAUD et al. 1963). Thus the picture was similar to that of a thymoma, thymic cyst, or other tumor. It should be possible with CT to show daughter cysts and thus restrict the differential diagnosis.

9.3 Tuberculoma of the Thymus

Tuberculous inflammation of the thymus has been reported in literature on pathologic anatomy (TESSERAUX 1953; DUPREZ et al. 1962). These authors describe a histologically proven tuberculoma of the thymus of approximately 10 cm in diameter.

Chest radiography in two planes showed a sharply edged tumor of homogeneous density in the anterior mediastinum in projection to the aortic arch. Conventional tomography showed no calcifications, and kymography showed no pulsation (DUPREZ et al. 1962). Experiences with modern radiologic techniques are not available.

9.4 Histiocytosis X of the Thymus

Histiocytosis X embraces a group of rare diseases (Hand-Schüller-Christian disease, Letterer-Siwe disease, and eosinophilic granuloma) which are connected with immunologic abnormalities, and possibly an insufficiency of the thymus (CONSOLINI et al. 1987). The pathologic anatomy shows the cause to be a proliferation of the macrophages. All organs containing reticuloendothelial cell components are involved. Clinical symptoms for this group of diseases (SHUANGSHOTI and SEKSARN 1987) include, in descending order of frequency: osteolytic bone disorders, fever, flush, hepatomegaly, swelling of soft tissues, otitis media, splenomegaly, lymphadenopathy, growth disturbances, hemorrhage, and interstitial and alveolar pulmonary infiltration.

According to a review by PESCARMONA et al. (1989) there have to date been five reported cases of a primary manifestation in the thymus. Only in the case described by BRAMWELL and BURNS (1986) was there concurrent myasthenia gravis. The four histiocytosis X foci were discovered by chance on thymectomy. BRAMWELL and BURNS (1986) regard it as possible that the concurrent presence of myasthenia gravis and histocytosis X in the thymus was coincidental. However, in 84 % of children suffering from histiocytosis X, HAMOUDI et al. (1982) observed pathologic changes to the thymus such as dysplasia, dysmorphia, and involution disturbances which were in part associated with an immunodeficiency of the T cells (HAMOUDI et al. 1982; NEWTON et al. 1987; CONSOLINI et al. 1987). Similar histologic results are reported by SIEGAL et al. (1985) and SHUANGSHOTI and SEKSARN (1987).

Radiologic results are reported by FASANELLI et al. (1987) and SHUANGSHOTI and SEKSARN (1987). On chest radiography in two planes both children described by FASANELLI et al. (1987) showed enlarged mediastinal lymphoma with a corresponding enlargement of the mediastinum and spreading of the carina tracheae. Conventional tomography showed dorsal displacement of the trachea and thymomegaly. This could be confirmed by CT. An enlargement of the thymus was also observed by SHUANGSHOTI and SEKSARN (1987) in both of the children they examined.

References

Allee G, Logue B, Mansour K (1973) Thymic cyst simulating multiple cardiovascular abnormalities and presenting with pericarditis and pericardial tamponade. Am J Cardiol 31: 377

Barat M, Sciubba JJ, Abramson AL (1985) Cervical thymic cyst: case report and review of literature. Laryngoscope 85: 89

Baron RL, Lee JKT, Sagel SS, Peterson RR (1982) Computed tomography of the normal thymus. Radiology 142: 121

Benveniste GL, Holoyda A, Hamilton DW (1980) Cervical thymic cyst: report of an unusual presentation of a rare lesion. Aust NZ J Surg 50: 309

Bhaskar SN, Bernier JL (1959) Histogenesis of branchial cysts. Am J Pathol 35: 407

Bieger CA, Mc Adams AJ (1966) Thymic cysts. Arch Pathol 82: 535

Bramwell NH, Burns BF (1986) Histiocytosis X of the thymus in association with myasthenia gravis. Am J Clin Pathol 86: 224

Brown LR, Muhm JR, Sheedy PF, Unni KK, Bernatz PE, Hermann RC (1983) The value of computed tomography in myasthenia gravis. AJR 140: 31

Castleman B, Iverson L, Menendez VP (1956) Localized mediastinal lymph-node hyperplasia resembling thymoma. Cancer 9: 822–830

Ceuppens H (1984) Thymic cyst in an unusual site. Neth J Surg 36: 17

Claus D, Coppens JP (1984) Sonography of mediastinal masses in infants and children. Ann Radiol (Paris) 27: 150

Consolini R, Cini P, Cei B, Bottone E (1987) Thymic dysfunction in histiocytosis-X. Am J Pediatr Hematol Oncol 9: 146

Cuasay RS (1977) Thymic cysts of the mediastinum. J Med Soc NJ 74: 425

Danylewicz-Wytrychowska T (1981) Zur Röntgendiagnostik und Differentialdiagnose der Thymuserkrankungen im Kindesalter. Radiologe 21: 542

Day DL, Gedgaudas E (1984) The thymus. Radiol Clin North Am 22: 519

de Geer G, Webb WR, Gamsu G (1986) Normal thymus: assessment with MR and CT. Radiology 158: 313

Dehner LP, Martin SA, Sumner HW (1977) Thymus related tumors and tumor-like lesions in childhood with rapid clinical progression and death. Hum Pathol 8: 53

Duprez A, Cordier R, Schmitz P (1962) Tuberculoma of the thymus. First case of surgical excision. J Thorac Cardiovasc Surg 44: 115

Düx A (1977) Mediastinum. In: Teschendorf W, Anaker H, Thurn P (eds) Röntgenologische Differentialdiagnostik, vol I/2, 5th edn. Thieme, Stuttgart

Fahmy S (1974) Cervical thymic cysts: their pathogenesis and relationship to branchial cysts. J Laryngol Otol 88: 47

Fasanelli S, Barbuti D, Graziani M, Donfrancesco A (1987) Thymic involvement in acute disseminated histiocytosis-X Rays (Roma) Diagn Radiol 12: 39

Fungi EG, Gotlieb E, Veamonde CA et al. (1957) Myasthenia gravis following excision of a thymic cyst. Study of electrolytes during a myasthenic attack. Prensa Med Argent 44: 3754

Givel JC, Merlini M, Clarke DB, Dusmet M (1990) Surgery of the thymus. Springer, Berlin Heidelberg New York

Giraud G, Negre E, Thevenet A, Beraud P (1963) Kyste hydratique du thymus. Presse Med 27: 1375

Goske Rudick M, Wood BP (1980) The use of ultrasound in the diagnosis of a large thymic cyst. Pediatr Radiol 10: 113

Graeber GM, Thompson LD, Ronnigen LD, Jaffin JZ, Zajtchuk R (1984) Cystic lesion of the thymus. J Thorac Cardiovasc Surg 87: 295

Hamoudi AB, Newton WA, Mancer K, Penn GM (1982) Thymic changes in histiocytosis. Am J Clin Pathol 77: 169

Hurley MF (1977) Cervico-mediastinal thymic cyst: cyst puncture and contrast radiographic demonstration. Br J Radiol 50: 676

Johnsen NJ, Bretlau P (1976) Cervical thymic cysts. Acta Otolaryngol 82: 143

King RM, Telander RL, Smithson WA, Banks PM, Mao-Tang Han (1982) Primary mediastinal tumors in children. J Pediatr Surg 17: 512

Krech WG, Storey CF, Umiker WC (1954) Thymic cysts. J Thorac Surg 27: 477

Kuhlman JE, Fishman EK, Wang KP, Zerhouni EA, Siegelman SS (1988) Mediastinal cysts: diagnosis by CT and needle aspiration. AJR 150: 75

Lackner J (1960) Mediastinaltumoren im Kindesalter. ROFO 93: 429

Leong ASY (1990) Thymic cysts. In: Givel J-C (ed) Surgery of the thymus. Pathology, associated disorders and surgical technique. Springer, Berlin Heidelberg New York, pp 71–77

Le Roux BT, Kallichurum S, Shama DM (1984) Mediastinal cysts and tumors. Curr Probl Surg 21: 25

Levine C (1988) Cervical presentation of a large thymic cyst: CT appearance. J Comput Assist Tomogr 12: 656

Livesay JJ, Mink JH, Fee HJ, Bein ME, Sample WF, Mulder DG (1979) The use of computed tomography to evaluate suspected mediastinal tumors. Ann Thorac Surg 27: 305

Lyons TJ, Dickson JAS, Variend S (1989) Cervical thymic cysts. J Pediatr Surg 24: 241

Marchevsky AM (1990) Mediastinal tumor-like conditions and tumors that can simulate thymic neoplasms. In: Givel J-C (ed) Surgery of the thymus. Springer, Berlin Heidelberg New York, pp 151–162

Mikal S (1974) Cervical thymic cyst: case report and review of the literature. Arch Surg 109: 558

Moskowitz PS, Noon MA, McAlister WH, Mark JBD (1980) Thymic cyst hemorrhage. A cause of acute symptomatic mediastinal widening in children with aplastic anemia. AJR 134: 832

Newton WA, Hamoudi AB, Shannon BT (1987) Role of the thymus in histiocytosis X. Hematol Oncol Clin North Am 1: 63

Ngovan P, Goudard J, Renouard C, Benichou JJ, Labrune B (1985) Cyste thymique cervical congénital. Arch Fr Pédiatr 42: 785

Otto HF (1984) Pathologie des Thymus. In: Doerr W, Seifert G (eds) Spezielle pathologische Anatomie, vol 17. Springer, Berlin, Heidelberg, New York

Otto HF, Hüsselmann H (1978) Klinisch-pathologische Studie zur Klassifikation und Prognose von Thymustumoren. Teil I. Histologische und ultrastrukturpathologische Untersuchungen. Z Krebsforsch 91: 81

Pescarmona E, Rendina EA, Ricci C, Baroni CD (1989) Histiocytosis X and lymphoid follicular hyperplasia of the thymus in myasthenia gravis. Histopathology 14: 465

Podolsky S, Ehrlich EW, Howard JM (1962) Congenital thymic cyst attached to the pericardium. Dis Chest 42: 462

Radhnakrishna K, Dhope S, Ramnarayan K, Rao PLNS (1989) Thymic cysts of the neck. Pediatr Surg Int 4: 351

Raila FA, McKerchar B (1977) Thymic cysts simulating loculated pneumomediastinum in the newborn. Br J Radiol 50: 286

Raines JM, Rowe LD (1981) Progressive neonatal airway obstruction secondary to cervical thymic cyst. Otolaryngol Head Neck Surg 89: 723

Rastegar H, Arger P, Harken AH (1980) Evaluation and therapy of mediastinal thymic cyst. Am Surg 46: 236

Ratnesar P (1971) Unilateral cervical thymic cyst. I. Laryngol Otol 85: 293

Reiner M, Beck AR, Rybak B (1980) Cervical thymic cysts in children. Am J Surg 139: 704

Rosai J, Levine ED (1976) Tumors of the thymus. In: Atlas of Tumor Pathology, second series, fascicle 13. AFIP, Washington DC, pp 207–211

Rosevear WH, Singer MI (1981) Symptomatic cervical thymic cyst in a neonate. Otolaryngol Head Neck Surg 89: 738

Rösslein R, Herzog B, Oberholzer M, Ohnacker H, Signer E (1988) Zervikale Thymuszyste im Kindesalter. Z Kinderchir 43: 334

Schillhammer WR, Tyson MD (1962) Mediastinal thymic cysts. Arch Surg 85: 410

Schluger J, Scarpa WJ, Rosenblum DJ, Pinck RL, Giustra FX (1968) Thymic cyst simulating massive cardiomegaly. Report of a case and review of the literature. Dis Chest 53: 365

Schnyder P, Candardjis G (1987) CT thymic abnormalities. Eur J Radiol 7: 107

Seltzer RA, Mills DS, Baddock SS, Felson B (1968) Mediastinal thymic cyst. Dis Chest 53: 186

Shin C-S, Levowitz BS (1973) Cervicomediastinal thymic cyst. NY State J Med 73: 2695

Shuangshoti S, Seksarn P (1987) Histiocytosis-X: Overlapping form between Letterer-Siwe disease and Hand-Schüller-Christian disease with advanced thymic involvement and obstructive jaundice. J Med Assoc Thai 70: 344

Siegal GP, Dahner LP, Rosai J (1985) Histiocytosis X (Langerhans cell granulomatosis) of the thymus. Am J Surg Pathol 9: 117

Siegel MJ, Glazer HS, Wiener JI, Molina PL (1989) Normal and abnormal thymus in childhood: MR imaging. Radiology 172: 367

Siegelmann SS, Scott WW Jr, Baker RR, Fishmann EK (1984) CT of the thymus. In: Siegelmann SS (ed) Computed tomography of the chest. Churchil Livingstone, Philadelphia, pp 233 ff.

Strome M, Eraklis A (1977) Thymic cysts in the neck. Laryngoscope 87: 1645

Tesseraux H (1953) Physiologie und Pathologie des Thymus unter besonderer Berücksichtigung der pathologischen Morphologie. Barth, Leipzig

Ugon VA, Piovano S, Tomalina D (1959) Quiste hidatico del timo. Primera observacion mundial. Thorax 8: 48

van Schil P, Jorens P, Schoofs E, De Backer W, Goovaerts G (1988) Mediastinal thymic cyst. Thorac Cardiovasc Surg 36: 159

Wagner CW, Vinocur CD, Weintraum WH, Golladay ES (1988) Respiratory complications in cervical thymic cysts. J Pediatr Surg 23: 657

Walter E (1982) Computertomographische Diagnostik des Thymus. In: Lissner J, Doppman JL (eds) CT 82, Internationales Computertomographie Symposium, Seefeld/Tirol. Schnetztor, Konstanz

Walter E, Hübener K-H (1980) Computertomographische Charakteristika raumfordernder Prozesse im vorderen Mediastinum und ihre Differentialdiagnose. ROFO 133: 391

Webb WR (1989) MR imaging of treated mediastinal Hodgkin disease. Radiology 170: 315

Webb WR, Gamsu G, Stark DD et al. (1984) Evaluation of magnetic resonance sequence in imaging mediastinal tumors. AJR 143: 723

Welch KJ, Tapper D, Vawter GP (1979) Surgical treatment of thymic cysts and neoplasms in children. J Pediatr Surg 14: 691

Whittaker LD, Lynn HB (1973) Mediastinal tumors and cysts in the pediatric patient. Surg Clin North Am 53: 893

Wychulis AP, Payne WS, Clagett OT, Woolner LB (1971) Surgical treatment of mediastinal tumors. A 40 years experience. J Thorac Cardiovasc Surg 62: 379

Young R, Pochaczevsky R, Pollak L, Bryk D (1973) Cervico-mediastinal thymic cysts. AJR 117: 855

Zanca P, Chuang TH, DeAvila R, Galindo DL (1965) True congenital mediastinal thymic cyst. Pediatrics 36: 615

10 Trauma and Hemorrhage of the Thymus

E. WILLICH

10.1 Trauma

Severe thoracic trauma can also cause an injury to the thymus. However, this has been described very seldom (BARON et al. 1982).

LABITZKE and SCHRAMM reported in 1981 on a 5-year-old boy who suffered from severe circulatory disturbances, hypovolemic shock, and also upper vein congestion, after an accident that resulted in multiple contusions and fractures. Radiologically a considerable mediastinal enlargement was observed ventrally and to the left, suggesting a rupture of the heart and aorta or a pericardial tamponade. This was, however, excluded by angiography. Thoracotomy showed a rupture of the left thymic lobe. After extirpation of the lobe the mediastinal compression disappeared immediately.

A pneumomediastinum sometimes results from microtrauma, such as (a) rupture of emphysematous alveoli in the pulmonary marginal zones during artificial respiration of premature infants and newborns, and (b) emphysematous expansion of the lung in staphylococcal or acute interstitial pneumonia in babies and small infants and also in obstructive bronchitis and bronchopneumonia (Fig. 10.1). However, pneumomediastinum has also been observed in early childhood without any apparent cause or due only to forced coughing, e. g., in cases of foreign body aspiration with valvular stenosis (RUPPRECHT 1973).

In schoolchildren, traumatic pneumomediastinum is well-known. Air insufflation into the mediastinum for diagnostic reasons has been discontinued since the advent of CT.

With a view to explaining the mechanism and topography of pneumomediastinum, QUATTROMANI et al. (1981) studied two groups: nine dead newborns with normal mediastinal conditions and eight premature infants with pneumomediastinum. Postmortems were performed in all of the nine dead newborns and in the two members of the latter group who died; pathoanatomic findings were correlated with the radiologic signs. They found an embryologic mesenchymal capsule which participates in the fetal migration of the thymus and matures into a real fascia attaching the lower poles of both lobes of the thymus to the pericardium. In this way potential fissures can develop that contribute to our understanding of the normal X-ray appearance. Upon microscopic exploration a semitransparent, whitish, glistening connective tissue membrane is found which spreads over the anterior surface of the thymus and pericardium. If any air dissects from the lungs and reaches one of these fissures, a specific radiographic appearance will result.

Radiodiagnosis: In the 1st year of life the thymus is positioned laterally, and in the lateral view anteriorly, in the form of a "butterfly sign" (Fig. 10.1), or a "spinnaker sign" if the gland shows a crescentic configuration and paramediastinal air lucency (MOSELEY 1960; Figs. 5.1, 5.7). One or both lobes of the thymus can be lifted and below them lies the ribbon-like area of increased transparency caused by incoming air (KLEMENCIC et al. 1969; Fig. 10.1).

In toddlers (1–5 years old) and schoolchildren a lifted thymic tip projecting toward the pulmonary concavity often exists in conjunction with the paramediastinal air lucency. This proves, that the "effaced heart waist" or "prominent pulmonary segment" in these age groups often represents nothing more than persisting thymic tissue (Fig. 10.2), as was already revealed by diagnostic pneumomediastinography in the 1960s (LISSNER 1963; POHLENZ 1968). For the differentiation of real congenital heart diseases see Sect. 7.3.5.

Another important radiodiagnostic sign is the cervical soft tissue emphysema that frequently accompanies pneumomediastinum, or the combination with pneumothorax (Fig. 10.2, upper right border).

In the newborn reported by RAILA and McKERCHAR (1977), the air in the two lobes of a thymic cyst simulated pneumomediastinum.

Course of disease: After removal of the cause in cases of disease or after trauma, the air absorbs within a few days and the thymus returns to its normal position.

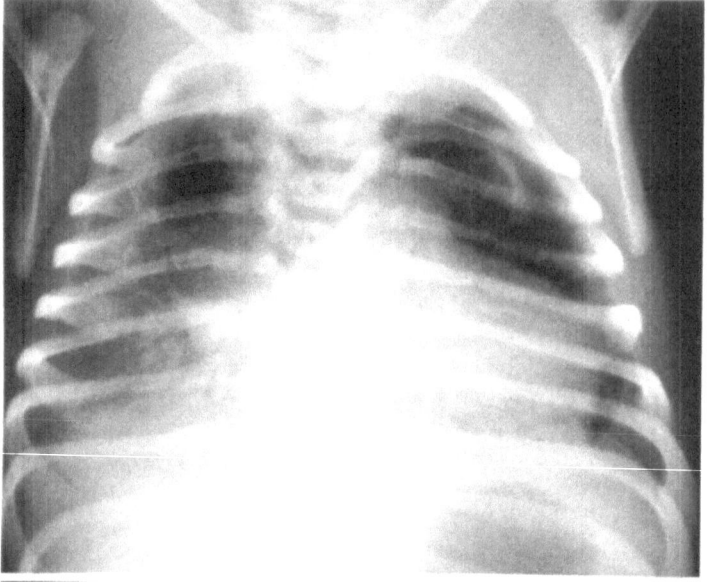

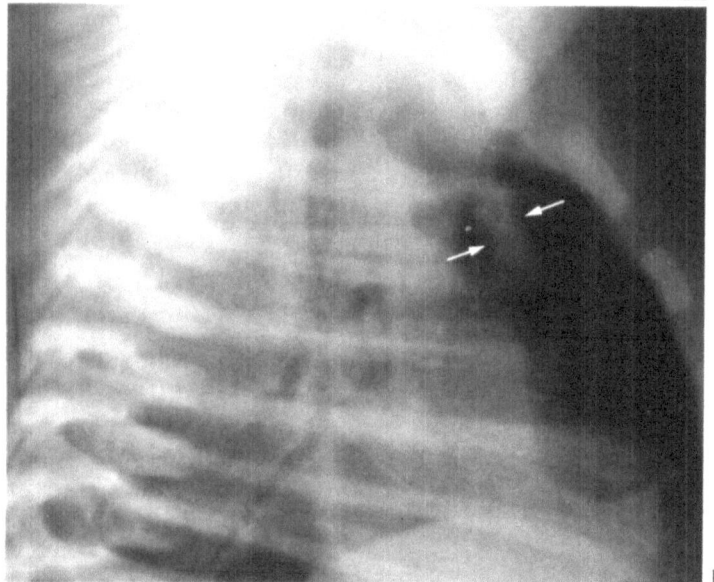

Fig. 10.1 a, b. Thymus in a 2-day-old female with pneumomediastinum. **a** Anteroposterior radiograph of the chest: The left lobe of the thymus is lifted in a semicircular fashion (butterfly sign); the right lobe pushed off similar a marginal atelectasis. **b** Lateral view (spot film): Bill-shaped lifting of the thymus ventrally within an air depot anteriorly *(arrows)*. Total resorption had occurred after a few weeks

10.2 Hemorrhage

Thymic hemorrhage very rarely occurs without preceding trauma. It has been described:

- Spontaneously, without any apparent cause (= "idiopathic"), in infants (WOOLLEY et al. 1974) or adults (GOSHHAJRA 1977)
- As a secondary phenomenon in blood diseases in newborns (CAFFEY 1978; CARROLL and TA 1980; VAN SONNENBERG et al. 1983), infants (LE-MAITRE et al. 1989), and children (MOSKOWITZ et al. 1980)

- After open heart operations (FISHER and REIS 1969)
- In cystic thymomas and thymic cysts (BIEGER and McADAMS 1966; MISSIER et al., 1971; FAHMY 1974; DEHNER et al. 1977; MOSKOWITZ et al. 1980; VAN SCHIL et al. 1988; RADHAKRISHNA et al. 1989)

Depending on the extent of bleeding and the patient's age, *clinical symptoms* include acute dyspnea, chest pain, acute deterioration in condition, pallor, shock, tachypnea, coma, rectal bleeding, bloody stools, meteorism, and distended abdomen. Laboratory findings include low levels of hemo-

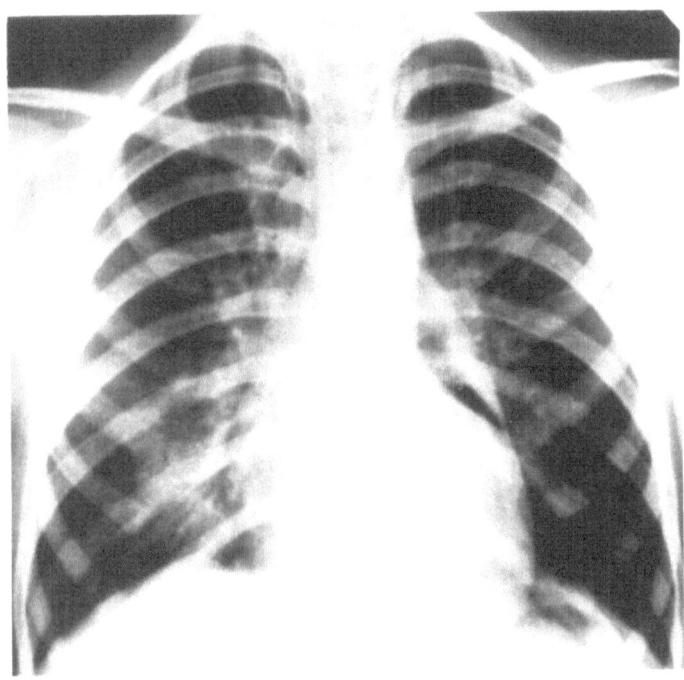

Fig. 10.2. Left sided traumatic pneumomediastinum in a 12-year-old boy with pneumonia of the right lower lung lobe. Cervical soft tissue emphysema *(right upper margin of the thorax)*

globin, erythrocytes, and thrombocytes, a reduced prothrombin time, and an increased partial thromboplastin time. There are also cases in which the above-mentioned symptoms are lacking and bleeding is only established histologically (THOMAS and GUPTA 1988).

Thymic hemorrhage must be excluded whenever acute mediastinal enlargement up to the level of a solid mass or "thymic enlargement" is verified radiologically in children with the aforementioned symptoms. Thymic hemorrhage is especially likely in newborns, in children with hemorrhagic diatheses, in trauma patients, and after thoracic operations, e. g., heart surgery. In some of the reported cases blood effusions were radiologically visible in the left pleural cleft, and consideration should therefore always be given to the possibility of hemorrhage into the thymus when thymic enlargement occurs in conjunction with a mediastinal or parietal pleural effusion (WOOLLEY et al. 1974; SIEGER et al. 1974).

Nowadays ultrasonography represents another method for recognizing intraparenchymal thymic hemorrhages and hematomas. Its use was first fully described by LEMAITRE et al. (1989) in a 2-month-old baby. In the follow-up changes can be well recorded with ultrasonography. The ultrasonographic findings in respect of a thymic hemorrhage can be compared with those in respect of a liver, spleen, or kidney hemorrhage owing to the simi-

larity in echo pattern. Smaller bleedings show linear, echogenic foci, while severe bleedings show round foci. After repeated hemorrhage into the thymus, one may at first find small, cystic interspaces in combination with echogenic structures. These reported findings, however, are not pathognomonic; they resemble those in lymphomas. If these ultrasonographic findings are detected in children with the above clinical symptoms or laboratory findings or in the presence of low vitamin K-dependent coagulation factors, thymic hemorrhage will certainly be present.

References

Baron RL, Lee JKT, Sagel SS, Peterson RR (1982) Computed tomography of the normal thymus. Radiology 142: 121–125

Bieger C, McAdams AJ (1986) Thymic cysts. Arch Pathol 82: 535–541

Caffey J (1978) Pediatric X-ray diagnosis. Year Book Medical, Chicago, p 510

Carroll BA, Ta HN (1980) Ultrasonographic appearance of extranodal abdominal lymphoma. Radiology 136: 419–425

Dehner LP, Martin SA, Summer HW (1977) Thymus related tumors and tumor like lesions in childhood with rapid clinical progression and death. Hum Pathol 8: 53–56

Fahmy S (1974) Cervical thymic cysts: their pathogenesis and relationship to branchial cysts. J Laryngol Otol 88: 47–60

Fisher RD, Reis RL (1969) Post-operative cardiac tamponade produced by thymic hematoma. Arch Surg 98: 204–205

Goshhajra K (1977) Spontaneous thymic hemorrhage in an adult. Chest 72: 666–667

Klemencic J, Kraus R, Kratz R (1969) Das Röntgenbild des symptomatischen spontanen Pneumomediastinums beim Neugeborenen, Säugling und Kleinkind. Radiologe 9: 278–281

Labitzke R, Schramm G (1981) Thymusruptur nach Thoraxtrauma. Z Kinderchir [Suppl] 33: 147–149

Lemaitre L, Leclerc F, Dubos JP, Marconi V, Lemaitre D (1989) Thymic hemorrhage: a cause of acute symptomatic mediastinal widening in an infant with late hemorrhagic disease. Sonographic findings. Pediatr Radiol 19: 128–129

Lissner J (1963) Die röntgenologische Diagnostik der Thymustumoren. Radiologe 1: 31–36

Missier PA, Kreps S, Nachtigall RH, Jaspin G, Fisher WW (1971) Hemorrhagic cysts of thymus. NY State J Med 71: 1930–1931

Moseley JE (1960) Loculated pneumomediastinum in the newborn, a thymic spinnaker sail sign. Radiology 75: 788–790

Moskowitz PS, Noon MA, McAlister WH, Mark JBD (1980) Thymic cyst hemorrhage: a cause of acute, symptomatic mediastinal widening in children with aplastic anemia. AJR 134: 832–836

Pohlenz O (1968) Röntgenologische Thymusdiagnostik. Med Klin 63: 1255–1259

Quattromani FL, Foley LC, Bowen A, Weisman L, Her-

nandez J (1981) Fascial relationship of the thymus: radiologic-pathologic correlation in neonatal pneumomediastinum. AJR 137: 1209–1211

Radhakrishna K, Khope S, Ramnarayan K, Rao PLNG (1989) Thymic cysts of the neck. Case reports and literature review. Pediatr Surg Int 4: 351–353

Raila FA, McKerchar B (1977) Thymic cysts simulating loculated pneumomediastinum in the newborn. Br J Radiol 50: 286–297

Rupprecht E (1973) Pneumothorax und Pneumomediastinum beim Neugeborenen. Kinderärztl Prax 41: 383–398

Sieger L, Higgins GR, von Adelsberg S, Isaars H (1974) Acute thymic hemorrhage: an unusual cause of respiratory distress in infancy. Am J Dis Child 128: 86–87

Thomas NB, Gupta SC (1988) Unilobar enlargement of normal thymus gland causing mass effect. Br J Radiol 61: 244–246

van Schil P, Jorens P, Schoofs E, De Backer W, Goovaerts G (1988) Mediastinal thymic cyst. Thorac Cardiovasc Surg 36: 159–160

van Sonnenberg E, Lin AS, Deutsch AL, Mattrey RF (1983) Percutaneous biopsy of difficult mediastinal hilar and pulmonary lesions by computed-tomographic guidance and a modified coaxial technique. Radiology 148: 300–302

Woolley MM, Isaacs H, Lindesmith G, Vollmer DM, van Adelsberg S (1974) Spontaneous thymic hemorrhage in the neonatal. Report of two cases. J Pediatr Surg 9: 231–233

11 The Thymus and Myasthenia Gravis

H. Wiethölter, E. Willich, and E. Walter

11.1 Definition of Myasthenia Gravis

H. Wiethölter

Myasthenia gravis (MG) is the best known organ-specific autoimmune disease; it is caused by a loss of functional acetylcholine receptors (AChR) at the neuromuscular junction, resulting in fatigable weakness of voluntary muscle. Diagnostically relevant serum antibodies against AChR are present in about 90% of patients with generalized MG.

The first reasonably complete accounts of MG were those by Erb (1879), who designated the disease as bulbar palsy. By the turn of the century the first observation of a relationship between MG and the thymus gland was described (Weigert 1901). The autoimmune nature was suspected by Simpson (1960) because of its association with other autoimmune diseases, and a further clue came from experiments on animals which were immunized with AChRs (from electric fish) – in order to raise antibodies – and developed myasthenia (Patrick and Lindstrom 1973).

11.2 Clinical Manifestation

11.2.1 Symptoms and Signs

Myasthenia gravis is characterized by painless muscle weakness after repeated or persistent activity, with good or at least partial restoration after a short rest. Eye muscles are particularly vulnerable and ocular symptoms such as ptosis and diplopia will occur at some stage in the illness in about 90%. The next most frequently affected muscles are those reflecting bulbar symptoms (about 30%), with difficulties of speech, facial expression, chewing, and swallowing followed by regurgitation of liquids. In generalized MG the proximal limb muscles are involved more than the distal ones.

Limb muscle weakness is usually symmetric but pronounced asymmetry may be observed. Involvement of respiratory and trunk muscles may sometimes be the first sign leading to medical attention. Weakness tends to increase as the day wears on and watching television in the evening may be a problem because of double vision. Some factors such as infections, physical stress, emotional disturbance, puerperium, and vaccination have been blamed for triggering a subclinical disease.

In MG there is evidence for heterogeneity of disease expression and patients can be grouped (Table 11.1) into five different clinical subgroups according to age of onset, thymic changes, and ocular versus generalized form (Compston et al. 1980).

Myasthenia gravis may occur at any age but in nearly 50% the age at onset is 20–30 years, when it is more common in females. A second peak of incidence is around 40–50 years, with males being preferably affected. In the latter cases purely ocular involment seems to be relatively higher. Thymomas are somewhat more frequent in patients over 40.

11.2.2 Classification

Clinical staging follows the classification introduced by Osserman (1958) (Table 11.2).

11.2.3 Clinical Examination

The history reveals the variable muscle weakness and fatigability and should be assessed by appropriate examination. Ptosis, which is often asymmetric, or diplopia can be provoked when patients are asked to look upwards (Simpson test) or to one side for 60 s. Closing the eyes for a few minutes may reduce ptosis. Bright light can increase the tendency towards ptosis. Diplopia should be quantified by orthoptic procedures (Maddox cross).

Table 11.1. Subgroups of MG patients

	Thymoma	Thymoma absent		Ocular MG	Anti-AChR neg.
		Young-onset	Old-onset		
Patients (%)	10–15	50	15	10–15	5–10
Age of onset (years)	20–70	2–40	40–70	10–70	5–50
Anti-AChR-titre (% positive patients)	High (100)	High (95)	Moderate (90)	Low (60)	(0)
Anti-striated muscle antibody (% positive patients)	90	20	50	20	(0)
Predominant HLA Association[a]	None	$A_1/B_8/DR_3$	$A_3/B_7/DR_2$	None	?
Sex (male/female)	~1.8	~0.3	~2.5	~1.6	3.6

[a] Demonstrated in Caucasian people (Newsom-Davis et al. 1987)

Table 11.2. Classification according to Osserman (1958)

I. *Ocular myasthenia*

II. A. *Mild generalized myasthenia* with slow progression; no crisis; drug-responsive

   B. *Moderate generalized myasthenia;* severe skeletal and bulbar involvement, but no crisis; drug response less than satisfactory

III. *Acute fulminating myasthenia;* rapid progression of severe symptoms with respiratory crisis and poor drug response; high incidence of thymoma; high mortality

IV. *Late severe myasthenia,* same as III but progression over 2 years from class I to II

Facial weakness leads to inability to whistle or to purse the lips. Defective swallowing is indicated by coughing after drinking a glass of water. Weakness of the neck or sternocleidomastoid muscle is tested by head lifting in supine position. This is normally possible for 2 min. Trunk and limb muscles are tested and scored by tonic muscle work against gravity. For example, healthy adults should be able to hold their arms stretched out horizontally for at least 3 min; legs should be raised to 45° in supine position for 2 min. Younger people should be able to squat fully and arise 20 times in a row; in older patients arising from a chair with the arms folded should be feasible. Weakness of respiratory muscles is measured by a decrease in vital capacity.

Mild muscle atrophy is found in only 10%–15% of patients with MG; there are no sensory disturbances, although paresthesias of hands and face are sometimes reported. Smooth and cardiac muscles are never involved. Tendon reflexes are normal and the Babinski sign is absent.

11.2.4 Prognosis

The onset of MG is usually insidious, but sometimes there is fairly rapid development. Once started, a slow progression follows with symptoms increasing during the first years and stabilization or improvements thereafter. In a retrospective study the natural course – without immunosuppressive treatment – reached a maximum severity during the first 7 years after onset and about 30% of the patients died. Spontaneous improvement or remission was unpredictable in the following years. Altogether, 22% of the patients were in complete remission, 18% improved considerably, 16% moderately, and 20% remained unchanged in this follow-up study (Oosterhuis 1989). Patients with ocular MG have a higher remission rate than those with generalized MG. Prognosis for patients with thymomas without special treatment is far worse. Without surgical removal more than 50% of such patients died (Oosterhuis 1981) and only in 30% did myasthenic symptoms improve.

Therapy with early thymectomy and immunosuppressive drugs has led to a far better prognosis. At least 90% of the patients are clinically stable and able to maintain work. In most patients a steady state is reached after 5–7 years (Schumm et al. 1985) and critical deterioration after that is rare.

11.3 Associated Thymic Changes

The thymus is the organ of T cell maturation. It reaches its full size at birth and undergoes involution after puberty. Thymic abnormalities are found in about 60%–70% of the myasthenic patients:

Table 11.3. Imaging detection of thymic abnormalities in MG

Author/year	No. of reported patients with MG	Hyperplasia	Thymoma	Normal	Other findings	Methods of detection/verification
Mink et al. (1978)	6	1	5	0		CT
Keesey et al. (1980)	20	7	6	7		Chest radiography, conv. tomogr., CT
Moore et al. (1982)	53	15	4	34		CT
Gürtler et al. (1982)	14	8	4	1	1 thymolipoma	CT
Fon et al. (1982)	57	23	16	18		CT
Brown et al. (1983)	19	6	6	4	1 cavernous hemangioma 2 thymogenic cysts	CT
Kaye et al. (1983)	36	21	10	4	1 thymogenic cyst	CT
Weiss et al. (1987)	23	7	2	14		CT
Batra et al. (1987)	16	7	2	7		CT, MRI
Thorvinger et al. (1987)	16	8	3	5		CT
Schnyder and Candardjis (1987)	6	2	4	0		CT
Emskötter et al. (1988)	14	9	4	1		CT, MRI
Glathe et al. (1989)	34	17	16	0	1 thymoma associated with teratoma	CT
	314 (100%)	131 (41.7%)	82 (26%)	95 (30.3%)	6 (1.9%)	

12% of the patients have a thymoma according Berrih-Aknin et al. 1987, in our analysis 26%, and about 40% have thymic hyperplasia (Table 11.3).

Thymomas are typically of lymphoepithelial type and local invasion is found in about 30%. Thymomas may occur at any age, although they seem to be more frequent between 40 and 60 years. Usually thymomas are otherwise asymptomatic and only detected by routine radiographs of the chest. Every patient with MG should have radiologic examination to exclude a thymoma. The incidence of thymomas is not exactly known; data from routine autopsy series suggest it is less than 0.1% (Namba et al. 1978). MG is reported in 10%–50% of patients with thymoma, and the real percentage is probably about 30%–50% (Namba et al. 1978).

"Thymic hyperplasia" does not necessarily refer to an increase in the size of the organ; rather it reflects the typical histologic picture with lymph node-like germinal centers. This is regularly found in patients with generalized young-onset MG (see Table 11.1), and cell suspensions from these thymuses produce anti-AChR antibodies in culture whose amount correlates quite well with the patients' serum antibody titer (Willcox and Vincent 1988). Germinal centers have also been found in 10%–13% of normal thymus glands (Oosterhuis 1985; Müller-Hermelink et al. 1986). In patients with ocular MG (Osserman type I) there is only little experience with thymic histology, although hyperplastic changes have been observed (Schumm et al. 1985). Myasthenics over the age of 40 often have thymic atrophy.

11.3.1 Association of Thymic Changes with Other Diseases

Thymic hyperplasia is not restricted to MG, and formation of germinal centers has been described in other autoimmune diseases, e.g., autoimmune thyroid disease, systemic lupus erythematosus, rheumatoid arthritis, Behçet's disease, and ulcerative colitis (see Oosterhuis 1984).

Thymomas are associated not only with MG but also with pure red cell aplasia, pancytopenia, hypogammaglobulinemia, systemic lupus erythemato-

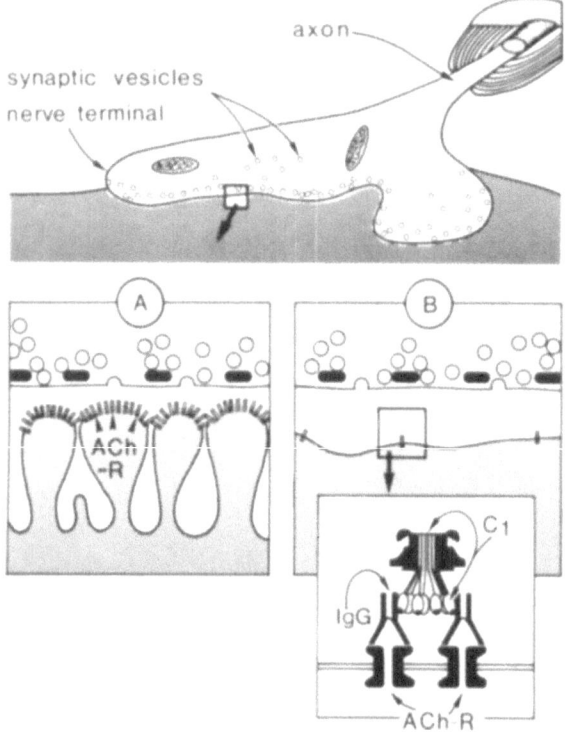

Fig. 11.1. Drawing of a normal (*A*) and a myasthenic (*B*) neuromuscular junction. *C1* = complement, activated by IgG. (M. Poremba).

sus, and pemphigus, diseases that might be due to developmental aberrations of the T cell system. About 90% of patients with thymoma and MG have autoantibodies against striated muscle proteins other than AChR.

11.4 Pathogenesis

Acetylcholine (ACh) is the transmitter of the neuromuscular junction. It is mainly synthesized in the motor nerve terminal, stored in vesicles, and released into the synaptic cleft when an impulse arrives at the nerve terminal. Nicotinic AChRs are located at the top of the deep foldings of the postsynaptic membrane (Fig. 11.1), each of these ligand-gated receptors forming an ion channel that opens for 1 ms after binding ACh. As sodium ions enter the muscle fiber, a depolarization, the endplate potential, results. After another millisecond ACh is hydrolyzed by a membrane-bound esterase and the membrane potential returns to normal. Normally the amount of released transmitter and AChRs is in vast excess so that further voltage-

gated sodium channels in the muscle membrane are activated and subsequently propagate an action potential along the muscle fiber.

Autoradiographic and immunohistochemical studies with α-bungarotoxin, a snake venom that binds specifically to active sites on the AChR, have shown that the number of receptors per synapse is reduced by 70%–90% in MG. Also, the postjunctional folds are degenerated, simplified, and therefore reduced in area. The reduction in AChRs leads to diminished sensitivity to ACh and a reduced safety factor, which, in turn, results in fatigability and muscle weakness.

The immunologic processes responsible for the above mechanisms are caused by the IgG autoantibodies which lead to (a) direct immunopharmacologic block of AChR (which surprisingly seems to be the least important mechanism), (b) increased degradation of AChR due to cross-linking of divalent antibodies, and (c) complement-dependent lysis.

11.5 Autoimmune Origin

The circulating anti-AChR antibodies are T cell dependent and the primary event in the pathogenesis is probably a sensitization of autoreactive T helper cells in the abnormal thymus (WEKERLE et al. 1981). Normal mammalian thymuses contain muscle-like "myoid cells" which express AChR and these may accidentally provide the local source of antigen (SCHLUEP et al. 1988). Only recently AChR-specific T cells could be detected in hyperplastic thymuses and thymomas from MG patients but not in non-MG thymuses (MELMS et al. 1988; SOMMER et al. 1988).

11.6 Diagnosis

When MG is suspected on clinical grounds, additional tests should be performed to confirm the diagnosis. The most specific and sensitive test is the demonstration of circulating IgG antibodies (sometimes IgM antibodies at the beginning of disease) against AChR. In most centers a radioimmunoassay is used which is positive in about 90% of the patients with generalized MG and 50%–70% of the ocular cases. False-positive tests are only seen in patients with thymoma without MG and in some healthy relatives of MG patients. Although a positive text makes MG almost certain, a negative test does not exclude it.

The typical electromyographic finding in MG is a decrement of the muscle action potential after supramaximal repetitive (3–5 Hz) nerve stimulation. Thenar and trapezius muscles are mainly tested. Single fiber electromyography is a time-consuming procedure which is also a very sensitive but not entirely specific method to detect a defect of neuromuscular transmission.

Anticholinesterase agents inhibit the hydrolyzation of ACh in the synaptic cleft, resulting in a relative increase in the locally available transmitter. Edrophonium chloride is given intravenously at a dose of 10 mg (2 mg initially plus 8 mg) to demonstrate a dramatic increase in muscle strength in myasthenics a few minutes after injection. Unpleasant cholinergic side-effects like bradycardia or nausea should be controlled with atropine, if necessary.

11.6.1 Radiologic Diagnosis

E. WILLICH and E. WALTER

It has long been recognized clinically that a close relationship exists between MG and changes to the thymus that are evident macroscopically and thus can also be visualized by means of imaging procedures. Consequently there have been many reports in the literature of investigations concerned with furnishing morphologic proof of changes by means of imaging techniques. According to data pertaining to the pathologic anatomy (LEVINE and ROSAI 1978), 65% of patients with MG display thymic hyperplasia, 10% a thymoma, and 25% a normal thymus. A survey of literature reports on thymic findings using imaging procedures reveals that of 314 patients with MG, 41.7% showed thymic hyperplasia, 26% a thymoma, and 30.3% a normally sized thymus (cf. Table 11.3). This survey could not take into account the findings of ELLIS et al. (1988) and OOSTERHUIS (1989) since, despite their large number of cases (154 and 73 respectively), they only reported on the incidence of thymoma; the same is true for the 114 cases reported by BERRIH-AKNIN et al. (1987) since these were diagnosed by immunohistologic methods.

Looking at the converse situation, MG is found in up to 46% of patients with proven thymoma (BERNATZ et al. 1961; BROWN et al. 1980, 1983; and others), and WILKINS et al. (1966) even reported an incidence of 58.7%.

As regards the demonstration of thymoma, in patients up to the age of about 20 years CT appears to offer at best only a slight advantage over plain chest radiography (3%), whereas in older patients (40/45 years) there is a distinct advantage (35%) due to the greater fat content of the thymus (FON et al. 1982; ELLIS et al. 1988). GLATHE et al. detected a thymoma in 44% of their adult MG patients using plain chest radiography, and in 78% using CT. In patients less than 40 years old, magnetic resonance imaging permits more reliable diagnosis of the tumor and better assessment of its status (EMSKÖTTER et al. 1988).

Since in approximately 90% of patients with MG and a thymoma antibodies against striated muscle can be demonstrated with immunofluorescence, the decision on whether to employ imaging procedures is facilitated.

For further detail on thymic hyperplasia and MG the reader is referred to Sect. 7.4.4. As regards MG in conjunction with thymoma, see Sect. 8.2.2.1.2 and 8.2.2.2.1; Sect. 8.2.1.5.3 deals with the pathologic anatomy.

11.7 Treatment

H. WIETHÖLTER

The treatment of MG involves careful use of three groups of drugs (antiacetylcholinesterases, immunosuppressants, and corticosteroids), thymectomy and plasmapheresis; see Table 11.4.

Table 11.4. Therapeutic regimen in myasthenic patients

1. Therapy with acetylcholinesterase inhibitors:
   Pyridostigmine up to 4×60 mg/day
   Pyridostigmine time span 90–180 mg at night
   Parenteral equivalent: 2 mg (i.m. or i.v.) is equivalent to 60 mg orally

   Neostigmine (Prostigmin): 15 mg orally before breakfast is possible
   Parenteral equivalent: 0.5 mg (i.v. or s.c.) is equivalent to 15 mg orally

   Cholinergic (muscarinergic) side-effects can require atropine sulfate 4–$5 \times 1/8$ mg

2. Thymectomy:
   Thymectomy by median sternotomy is necessary in patients with suspected thymoma (CT) and in patients up to 65 years irrespective of CT, if patients are suitable candidates for surgery

3. Immunosuppressive treatment with drugs:
   Glucocorticosteroids (for example Decortin H, Urbason) after a short increasing dosage (3 days 25 mg, 3 days 50 mg) up to 1–1.5 mg/kg body weight. After improvement or stabilization, change to an alternating treatment with slowly tapering dosage to long-term therapy with 10–15 mg prednisone every other day

   Additionally azathioprine (Imurek) 2–3 mg/kg body weight

   Alternative: cyclophosphamide (Endoxan) 2 mg/kg body weight. Only use in a therapeutically resistant course of disease

   Alternative: cyclosporine (Sandimmun) 5 mg/kg body weight

   Combined immunosuppressive treatment in severe generalized MG

   After thymectomy, if no definite improvement is evident 6 months later

   In patients who refuse thymectomy or are unfit for surgery

4. Plasmapheresis:
   In acute severe MG and myasthenic crisis; possibly also before or after thymectomy if respiratory insufficiency is present; 3–5 separation procedures every other day with 2–4 l plasma exchange in combination with immunosuppressive drugs (corticosteroids)

References

Batra P, Hermann C, Mulder D (1987) Mediastinal imaging in myasthenia gravis: correlation of chest radiography, CT, MR and surgical findings. AJR 148: 515

Bernatz PE, Harrison EG, Clagett OT (1961) Thymoma: A clinicopathologic study. J Thorac Cardiovasc Surg 42: 424

Berrih-Aknin S, Morel E, Raimond F et al. (1987) The role of the thymus in myasthenia gravis: immunohistological and immunological studies in 115 cases. Ann NY Acad Sci 505: 50

Brown LR, Muhm JR, Gray JE (1980) Radiographic detection of thymoma. AJR 134: 1181

Brown LR, Muhm JR, Sheedy II PF, Unni KK, Bernatz PE, Hermann RC (1983) The value of computed tomography in myasthenia gravis. AJR 140: 31

Compston DAS, Vincent A, Newsom-Davis J, Batchelor JR (1980) Clinical, pathological, HLA antigen and immunological evidence for disease heterogeneity in myasthenia gravis. Brain 103: 579

Drachman DB (ed) (1987) Myasthenia gravis: biology and treatment. Ann NY Acad Sci 505

Ellis K, Austin JHM, Jaretzki A (1988) Radiologic detection of thymoma in patients with myasthenia gravis. AJR 151: 873

Emskötter T, Trampe H, Lachenmayer L (1988) Kernspintomographie bei Myasthenia gravis. Dtsch Med Wochenschr 113: 1508

Erb W (1879) Zur Kasuistik der bulbären Lähmungen: Über einen neuen wahrscheinlich bulbären Symptomen-Komplex. Arch Psychiatr Nervenkrankh 9: 336

Fon GT, Bein ME, Manouso AA, Keesey JC, Lupetin AR, Wong WS (1982) Computed tomography of the anterior mediastinum in myasthenia gravis. Radiology 142: 135

Glathe S, Neufang KF, Haupt FW (1989) Was leistet die radiologische Thymusdiagnostik bei der Myasthenia gravis? Röntgenblätter 42: 455

Goldstein G, Mackay IR (1969) Thymic tumours and systemic diseases associated with thymomas. In: Goldstein G, Mackay IR (eds) The human thymus. William Heinemann Medical Books, London, pp 194–227

Gürtler KF, Janzen RWC, Hagemann J, Otto HF (1982) Computertomographie des Mediastinums bei Myasthenia gravis pseudoparalytica. ROFO 136: 35

Kaye AD, Jenssen R, Arger PH et al. (1983) Mediastinal computed tomography in myasthenia gravis. J Comput Tomogr 7: 273

Keesey J, Bein M, Mink J et al. (1980) Detection of thymoma in myasthenia gravis. Neurology 30: 233

Levine GD, Rosai J (1978) Thymic hyperplasia and neoplasia: a review of current concepts. Hum Pathol 9: 495

Melms A, Schalke BCG, Kirchner T, Müller-Hermelink HK, Albert E, Wekerle H (1988) Thymus in myasthenia gravis. Isolation of T-lymphocyte lines specific for the nicotinic acetylcholine receptor from thymuses of myasthenic patients. J Clin Invest 81: 902

Mink JH, Bein ME, Sukov R, Herrmann C, Winter J, Sample WF, Mulder D (1978) Computed tomography of the anterior mediastinum in patients with myasthenia gravis and suspected thymoma. AJR 130: 239

Moore AV, Korobkin M, Powers B et al. (1982) Thymoma detection by mediastinal CT: patients with myasthenia gravis. AJR 138: 217

Müller-Hermelink HK, Marino M, Palestro G (1986) Pathology of thymic epithelial tumors. Curr Top Pathol 75: 207

Namba T, Brunner NG, Grob D (1978) Myasthenia gravis in patients with thymoma with particular reference to and after thymectomy. Medicine 57: 411

Newsom-Davis J, Willcox N, Schluep M et al. (1987) Immunological heterogeneity and cellular mechanisms in myasthenia gravis. Ann NY Acad Sci 505: 12

Oosterhuis HJGH (1981) Observations of the natural history of myasthenia gravis and the effect of thymectomy. Ann NY Acad Sci 377: 678

Oosterhuis HJGH (1984) Myasthenia gravis. Churchill Livingstone, Edinburgh

Oosterhuis HJGH (1989) The natural course of myasthenia gravis: a long term follow up study. J Neurol Neurosurg Psychiatry 52: 1121

Osserman KE (1958) Myasthenia gravis. Grune & Stratton, New York

Patrick J, Lindstrom JM (1973) Autoimmune response to acetylcholine receptor. Science 180: 871

Schluep M, Willcox N, Ritter MA, Newsom-Davis J, Larche M, Brown AN (1988) Myasthenia gravis thymus: clinical, histological and culture correlations. J Autoimmunol 82: 1295

Schnyder P, Candardjis G (1987) Computed tomography of thymic abnormalities. Eur J Radiol 7: 107

Schumm F, Wiethölter H, Fateh-Moghadam A, Dichgans J (1985) Thymectomy in myasthenia with pure ocular symptoms. J Neurol Neurosurg Psychiatry 48: 332

Simpson JA (1960) Myasthenia gravis. A new hypothesis. Scott Med J 5: 419

Sommer N, Harcourt G, Willcox N, Newsom-Davis J (1988) Acetylcholine receptor-specific T-lymphocyte responses in thymus, thymoma and lymph nodes from patients with myasthenia gravis. J Neurol Neurosurg Psychiatry 51: 1358

Thorvinger B, Lyttkens K, Samuelsson L (1987) Computed tomography of the thymus gland in myasthenia gravis. Acta Radiol 28: 399

Tola MR, Granieri E, Paolino E, Caniatti L, Quatrale R, Mazzanti B, D'Alessandro R (1989) Epidemiological study of myasthenia gravis in the province of Ferrara, Italy. J Neurol 236: 388

Weigert C (1901) Pathologisch-anatomischer Beitrag zur Erb'schen Krankheit (Myasthenia gravis). Neurologisches Zentralblatt 20: 597

Weiss C, Dinkel E, Wimmer B, Schildge J, Grosser G (1987) Der Thymus im Computertomogramm. Radiologe 27: 414

Wekerle H, Hohlfeld R, Ketelsen UP, Kalden JR, Kalies J (1981) Thymic myogenesis, T-lymphocytes and the pathogenesis of myasthenia gravis. Ann NY Acad Sci 377: 455

Wilkins EW, Edmunds LH, Castleman B (1966) Cases of thymoma at the Massachusetts General Hospital. J Thorac Cardiovasc Surg 52: 322

Willcox N, Vincent A (1988) Myasthenia gravis as an example of organ-specific autoimmune disease. In: Bird G, Calvert JE (eds) B-Lymphocytes in human disease. Oxford University Press, Oxford, p 469

Willcox N, Schluep M, Sommer N, Campana D, Janossy G, Brown AN, Newsom-Davis J (1989) Variable corticosteroid sensitivity of thymic cortex and medullary peripheral-type lymphoid tissue in myasthenia gravis patients: structural and functional effects. Quart J Med 73: 1071

Subject Index

abdominal carcinosis 146, 151, 183
abnormalities (thymic) 63 ff.
abscess 30, 67, 68
accessory thymic tissue 64, 66
acetylcholine 212
– receptors 209
– receptor antibodies 137
acetylcholine-esterase 13
– inhibitors 214
acromegaly 82, 90
ACTH 40, 94, 148, 149, 151
acute lymphoblastic leukemia 59
Addison's disease 82, 90
adrenal gland metastasis 125, 183
agammaglobulinemia 63, 126
agranulocytosis 126
alpha
– bungarotoxin 212
– glycerophosphate dehydrogenase
  149
– MSH 149
– naphythylacetat esterase 80
alymphoblasia (thymic) 63
anencephaly 82, 90
aneurysma 67, 130, 136, 171, 178
angiocardiography 26, 31
– thymolipoma 176
– thymus persistens 73, 76
antikeratin antibody 137
antikeratin antiserum 116
angiofollicullar lymphonode hyperplasia 83, 195
antiacetylcholinesterase 213
antibodies 209
– monoclonal 6, 118, 159
– striated muscles 212, 213
antidiuretic hormone 151
antigen 7 ff.
– class II 7, 8
– recognition 16
– soluble 16
aplasia
– endogen 57, 58
– red cell 125, 126, 151
– thymic 35, 63
aphthous ulcer 126
aplastic anemia 126, 174, 176, 196, 197
arteriography 30 f., 50
– carcinoid 152
– Hodgkin's disease 160
– normal thymus 50
– seminoma 183
– technique 30
– thymic carcinoma 146
– thymic cyst 197

– thymic lymphoma 171
– thymic renal metastasis 136
– thymolipoma 176
– thymoma 135 f.
aryepiglottic fold 174
atelectasis 1, 40, 84, 88, 102, 103
atrophy
– lipomatous 9, 44, 70
– thymic 11, 211
attenuation values see CT of each
  disease
autoimmune anemia 82
autoimmune disease 77, 82, 125, 211
autopsy 211
azathioprine 214

Babix casing 23
basal cell carcinoma 126
basaloid cell carcinoma 111, 112,
  116, 140, 145
B-cell-lymphoma 156, 159
Beckwith-Wiedemann-Syndrome 81
Bednar's cyst 195
Behçet's disease 82, 211
beta-endorphin 149
biopsy 26
– contraindication 139
– dystopic thymic tissue 66
– hyperplasia 103, 104
– pneumothorax 139
– thymic dystopia 66
– thymic lymphoma 170
– thymolipoma 178
– thymoma 139
birth 92
B-lymphocytes 15, 16, 80, 82
Bochdalek's space 124
bone 24, 100, 188
bone marrow 18
bone metastasis
– carcinoid 148, 151, 152
– germ cell tumors 183, 186, 187, 190
– seminoma 183
– thymic carcinoma 146
– thymoma 124
brain metastasis
– carcinoid 151
– germ cell tumors 183, 186, 187, 190
– seminoma 183
– thymoma 124
branchial cleft 146
– cyst 65, 201
– pouches 5
breast carcinoma 29
bronchial stenosis 127, 175

bronchoesophageal cyst 67
bronchogenic carcinoma 29, 30
bronchogenic cyst 68, 200
bronchography 32
bronchoscopy 32, 124
Bucky film 176
burns 57, 81, 92
butterfly sign 205

Calcification 40, 95, 100
– aneurysma 171
– carcinoid 148, 152, 154
– conventional tomography 24
– germ cell tumors 183, 185, 188, 190
– hemangioma 192
– Hodgkin's disease 160
– NHL 171
– thymic carcinomas 146
– thymic cyst 197, 199
– thymolipoma 178
– thymoma 24, 127, 128, 132, 133,
  137, 138
– tuberculoma 199
calcitonin 148, 149, 151
carcinoma (thymic) 109, 111, 145 ff.
– arteriography 146
– chemotherapy 146
– classification 111
– clinical symptoms 146
– chest radiography 146
– computed tomography 146
– conventional radiography 146
– conventional tomography 146
– differential diagnosis 147
– histogenesis 146
– histology 145, 146
– imaging procedures 146, 147
– metastasis 146
– MRI 147
– nuclear medicine 147
– occurrence 145
– pathology 145, 146
– prognosis 147
– radiotherapy 147
– therapy 147
– surgery 146
– ultrasonography 146
Carcinoid 80, 109, 148 ff.
– arteriography 152
– bronchial carcinoid 152
– chemotherapy 155
– chest radiography 152
– clinical symptoms 151
– computed tomography 152
– conventional radiography 152

Carcinoid
- differential diagnosis 137, 154
- Eaton-Lambert-Syndrome 151
- histochemical results 148
- histogenesis 148
- histology 148
- hormones 148, 149, 151
- imaging procedures 152, 155
- immunhistologic results 148, 149
- infiltration 148, 152
- localization 149, 151
- MEN I, II 149, 151
- metastasis 148, 151, 152
- MRI 152
- nuclear medicine 152
- occurrence 149
- pathogenesis 148
- pathology 148
- pseudomyasthenia 151
- prognosis 155
- radiotherapy 155
- tumor spread 151
- ultrasonography 152
cardiac
- defect 57, 92, 176, 196
- murmur 124
- muscles 210
- symptoms (thymic hyperplasia) 84, 100
- tamponade 124
cardiomegaly
- hyperplasia 100
- normal thymus 35
- persistent thymus 72, 76
- thymic cyst 196, 197
- thymolipoma 176, 178
cardiothymic index 51
Castleman's disease 80, 83, 195
castration 90
category I of thymic epithelial tumors 111
category II of thymic epithelial tumors 116
cavography 31
- germ cell tumors 183, 187
- lymphoma 171
cerebral infarction 30
cervical fistulas 65
cervical thymus 5, 24, 65 f.
- clinical symptoms 65
- computed tomography 65
- conventional radiography 65, 66
- conventional tomography 66
- differential diagnosis 65
- esophagography 65
- ultrasonography 65
cervical thymic tissue 5
chemotherapy 11
- measurement of thymic size 51
- rebound hyperplasia 94
- technique 23
  see therapy of malignant tumors chest radiography
chromogranin 149
class II antigens 7, 8

clear cell carcinoma 111, 112, 116, 140, 145
clear cell lymphoma 156
cholecystokinin 148, 149, 151
cholinergic side effects 213, 214
choristoma 109, 193
chorioncarcinoma 182, 186
chromogranin A 148
colitis ulcerosa 82, 211
colloid cyst 190
computed tomography 25 ff.
- advantage of CT 26
- carcinoid 152
- cervical thymus 65
- configuration of thymus 42, 43
- dynamic CT 26
- dystopic thymus 65, 67
- fatty thymic degeneration 42
- germ cell tumors 183, 184, 190
- Hodgkin's disease 161
- Houndsfield units (HU) 26, 44
- localization of normal thymus 41
- radiation dose 26
- seminoma 183
- size of thymus 51
- thymic carcinomas 146
- thymic involution in CT 42, 44, 45
- thymic remnants 42
- thymogenic cyst 197
- thymolipoma 177
- thymoma 129
congenital heart disease 58, 72
contrast studies, CT 26
  see arteriography, computed tomography, phlebography, pyelography etc.
conventional diagnostics
- carcinoid 152
- cervical thymus 65, 66
- Hodgkin's disease 160
- NHL 164
- normal thymus 35
- seminoma 183
- thymic carcinomas 146
- thymogenic cyst 197
- thymolipoma 176
- thymoma 127
conventional tomography 24
- carcinoid 152
- carcinomas (thymic) 146
- cervical thymus 66
- dystopic thymus 66
- germ cell tumors 183, 187
- Hodgkin's disease 160
- NHL 164
- seminoma 183
- technique 24
- thymic hyperplasia 91
- thymic persistens 70
- thymogenic cyst 197
- thymolipoma 176
- thymoma 127 f., 139
corticosteroids 11, 213, 214
corticosteroid therapy 11, 80, 81
corticotropin 151

Cushing's syndrome 94, 149, 151, 155, 160
cyclophosphamide 214
cyclosporin A 214
cyst
- Bednar's 195
- branchial 65, 201
- bronchogenic 200
- colloid cyst 190
- dermoid cyst 178, 186, 188
- hydatide cyst 201 f.
- pericardial cyst (see there)
- teratogenic cyst 178, 190
- thoracic duct cyst 67
- thymic cyst 24, 88, 127, 171, 188, 190, 195 ff., 206
- thyroglossal cyst 65
- within epithelial tumors 110
- within thymoma 131
cystic degeneration 29, 65
- carcinoid 154
- cervical thymus 65
- germ cell tumor 183, 185, 188
- malignant thymic lymphoma 161, 162, 164, 201
- thymic carcinomas 146
- thymic cyst 201
- thymoma 127, 131, 132, 137, 138, 154, 201, 206
cystic softening 130
cytokeratin 148
cytology 139, 178
cytostatics 40, 58
  see therapy, chemotherapy of each malignant tumor

Dermatologic diseases 126
dermatomyositis 126
dermoid cyst 65, 178, 186, 188
descensus thymi 5
developmental abnormalities of thymus 63 ff.
dextrocardia 38
diabetes mellitus 82
Diamond-Backfan-Anemia 126
diaphragma-metastasis 146
Di George-Syndrome 20, 63
digital radiography 127, 129
diplopia 209
Dubois' abscess 195
dynamic CT 26
  see CT of each disease, contrast studies
dysfunction 80
dysgenesis
- reticular 63
- thymic 11
dysgerminoma 182
dysplasia 63
- red cell 151
dystopia (thymic) 5, 23, 24, 30, 59, 63 ff., 88
- cervicalis 5, 65 f.
- esophagography 136
- germ cell tumor 183

– intrapulmonary thymoma 121–123, 125
– middle mediastinum 66
– posterior mediastinum 66
– superior mediastinum 65
– thymogenic cyst 195 ff.
– thymomas 110, 121
– tracheal thymoma 122
– tympanic cavity 5

Ear malformation 68
Eaton-Lambert-Syndrome 151
ectopia of thymus 63, 64
ectopic gastric mucosa 30
ectopic thymic tissue 5, 23, 59
endophonium-chlorid 213
embryology of thymus 5
embryonal carcinoma 182
endocarditis 176
endocrine function 15
endocrinologic disease 78, 81, 82, 90, 125, 126, 151
    see special endocrinologic diseases as well
endodermal sinus tumor 182
endplate potential 212
endplates 209
enteroglucagon 151
eosinophilic granuloma 202
epitheloid cells 110
epitheloid cell typ thymoma 110 ff.
– cortical type 117
– medullary type 117
    see thymoma
erythroblastic hypoplasia 126
erythropoietin 126
esophageal
– carcinoma 30
– compression 88
– cyst 67
– displacement 177
esophagography 26, 30, 65, 197

Fatigability 209
fatty thymic degeneration 42 ff., 53
fetoprotein 186, 190
fibroma (thymic) 192
fibrosis
– endocardium 151
– malignant lymphoma 162
– postradiation 133
fine needle biopsy see biopsy
fistula cervical 65
flush-syndrome 151
follicular hyperplasia 209
foregut 148, 200
fungal infection 126
fluorescence, formalin-induced 149
fluoroscopy 23
– normal thymus 23
– persistent thymus 70
– technique 23
– thymic hyperplasia 91
– thymic malignant lymphoma 171
– thymogenic cyst 197

– thymolipoma 176
– thymoma 127, 128, 139
function (thymic) 15

Gallium-67-citrate 29 f.
– bone metastasis of thymoma 29
– dystopia 68
– Hodgkin's disease 29
– malignant tumors 29 f., 135
– meningitis 29
– neuroblastoma 29
– seminoma 185
– teratoma 29
– thymic cyst 29
– thymic hyperplasia 29
– thymoma 29, 135
– Wilms' tumor 29
gastric mucosa 200
gastric mucous membrane 30
gastric duplicatures 30
gastrin 151
giant thymus 35
germ cell tumors 80, 81, 109, 137, 180 ff.
– embryogenesis 180
– metastasis 183, 186, 187, 190
– non seminomatous germ cell tumors 186 ff.
– pathologic features 180
– recurrence 186
– seminoma 182 ff.
germinal centers 77, 82, 211
glucagon 151
glucocorticoids in thymoma 140
goiter 1, 190
granulomatous mediastinitis 195
– myocarditis 126
– thymoma 156, 161
Graves's disease see thyrotoxicosis
gravida 59
grimelius 148
growth disturbances 202
gonadal hypofunction 82
gynecologic malignancies 127
gynecomastia 183, 186, 190

Hand-Schueller-Christian-Disease 202
Hashimoto's thyroiditis 82
Hassal's corpuscles 6, 11, 113, 114, 174, 178
hCG 186
heart
– defect 63, 76
– disease 70, 72
– metastasis 186
heat injuries see burns 192
hemangioma 65, 109, 192, 195
hemangiopericytoma 114
hematoma (see hemorrhage) 207
hematologic disease 125
    see single types too
hemolytic anemia 126
hemopoietic insufficiency (thymoma) 125

hemopoietic stem cell markers 18
hemorrhage of thymus 206
– etiology 206
– clinical symptoms 206
– injury 205
– ultrasonography 207
hepatic cirrhosis 82
hepatoma 30
hepatomegaly 78
heterodimers 16, 18
histiocytic thymic tumors 174
histiocytosis 90
histiocytosis X 30, 202
HLA-system 16, 17
Hodkin's disease see Morbus Hodgkin
HU see Houndsfield units (CT)
hydatidosis 195, 201
hygroma 65
hyperfunction 80
hyperparathyroidism 63, 149
hyperpigmentation 151
hyperplasia 24, 29, 30, 40, 58, 63, 68, 76, 77 ff., 94, 139, 171, 195
– associated diseases 89
– classification 78
– clinical features 78 f.
– dystopia 68
– follow up 104
– imaging procedures 90 f.
– incidence 78
– lymphofollicular hyperplasia 82
– myasthenia gravis incidence 211, 213
– pathologic features 78
– radiotherapy 103
– rebound thymic hyperplasia 81, 92, 164, 170
– therapy 103
– true thymic hyperplasia 78 f., 81
hyperthyroidism 176
hypogammaglobulinemia 80, 126, 151, 174, 211
hypothyreoidism 81, 90

I-131 200
imaging normal thymus 35 ff.
– computed tomography 41
– conventional diagnostics 35
– invasive procedures 50
– measurement of size 51
– MRI 46
– size of thymus 51
– ultrasonography 40
imaging procedures (principles) 23 ff.
I-131-MIBG 137, 152
immundeficiency 20
– diseases 63
immune system 5, 16
immunhistology
– epithelial thymic tumors 116
– hyperplasia 82
immunofluorescence 213
immunologic functions 77, 92
– phenomens (thymoma) 125
– response 9

immunosuppressants 213
immunosuppressive treatment 210, 214
infection 40
infant death syndrome 84
infiltration local
– carcinoid 148, 151
– germ cell tumors 186
– thymic carcinoma 146
– thymoma 124
insulin 151
interleukin-2-receptor complex 17
interlobar involvement of normal thymus 40
internal thoracic artery 31
intrapulmonary thymoma 133
involution (thymic) 9 ff., 15, 57 ff.
– acute endogenous 57
– endogenous 57
– exogenous 57
– transplacentar 59
– irradiation 57

Kallikrein 151
Klinefelter's syndrome 186
kymography 32
– thymogenic cyst 197, 201
– thymoma 136
kidney metastasis
– germ cell tumor 186
– intravenous urography 136
– malignant thymic lymphoma 136
– thymoma 124, 129, 136

Laryngeal malformation 88
leu-enkephalin 149
leukemia 20, 81, 90, 93, 95, 100, 109, 156, 162, 165 ff.
– acute lymphatic 59, 168
– chemotherapy 170
– chronic myeloic 168
– clinical symptoms 168
– computed tomography 169
– differential diagnosis 170
– imaging procedures 168, 171
– MRI 162
– myoblastic 157
– plain film radiography 168
– pleural effusion 168
– radiotherapy 170
– therapy 170
– ultrasonography 160, 169
leukemia thymica 168
leukocytosis in thymic hyperplasia 80
leukosarcomatosis 157
Letterer-Siwe-Disease 202
lichen planus 126
limbic encephalitis 127
lipoma/lipomatosis
– mediastinal 174, 175, 178
– pharynx 176
– thymic 66, 174
– thyroid 176
liposarcoma 178
lipothymoma 175

liver disease 82
liver metastasis
– carcinoid 148, 151
– germ cell tumors 183, 186
– seminoma 183
– thymic carcinoma 146
– thymoma 124
localization of normal thymus 5
Louis-Bar-Syndrome 63
lues 195
lung metastasis
– carcinoid 148, 151
– germ cell tumor 183, 186
– thymoma 124, 125, 151
lupus erythematodes 82, 90, 126, 211, 212
lymphadenoma 65
lymphadenopathy 59, 78, 100, 202
lymphangioma 65, 195
lymph node enlargement 46, 162
lymph node metastasis 65
– carcinoid 148, 151
– germ cell tumors 186
– seminoma 183
– thymic carcinoma 146
– thymoma 124
lymphoid germinal centers 77
lymphogenic cyst 201
lymphoepithelioma like carcinoma 111, 112, 116, 145

Magnetic resonance imaging (MRI) 26 ff.
– carcinoid 152
– dystopic thymus 68
– ECG gating 28
– germ cell tumors 185, 190
– Hodgkin's disease 162
– image contrast 27
– image production 27
– NHL 162 f.
– normal appearance of anatomic structures 27
– normal thymus 46 ff.
– – in adults 48
– – in children 46
– persistent thymus 70
– size of thymus 53 f.
– spin-echo-technique 27
– technique 26
– thymic carcinoma 147
– thymic hyperplasia 92
– thymogenic cyst 200
– thymolipoma 178
– thymoma 133 ff.
– T1-weighted image 27 ff.
– T2-weighted image 27 ff.
maldevelopment 110
malignant melanoma 126
malignant lymphoma 24, 29, 30, 58, 59, 67, 81, 93, 100, 109, 156
    see Hodgkin's disease, leukemia, Non-Hodgkin's lymphoma
malignomas associated with thymoma 125

malnutrition 11
measurement of thymic size 51 ff.
mediastinal masses 46
mediastinoscopy 32
melanocytes 151
melanoma 126
meninges metastasis 124, 129
meningoceles 67
mesenchymal thymic tumors 67, 109, 174 ff.
metastasis
– abd. carcinosis 146, 151, 183
– adrenal gland 183
– bone 124, 146, 148, 151, 183, 186
– brain 124, 151, 183, 186, 187, 190
– carcinoid 148, 151
– diaphragma 146
– germ cell tumors 183, 186, 187, 190
– intestine 186
– kidney 124, 129, 136, 186
– liver 124, 146, 148, 151, 183, 186
– lung 124, 125, 133, 148, 151, 183, 186
– lymph nodes 65, 124, 146, 148, 151, 183, 186
– meninges 124, 129
– pancreas 186
– pericard 132, 133, 148, 186
– pleura 124, 131 ff., 146, 186
– renal thymic 136
– skin 148, 183
– spinal cord 151, 183
– spleen 124, 151, 183
– thymic carcinoid 148, 152
– thymic carcinoma 146
– thymoma 124, 125, 131 ff.
– thyroid 183
– tonsilles 183
– within the thymus 109, 193
met-enkephalin 149
MHC class II antgens 7 ff.
MHC complex 17
MIBG 152
migration of the thymus 5, 63
mitral valve defect 176
mixed cell type thymoma 111
monoclonal antibodies 52, 71
Morbus Hodgkin 29, 58, 81, 91, 156, 159 ff.
– angiography 160
– calcification 160
– chemotherapy 164
– chest radiography 160
– clinical symptoms 160
– computed tomography 161
– conventional radiography 160
– conventional tomography 160
– follow up 163
– hyperplasia (reactive) 164
– imaging procedures 160, 171
– MRI 162
– nuclear medicine 164
– occurrence 159
– pathologic features 156
– prognosis 159

– radiotherapy 164
– recurrence 164
– therapy 163, 164
– ultrasonography 160
Morgagni's foramen 124
mors thymica 1, 84
MRI see magnetic resonance imaging
mucoepidermoid carcinoma 111,
    113, 116
multiple endocrine neoplasia
    (MEN I, II) 149, 151, 155
multiple sclerosis 82
Myasthenia gravis 15, 209 ff.
– associated thymic changes 210
– carcinoid 151
– classification 209, 210
– clinical examination 209
– diagnosis 213
– ectopic lung thymoma 125
– Hodgkin's disease 160
– incidence
– – thymoma 211, 213
– – hyperplasia 211, 213
– – normal thymus 211, 213
– malignant thymic lymphoma 160
– pathogenesis 212
– prognosis 210
– radiologic diagnosis 213
– symptoms 209
– therapy 210
– thymic cyst 196
– thymic hyperplasia 77, 82, 88, 90, 92
– thymic persistens 70, 72
– thymolipoma 174, 176
– thymoma 119, 125, 137, 140
– treatment 213
– tumorlike lesion 196
myasthenic crisis 214
myocarditis (thymoma) 126
myoblastic leukemia 157
myeloic leukemia (chronic) 168
myocardium infiltration in thymic
    carcinoma 146
myoid cells 82, 174, 212
myoid cell sarcoma 174
myosarcoma 174

Na + -channels 212
necrosis 110
necrotic liquefaction
– NHL 165
– thymoma 132
needle biopsy see biopsy
neostigmin 214
neuroblastoma 29, 67
neurofilament reactivity 148
neurogenic tumor 127
neuromuscular junction 212
neuron-spezific enolase 148, 149
neurotensin 148, 149
Nezelof syndrome 63
Non-Hodgkin-Lymphoma 20, 80, 90,
    95, 156, 164 ff.
– cavography 171
– chemotherapy 170

– clinical symptoms 164
– computed tomography 164
– conventional radiography 164
– differential diagnosis 170
– extrathymic lymphoma 171
– imaging procedures 164, 171
– MRI 162 f.
– necrotic liquefaction 165
– pathologic features 156
– radiotherapy 170
– therapy 170
– ultrasonography 160, 164
Non-seminomatous germ cell tumors
– clinical symptoms 186
– conventional radiography 187
– chest radiography 187
– CT 188
– differential diagnosis 190
– hormonal production 186
– imaging procedures 187 ff., 190
– MRI 190
– nuclear medicine 190
– occurrence 186
– osseous metastasis 187, 190
– prognosis 190
– therapy 190
– tumor spread 186
– ultrasonography 187
normal appearance of tissue in MRI
    27
normal thymus
– anatomy 5 ff.
– arterial supply 30
– embryology 5
– imaging procedures 35
– immunologic function 15 ff.
– incidence of myasthenia gravis
    213
– interlobar involvement 40
– involution 9
– venous anatomy 31
notch sign 37
nuclear medicine 29 ff.
– carcinoid 152
– Gallium-67-citrate 29, 68
– Hodgkin's disease 164
– non seminomatous germ cell
    tumors 190
– principles 29 ff.
– selenium-75-methionine 30
– technique 29
– seminoma 185
– thymic carcinoma 147
– thymogenic cyst 200
– thymoma 135
– technetium-99m-gluceptate 30
– – pertechnetate 30, 135
– – polyphosphate 29, 190, 200

oblique views 127
ocular myasthenia gravis 127, 209,
    210, 211
onychomycosis 126
Osserman 209
ossification (sternum) 24

osteoarthropathia 151, 152
osteosarcoma 81
otitis media 202

pancreatic metastasis 186
pancytopenia 126
paranasal sinus carcinoma 30
parathormone 149
parathymic syndromes 125
parathyroid
– adenoma 171
– carcinoma 30
– gland 5, 65, 171, 197
parenchyma of the thymus 6
parotid cyst 65
pemphigus 212
periarteritis nodosa 82
pericardial
– cyst 138, 176, 178, 200
– effusion 160, 178
– metastasis 132, 133, 148, 186
– infiltration 122, 146
– tumor 178
pericarditis 124, 140
peritoneal tumor infiltration 146
pernicious anemia 126
persistent thymus 40, 70 ff., 199
– clinical features 70
– differential diagnosis 70
– imaging procedures 70
– pathology 70
– pathophysiology 70
pharyngeal pouches 5
pharynx (lipoma) 68, 176
phlebography 31
– normal thymus 30
– technique 31
– thymoma 136
pituitary gland 82
plasmapheresis 213, 214
plastic casing 23
pleural effusion 95, 160, 164, 167
pleuritis (mediastinalis, interlobaris)
    1, 100
pleurisy (interlobar) 100
pleura metastasis
– germ cell tumor 186
– thymic carcinoma 146
– thymoma 124, 131 ff.
pneumomediastinography 26, 32, 50
– persistent thymus 70
– thymic hyperplasia 92
– thymoma 136
pneumomediastinum (trauma) 205
pneumonia 29, 30, 40, 57, 202
pneumothorax 139, 205
polyarthritis 126
polymyositis 126
posterior mediastinum 110, 127
premature infants 60
prevenous thymus 66
pseudomyasthenia 151
ptosis 209
pulmonary
– maturity 59

pulmonary
– segment 40, 70, 205
– stenosis 76, 124
– trunk 129
– vessels (thymoma) 132
pure red cell anemia 125, 126, 211
pyelography (retrograde) 136
pyridostigmin 214

Radiation 133
radio-immuno-assay 212
radiotherapy 11, 57, 197
– esophagitis 140
– pericarditis 140
– pneumonitis 140
– side effects 140
– thymic cyst 201
– thymic hyperplasia 84
– thymoma 140
rebound hyperplasia 92 ff.
red cell aplasia 111
– carcinoid 151
– thymoma 125, 126
regenerative hyperplasia 92 ff.
renal metastasis 136
repetitive (3–5 Hz) nerve stimulation
     213
respiratory distress syndrome 35, 59, 60
reticular dysgenesis 63
retrovenous thymus 66
rhabdomyosarcoma 58, 81
rheumatoid arthritis 82, 126, 140, 211

Saccharomycosis 126
sagittal imaging MRI 29
sail sign 36, 41
sarcoidosis 30, 81
sarcoma 100
sarcomatoid thymic carcinoma 111,
     112, 116, 140, 145
schwannoma 127
scleroderma 82, 126
sclerosing mediastinitis 195
sebaceous matter 188
seborrheal keratosis 126
selenium-75-methionine 30
– bronchogenic carcinoma 30
– malignant lymphoma 30
– parathyroid carcinoma 30
– thymic hyperplasia 30
– thymoma 30, 135
– thyroid carcinoma 30
seminoma 180 ff.
– angiography 183
– clinical symptoms 182
– computed tomography 183
– conventional radiography 183
– conventional tomography 183
– differential diagnosis 186
– imaging procedures 183, 186
– metastasis 183
– MRI 185
– nuclear medicine 185
– occurrence 182
– plain film radiography 183

– prognosis 186
– radiosensitivity 186
– therapy 186
– ultrasonography 183
– vena cavography 183
seminomatous thymoma 182
sepsis 57
serotonine 149, 151, 152, 153
Simpson test 209
single fibre electromyography 213
size of thymus 51 ff.
Sjögren's syndrome 82, 126
skin metastasis 14, 183
small cell carcinoma 145, 146
somatostatin 149
spinal cord metastasis
– carcinoid 151
– germ cell tumor 183
spindle cell typ thymoma 111
spin-echo-technique (MRI) 27
spinnacker sign 38, 205
spleen metastasis
– carcinoid 151
– germ cell tumors 183
– thymoma 124
splenomegaly 78, 202
squamous cell carcinoma 109, 112,
     116, 145, 146 ff.
– clinical symptoms 146
– radiology 146 ff.
starry sky macrophages 82
status thymolymphaticus 1, 15
substance P 151
synaptophysin 148, 149
steroid
– production 58
– test 57, 58, 68, 95, 103, 164, 170
– therapy 51, 84, 88
– treatment 15
stomach carcinoma 30
stridor 1, 84, 88
stress involution (thymic) 57
stress situation 35, 57, 92
submandibular swelling 65
surgery 40, 57
systemic lupus erythematodes
     see lupus erythematodes

T-cell-antigen receptor 16
T-cell leukemia 168
T-cells 9, 17, 18
Technetium-99m-gluceptate 30
Technetium-99m-pertechnetate 30,
     135
– dystopic thymic tissue 30
– gastric duplicatures 30
– gastric mucous membrane 30
– gastroenteric cysts 30
– thymoma 135
Technetium-99m-polyphosphate
– germ cell tumors 190
– thymic bone metastasis 29
– thymogenic cyst 200
teeth 24, 100, 188
teratocarcinoma 182, 186

teratoma 24, 29, 66, 100, 186
testicular carcinoma 59, 100
T-helper-cells 8, 15, 17, 82, 212
teratogenic cyst 178, 190
thermal burns see burns
thoracic duct 67
– cyst 67
thoracotomy 59, 68, 104
thymectomy 15, 16, 80, 88, 126, 202,
     210, 213
thymic
– aplasia 35
– arteries 31
– atrophy 11, 57, 211
– carcinoma see carcinoma of the thy-
     mus
– carcinoid see carcinoid
– cyst 24, 29 see thymogenic cyst too
– death 1, 15
– dysfunction 80
– dysgenesis 11
– enlargement 59, 207
– endocrine function 15
– heart 1
– hyperplasia see hyperplasia
– hormones 8, 19
– involvement 57 ff.
– lipoma 66
– parenchyma 6
– remnants (CT) 42 ff.
– size 51 ff.
– thickness 51
thymitis 83
thymocytes (stage I, II, III) 9
thymocyte precursors 18
thymogenic cyst 88, 127, 137, 171,
     188, 190, 195 ff., 206
– angiography 197
– associated diseases 196
– bleeding 197
– clinical symptoms 196
– computed tomography 197
– conventional radiography 197
– conventional tomography 197
– differential diagnosis 137, 197
– dystopic 197
– fluoroscopy 197
– imaging procedures 197, 201
– localization 196
– MRI 200
– myasthenia gravis 196
– nuclear medicine 200
– occurrence 195
– pathologic features 195
– plain film radiography 197
– prognosis 201
– puncture 197, 201
– surgical removal 201
– therapy 201
– ultrasonography 201
thymolipoma 24, 109, 174 ff.
– arteriography 176
– biopsy 178
– clinical symptoms 175
– computed tomography 177

– conventional radiography 176
– conventional tomography 176
– differential diagnosis 178
– hyperthyroidism 176
– imaging procedures 176, 178
– MRI 178
– myasthenia gravis 176
– occurrence 174
– pathologic features 174
– pathogenesis 174
– plain film radiography 176
– prognosis 178
– systemic diseases 174, 176
– therapy 178
– ultrasonography 177
thymoliposarcoma 174
thymoma 29, 30, 40, 66, 80, 109,
  110 f., 121 ff.
– abdominal spread 121
– age distribution 121
– antikeratin antibody 116
– antikeratin antiserum 137
– arteriography 135
– associated diseases 125 ff.
– "benign" thymoma 111, 116, 130,
  139
– biopsy 139
– calcification 127, 128, 133
– caudal dystopia 124
– cervical dystopia 124
– chemotherapy 140
– classification 111, 114, 117
– clinical symptoms 122, 125
– computed tomography 129
– contrast studies 132
– conventional radiography 127
– conventional tomography 127, 139
– cystic thymoma 127, 130
– dermatomyositis 126
– differential diagnosis 137
– dystopia 122, 123, 124
– ectopic positions 121
– encapsulated thymoma 121, 130
– endocrinologic diseases 125
– esophagography 136
– epitheloid cell type thymoma 111,
  116, 131
– fluoroscopy 127, 139
– gallium-67-citrate 135
– granulomatous type 156
– hematologic diseases 125
– imaging procedures 127 ff., 139
– immunhistology 116
– immunologic phenomenes 125
– infections 125
– invasive thymomas 121, 131
– intrapulmonary thymoma 125,
  128, 133
– lymphocytic association 113
– local infiltration 124
– localization 121
– malignancies (other) 126
– "malignant" thymoma 111, 116,
  122, 132, 140
– metastasis 124, 125, 131

– mixed cell thymoma 111, 131
– MRI 133
– myasthenia gravis 119, 122, 125,
  140, 213
– neck localization 135
– needle biopsy 139
– nuclear medicine 135
– oblique views 127
– occurrence 121
– phlebography 136
– posterior mediastinal dystopia 122
– postradiation changes 133
– prognosis 118, 119, 139, 140
– pulmonary dystopia 122, 123
– pulmonary stenosis 124
– radiosensivity 140
– radiotherapy 140
– red cell aplasia 125
– selenium-75-methionine 135
– sex predilection 121
– spindle cell thymoma 111, 116,
  118, 131
– spread of thymoma 124, 132
– surgical treatment 139
– therapy 139
– thyroiditis 126
– tracheal dystopia 122
– tumor status 122
– ultrasonography 128
thymopoetin 19
thymopharyngeal duct 65, 195, 196,
  200
thymoptosis 68
thymosin α-1 19
thymosin β-4 19
thymulin 19
thymus (normal) 5 ff.
  see "normal thymus"
thymus-annularis 68
– cervicalis see cervical thymus
– persistens see persistent thymus
thyroiditis 90, 126, 211
thyrotoxicosis 81, 82, 90, 126, 211
thyroglossal cyst 65
thyroid
– arteries 31
– carcinoma 15, 30, 57, 151
– gland 65, 124, 125, 174, 176, 197, 201
– metastasis 183
thrombin time 207
thrombocytopenia 126
thromboplastin time 207
tinea capitis 126
tinea pedis 126
T-killer cells 16, 17
T-lymphoblastic NHL 156, 157
T-lymphocytes 8, 15, 16, 80, 118
tonsilles metastasis 186
toxoplasmosis 82
tracheal
– displacement 65
– obstruction 23
– stenosis 91, 139, 160, 197
– thymus 68
– tomography 197

tracheobronchial tomography 66
tracheobronchography 26
tracheomalacia 88
trauma 205 ff.
– pneumomediastinum 205
– radiography 205
T-suppressor/killer cells 16, 17
tuberculosis 30, 57, 81, 92, 195, 202
tumors of the thymus 109, 145, 192
– classification 109, 145, 192
– carcinoid 109, 148 ff.
– carcinoma 145
– epithelial tumors 109, 110 ff.
– epithelioma 192
– fibroma 192
– germ cell tumors 109, 180 ff.
– hemangioma 192
– histocytic 109
– Hodgkin's disease 109, 159 ff.
– lymphoid cells 109
– lymphoendothelioma 192
– lymphangioma 192
– lipoma 192
– myoid 109
– myxoma 192
– NHL 109, 164 f.
– neuroendocrine tumors 109
– reticuloma 192
– thymolipoma 109, 164 ff.
– thymoma 109, 121 ff.
T1-weighted images MRI 27 ff.
T2-weighted images MRI 27 ff.
tympanic cavity 5, 68

ulcerative colitis 211
ultrasonography 24
– access 24
– adults 24 ff.
– carcinoid 152
– cervical thymus 65
– children 24
– dystopia 65, 67
– echogenicity 41
– Hodgkin's disease 160
– hyperplasia 92
– leukemia 169
– NHL 164
– non seminomatous germ cell
  tumors 160
– normal 40 f.
– seminoma 183
– technique 24
– thymic carcinoma 146
– thymogenic cyst 197, 201
– thymolipoma 177
– thymoma 128, 135
undifferentiated thymic carcinoma
  112, 116
undifferentiated lymphoepithelioma
  like carcinoma 140
urogenital ridge 180

Valsalva's maneuver 196
Value of imaging procedures
  see imaging procedures

vasoconstricting substance 151
vena cavography 31, 183
vena cava superior obstruction 31
– germ cell tumors 183, 187
– malignant thymic lymphoma 171
– seminoma 183
– thymic carcinoma 146
– thymolipoma 176
– thymoma 122, 132, 136

ventricular obstruction 196
vessel
– aberrant 130
– anomalies 63, 88
– tumor infiltration 122, 124, 132,
   146 ff., 151
venous aneurysma 136
visualization of the thymus 23 ff.
vitamin K 207

wave sign 36
white cell aplasia 126
Wilms' tumor 29, 59, 81, 93, 100
Wiskott-Aldrich-Syndrome 63

Yolk sack tumor 182

Zollinger-Ellison-Syndrome
   149, 151

Medical Radiology

Diagnostic Imaging and Radiation Oncology

Series Editors:
L. W. Brady, M. W. Donner, H.–P. Heilmann, F. Heuck

This series recognizes the demand for an international state-of-the-art account of the developments reflecting the progress in the radiological sciences. Each volume conveys an overall picture of a topical theme so that it can be used as a reference work without taking recourse to other volumes.

The contents of the volumes concentrate on new and accepted developments in a manner appropriate for review by physicians engaged in the practice of radiology.

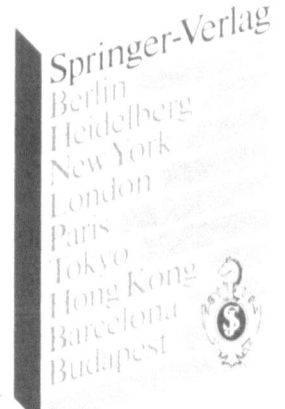

Springer-Verlag
Berlin
Heidelberg
New York
London
Paris
Tokyo
Hong Kong
Barcelona
Budapest

G. E. Laramore, University of Washington, Seattle, WA (Ed.)

Radiation Therapy of Head and Neck Cancer

1989. XII, 237 pp. 123 figs.
Hardcover ISBN 3-540-19360-X

J. H. Anderson, The Johns Hopkins University, Baltimore, MD (Ed.)

Innovations in Diagnostic Radiology

1989. XIII, 213 pp. 144 figs. some in color.
Hardcover ISBN 3-540-19093-7

R. R. Dobelbower Jr., Toledo, OH (Ed.)

Gastrointestinal Cancer

Radiation Therapy

1990. XV, 301 pp. 76 figs. 90 tabs.
Hardcover ISBN 3-540-50505-9

E. Scherer, C. Streffer, University of Essen; **K.-R. Trott,** London (Eds.)

Radiation Exposure and Occupational Risks

1990. XI, 150 pp. 32 figs. 55 tabs.
Hardcover ISBN 3-540-51174-1

S. E. Order, The Johns Hopkins University, Baltimore, MD; **S. S. Donaldson,** Stanford University, Stanford, CA

Radiation Therapy of Benign Diseases

A Clinical Guide

1990. VIII, 214 pp. 103 tabs.
Hardcover ISBN 3-540-50901-1

R. Sauer, University of Erlangen-Nürnberg, Erlangen (Ed.)

Interventional Radiation Therapy Techniques – Brachytherapy

1991. XII, 388 pp. 193 figs. 162 tabs.
Hardcover ISBN 3-540-52465-7

E. Scherer, C. Streffer, University of Essen; **K.-R. Trott,** Medical College of London (Eds.)

Radiopathology of Organs and Tissues

1991. X, 496 pp. 156 figs. 56 tabs.
Hardcover ISBN 3-540-19094-5

M. Rotman, C. J. Rosenthal, State University of New York, NY (Eds.)

Concomitant Continuous Infusion Chemotherapy and Radiation

1991. XIV, 304 pp. 42 figs.
Hardcover ISBN 3-540-52545-9

E. K. Lang, Louisiana State University, New Orleans, LA (Ed.)

Radiology of the Upper Urinary Tract

1991. IX, 370 pp. 418 figs. 14 tabs.
Hardcover ISBN 3-540-52546-7